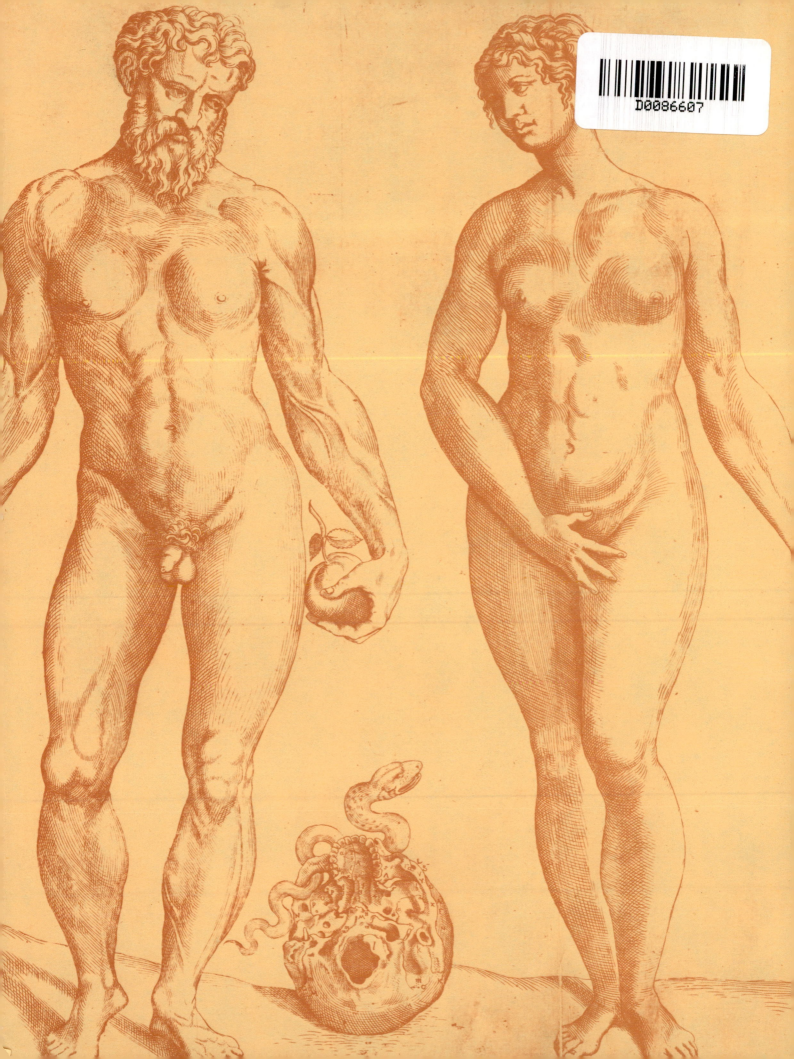

D0086607

Reconstruction and Rehabilitation of the Burned Patient

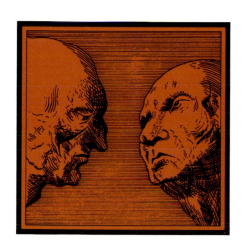

Irving Feller, M.D.
Clinical Professor of Surgery
Chief, Division of Burn Surgery
University of Michigan Medical Center
President, National Institute
for Burn Medicine
Ann Arbor, Michigan

William C. Grabb, M.D.
Professor of Surgery (Plastic)
Head of the Section of Plastic Surgery
University of Michigan Medical Center
Ann Arbor, Michigan

Published by the National Institute for Burn Medicine

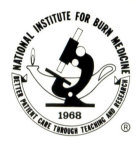

909 East Ann Street
Ann Arbor, Michigan 48104

Press of Thomson-Shore, Inc.
Dexter, Michigan

International Standard Book Number — 0 - 917478 - 50 - 9

Copyright, 1979, by the National Institute for Burn Medicine. Copyright under the International Copyright Union. All rights reserved. This book is protected by Copyright. No part of it may be duplicated or reproduced in any manner without written permission of the publisher. Made in the United States of America. Library of Congress Catalog Number — 78 - 61362.

DESIGN AND LAYOUT

Sandra Alexander Stone

To Reed O. Dingman, teacher, physician, colleague, and friend. For teaching us the art of surgery as few men could, healing our wounds, and encouraging us to look beyond the present limits of our profession to provide better care for our patients.

Portrait by Edgar L. Sherman,
Director of Medical Photography
University of Michigan Medical Center

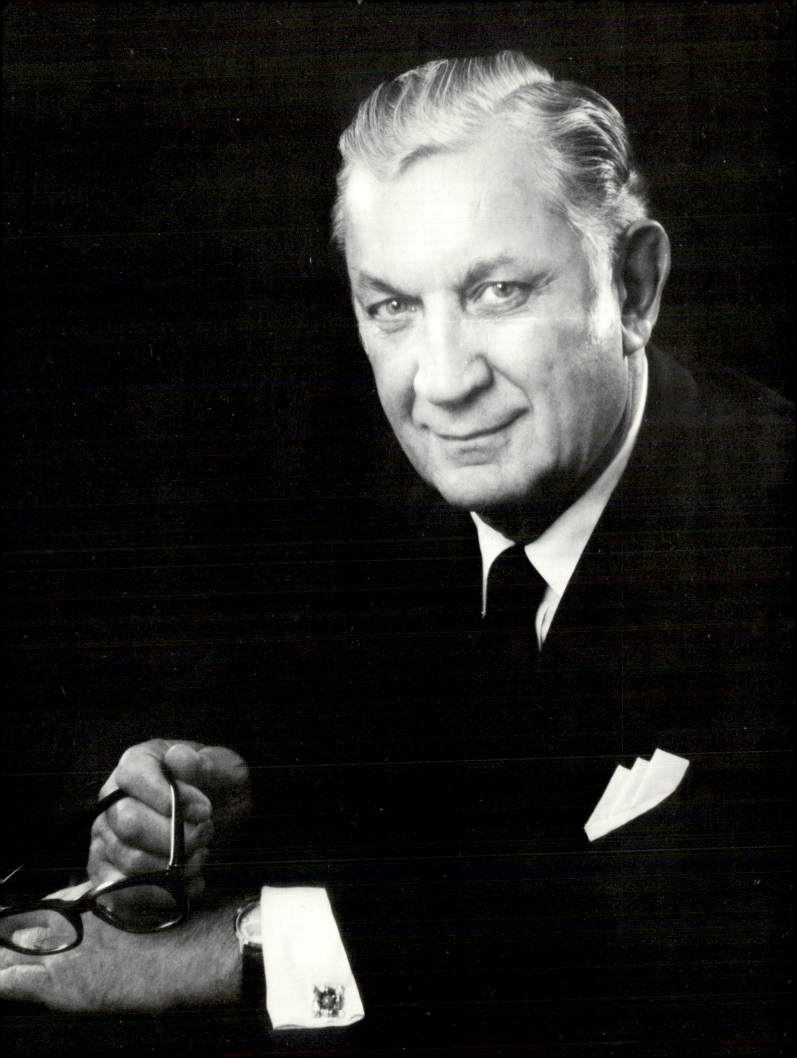

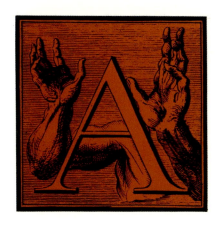

AUTHORS

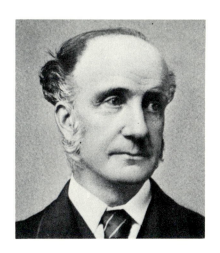

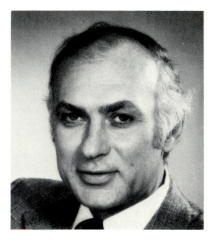

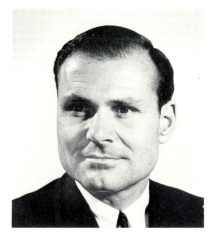

John Kelloch Barton, M.B.T.C.D., F.R.C.S.I.

Surgeon to the Adelaide Hospital
University Lecturer on Practical Anatomy
President, Royal College of Surgeons in
Ireland, 1882-1883, Dublin, *Ireland*

*Photo courtesy of the Board, Adelaide
Hospital, Dublin*

Robert W. Beasley, M.D.

Professor of Surgery (Plastic), New York
University, New York, New York

Roger Boles, M.D.

Professor of Otolaryngology, Chairman,
Department of Otolaryngology, University of California School of Medicine
Attending Staff, University of California
Medical Center
Attending Staff, San Francisco General,
San Francisco, California
Consultant, Letterman General (Army)
Consultant, U.S. Naval Hospital, Oakland, California

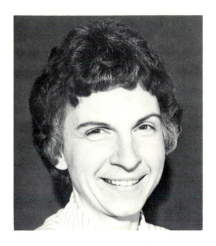

M.L. Bowden, M.S.W., A.C.S.W.

Director, Rehabilitation, National Institute for Burn Medicine, Ann Arbor, Michigan

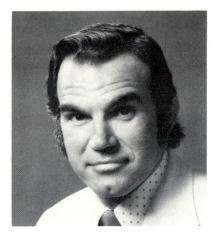

Angelo Capozzi, M.D., F.A.C.S.

Plastic and Reconstructive Surgery Center, Bothin Burn Center, Saint Francis Memorial Hospital, San Francisco, California

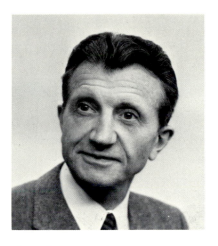

Pierre Colson, M.D.

Burns Unit, Hospital Saint Luc, Lyon, *France*

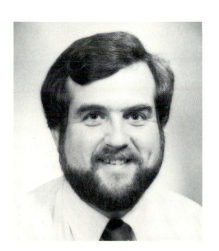

William L. Combs, M.S.

Staff Physical Therapist, Chelsea Community Hospital, Chelsea, Michigan

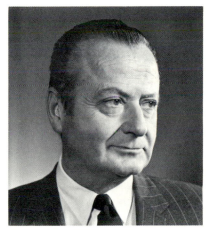

John Marquis Converse, M.D.

Director, Institute of Reconstructive Plastic Surgery, New York University Medical Center
Lawrence D. Bell Professor of Plastic Surgery, New York University Medical Center School of Medicine, New York, New York

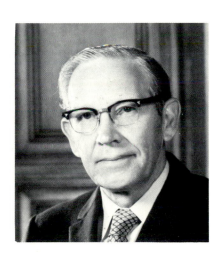

Thomas D. Cronin, M.D., F.A.C.S.

Clinical Professor of Plastic Surgery, Baylor College of Medicine
Director of Plastic Surgery, Residency Training Program, St. Joseph Hospital, Houston, Texas

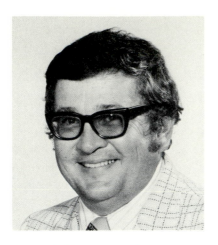

A.J. de la Houssaye, L.P.T.

Director, Biophysical Research, Shriners Burns Institute — Galveston Unit, Galveston, Texas

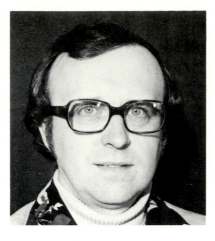

Terrence N. Davidson, Ph.D.

Assistant Research Scientist, Survey Research Center, Institute for Social Research, University of Michigan

Assistant Professor of Education, University of Michigan

Consultant, National Institute for Burn Medicine, Ann Arbor, Michigan

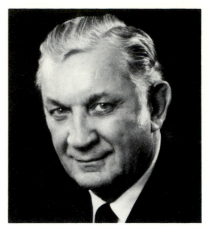

Reed O. Dingman, D.D.S., M.D., F.A.C.S.

Professor Emeritus, Surgery (Plastic and Reconstructive), University of Michigan Medical School, Ann Arbor, Michigan

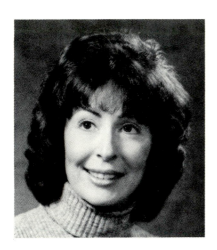

Sheryn S. Dungan, M.S.W., A.C.S.W.

Clinical Social Work Consultant, The Waltham Hospital, Waltham, Massachusetts

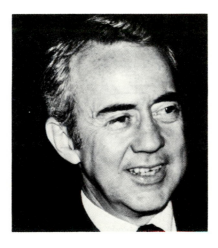

E. Burke Evans, M.D.

Professor of Surgery, Chief of Orthopaedic Surgery, University of Texas Medical Branch

Orthopaedic Surgeon-in-Chief, Attending Staff, University of Texas Medical Branch (John Sealy Hospitals), Galveston, Texas

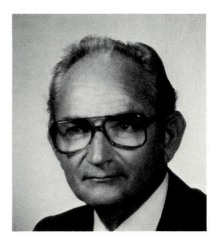

Irving Feller, M.D.
Editor

Clinical Professor of Surgery, Chief, Division of Burn Surgery, University of Michigan Medical Center

President, National Institute for Burn Medicine

Attending Surgeon, St. Joseph Mercy Hospital, Ann Arbor, Michigan

Attending Surgeon, Chelsea Community Hospital, Chelsea, Michigan

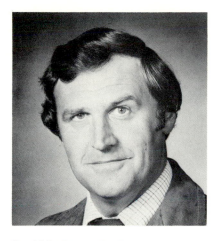

David P. Fisher, M.D.

Orthopedic Surgeon, St. Mary's Hospital
 and Medical Center, Grand Junction,
 Colorado
Assistant Clinical Professor, Department
 of Family Medicine and Department of
 Orthopedics, University of Colorado
 School of Medicine, Denver, Colorado

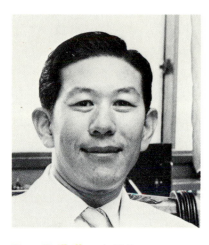

Ryosuke Fujimori, M.D.

Assistant Professor, Unit of Plastic Surgery, Faculty of Medicine, Kyoto University,   Kawahara-Machi,   Syogoin,
 Sakyo-Ku, Kyoto, *Japan*

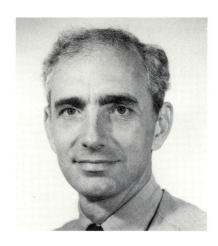

David W. Furnas, M.D.

Chief, Division of Plastic Surgery, Univer-
 sity of California, Irvine Medical Center
Professor and Chief, Division of Plastic
 Surgery, University of California, Irvine,
 Irvine, California

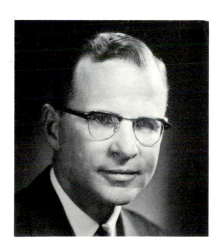

John C. Gaisford, M.D.

Chairman of the Department of Surgery
Director of the Burn Center, Western
 Pennsylvania Hospital, Pittsburgh,
 Pennsylvania

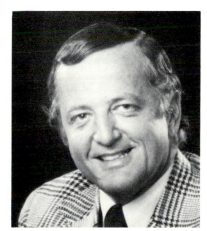

William C. Grabb, M.D.
Editor

Professor of Surgery (Plastic)
Head of the Section of Plastic Surgery,
 University of Michigan Medical Center,
 Ann Arbor, Michigan

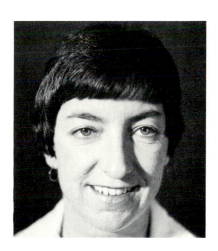

Mary E. Haab, R.N.

Burn Nurse Specialist, Michigan Burn
 Center, Ann Arbor, Michigan

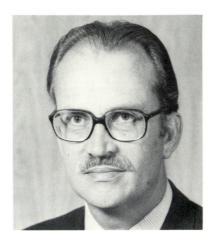

Shattuck W. Hartwell, Jr., M.D.

Department of Plastic Surgery, Cleveland
Clinic Foundation, Cleveland, Ohio

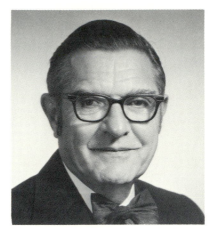

John W. Henderson, M.D.

Professor and Chairman, Department of
Ophthalmology, University of Michigan
Medical Center
Consultant, St. Joseph Mercy Hospital
Consultant, Ann Arbor Veterans Hospi-
tal, Ann Arbor, Michigan
Consultant, Wayne County General, El-
oise, Michigan

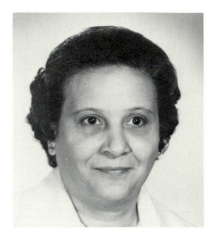

M. Phyllis Hill, M.S.W., A.C.S.W.

Senior Social Worker, University of Michigan Burn Center, Ann Arbor, Michigan

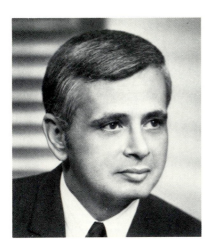

John E. Hoopes, M.D.

Professor of Surgery (Plastic), John Hop-
kins University School of Medicine
Plastic Surgeon-in-Charge, Johns Hopkins
Hospital, Baltimore, Maryland

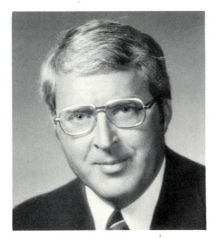

Thomas M. Hudak, M.D.

Chief of Plastic Surgery, St. Joseph's Hospital and Good Samaritan Hospital
Attending, Phoenix Plastic Surgery Program, Arizona Crippled Children's
Hospital, Phoenix, Arizona

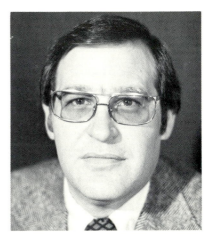

Michael H. James

Director, Program Development, National
Institute for Burn Medicine, Ann Arbor,
Michigan

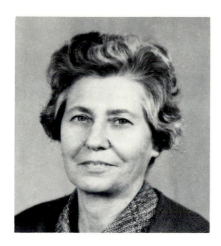

Heléné Janvier, M.D.

Burns Unit, Hospital Saint Luc, Lyon, *France*

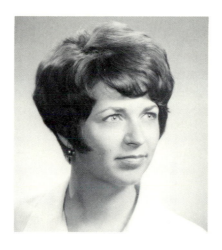

Claudella Archambeault-Jones, R.N.
Managing Editor

Director of Education, National Institute for Burn Medicine, Ann Arbor, Michigan

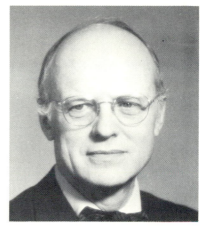

M.J. Jurkiewicz, M.D.

Professor of Surgery (Plastic), Emory University School of Medicine

Chief of Surgery, Grady Memorial Hospital, Attending Surgeon, Emory Affiliated Hospitals, Atlanta, Georgia

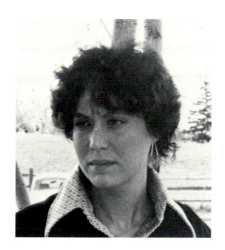

Leslie Kamil-Miller, M.S., O.T.R.

Acting Assistant Director, Occupational Therapy Division, Physical Medicine and Rehabilitation Department, University of Michigan Medical Center, Ann Arbor, Michigan

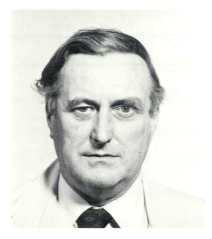

Desmond A. Kernahan, M.D.

Professor of Surgery, Northwestern University School of Medicine, Evanston, Illinois

Chief, Division of Plastic Surgery, Children's Memorial Hospital, Chicago, Illinois

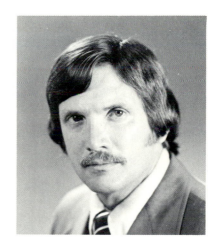

Lynn D. Ketchum, M.D.

Director, Hand Rehabilitation Center

Professor of Surgery (Plastic), University of Kansas Medical Center, Kansas City, Kansas

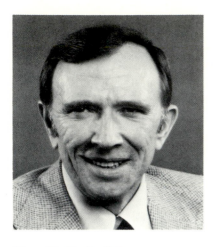

Glenn W. Kindt, M.D.

Professor, Department of Surgery (Neurosurgery), University of Michigan Medical Center, Ann Arbor, Michigan

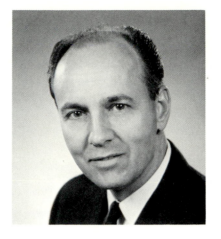

George H. Koepke, M.D.

Director, Physical Medicine and Rehabilitation, St. Mary's Hospital, Saginaw, Michigan

Former Professor and Acting Director of Physical Medicine and Rehabilitation, University of Michigan Medical Center, Ann Arbor, Michigan

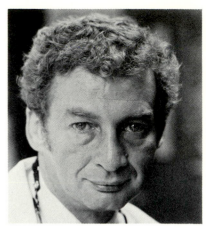

Thomas J. Krizek, M.D.

Professor of Surgery, Yale University School of Medicine

Chief, Section of Plastic and Reconstructive Surgery, Yale — New Haven Medical Center, New Haven, Connecticut

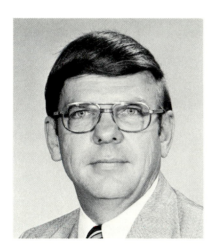

Duane L. Larson, M.D.

Director, University of Texas Burn Unit Chief of Staff, Shriners Burns Institute — Galveston Unit, Galveston, Texas

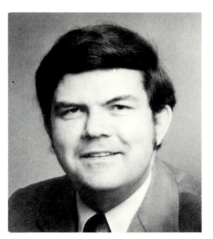

Denis C. Lee, Ph.D.

Associate Professor of Art, Associate Professor of Postgraduate Medicine

Director of Services, Medical and Biological Illustration

Director of Medical Sculpture, University of Michigan Medical Center, Ann Arbor, Michigan

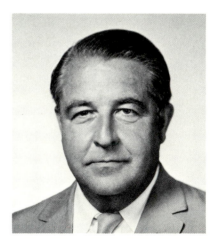

Jacob J. Longacre, M.D., Ph.D.

Late Associate Clinical Professor of Surgery (Plastic), University of Cincinnati, College of Medicine

Late Attending Plastic Surgeon, Cincinnati, Ohio

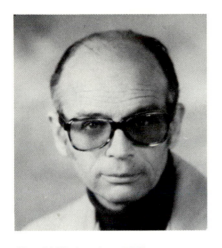

Harold W. Lueders, M.D.

West Contra Costa Plastic and Reconstructive Surgery Medical Group, Inc., Richmond, California

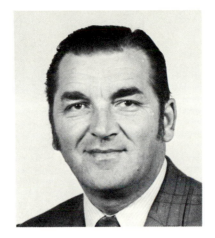

John B. Lynch, M.D.

Professor and Chairman, Department of Plastic Surgery, Vanderbilt University Medical Center

Chief of Plastic Surgery, Vanderbilt Affiliated Hospitals, Nashville, Tennessee

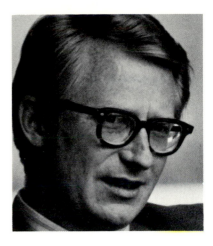

John W. Madden, M.D.

Clinical Professor, Department of Surgery (Hand), Clinical Professor, Department of Orthopedics (Hand Surgery), University of New Mexico, Albuquerque, New Mexico

Staff Surgeon, St. Joseph's Hospital

Staff Surgeon, Tucson Medical Center

Consultant, Davis Monthan Air Force Base Hospital, Tucson, Arizona

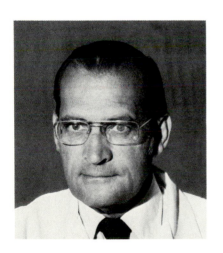

John E. Magielski, M.D., F.A.C.S.

Assistant Clinical Professor of Otorhinolaryngology, University of Michigan Medical Center

Attending Surgeon, St. Joseph Mercy Hospital, Ann Arbor, Michigan

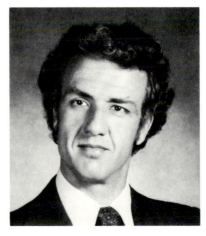

John M. Markley, Jr., M.D.

Assistant Clinical Professor of Surgery (Plastic), University of Michigan School of Medicine

Department of Plastic Surgery, St. Joseph Mercy Hospital, Ann Arbor, Michigan

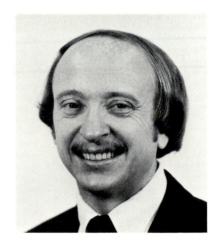

Roger F. Meyer, M.D.

Assistant Professor, Department of Ophthalmology

Director, Cornea Service, University of Michigan Medical Center, Ann Arbor, Michigan

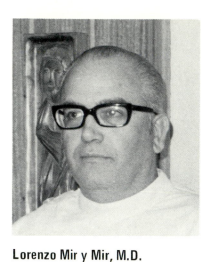

Lorenzo Mir y Mir, M.D.

Professor of Barcelona Faculty of
   Medicine (Retired)
Head, Plastic Surgery Department, Insti-
   tuto Policlinico de Barcelona
Expresident of the Catalan and Spanish
   Societies of Plastic Surgery, Barcelona
   Spain

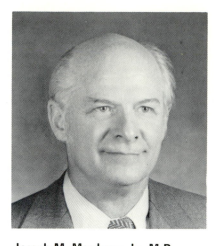

Joseph M. Meadows, Jr., M.D.

Consultant, St. Joseph Mercy Hospital
Psychiatric Director, Huron Valley Con-
   sultation Center, Ann Arbor, Michigan
Director, Psychiatric Services, Chelsea
   Community Hospital, Chelsea, Michigan

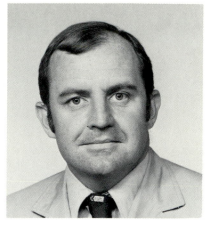

Joseph A. Moylan, M.D.

Associate Professor of Surgery
Chief, Trauma Service, Surgeon-in-
   Charge, Emergency Department, Duke
   University Medical Center, Durham,
   North Carolina

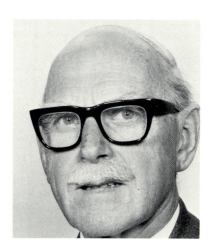

**John C. Mustardé, M.B., Ch.B..
D.O.M.S., F.R.C.S.**

Consultant Plastic Surgeon, West of Scotland Plastic Surgery Service (Retired),
   Canniesburn Hospital
Consultant Plastic Surgeon, Royal Hospital for Sick Children (Retired), Glas-
   gow, *Scotland*

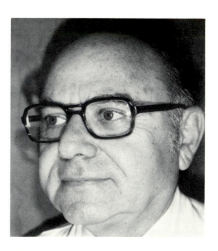

Zvi Neuman, M.D., F.A.C.S.

Late Professor of Plastic and Maxillofacial Surgery
Late Chief of the Department of Plastic
   and Maxillofacial Surgery, Hadassah
   Medical Organization, Jerusalem, *Israel*

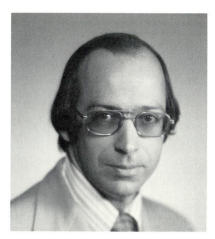

William B. Nickell, M.D., F.A.C.S.

Chief, Department of Plastic Surgery,
   East End Memorial Hospital, Baptist
   Medical Center Mont-Clair, Birming-
   ham, Alabama

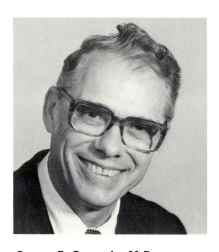

George E. Omer, Jr., M.D.

Professor and Chairman, Department of
Orthopaedics and Rehabilitation
Chief, Division of Hand Surgery, Depart-
ment of Surgery, University of New
Mexico School of Medicine, Albuquer-
que, New Mexico

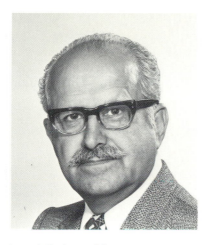

Joseph Paderewski

Medical Sculptor, Shriners Burn Institute
Galveston Unit, Galveston, Texas

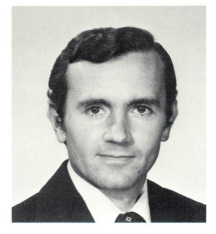

**Donald H. Parks, B.A., M.D.,
F.R.C.S. (C)**

Assistant Professor of Surgery (Plastic),
University of Texas Medical Branch
Chief, Division of Surgery, Shriners Burns
Institute — Galveston Unit, Galveston,
Texas

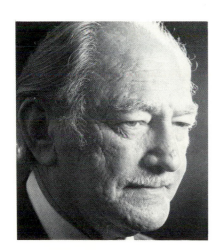

Jack Penn, M.D., F.R.C.S.

Professor of Plastic Maxillofacial and Oral
Surgery (Retired)
Consultant to University of Stellenbosch,
Cape Province
Consultant to S. African Army (Retired),
Clifton, Capetown, *South Africa*
Visiting Professor of Several Universities;
USA, *UK, Japan, Taiwan, Israel*

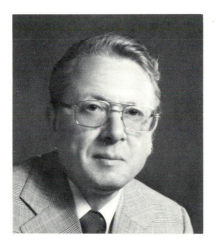

**Vincent R. Pennisi, M.D., D.D.S.,
F.A.C.S.**

Plastic and Reconstructive Surgery Cen-
ter, Bothin Burn Center, Saint Francis
Memorial Hospital, San Francisco,
California

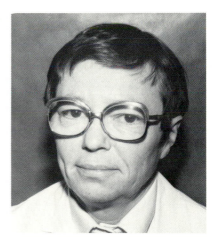

Kathryn E. Richards, M.D.

Assistant Clinical Professor of Surgery,
University of Michigan Medical School
Co-Director, Michigan Burn Center
Attending Surgeon, St. Joseph Mercy
Hospital, Ann Arbor, Michigan
Attending Surgeon, Chelsea Community
Hospital, Chelsea, Michigan

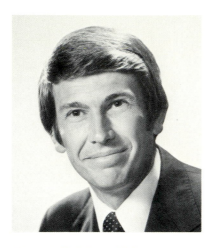

Kenneth E. Salyer, M.D.

Associate Professor, Chairman, Division of Plastic Surgery, Southwestern Medical School, University of Texas, Dallas, Texas

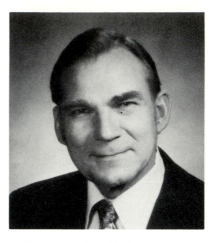

William S. Smith, M.D.

Professor and Head, Section of Orthopaedic Surgery, University of Michigan Medical Center, Ann Arbor, Michigan

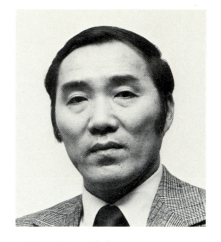

In Chul Song, M.D.

Professor of Plastic Surgery, Department of Surgery (Plastic), Downstate Medical Center, State University of New York, Kings County Hospital Center, Brooklyn, New York

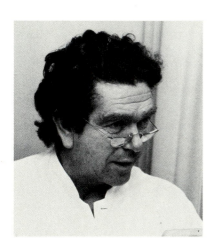

Bent Sørensen, M.D., D.M.Sc.

Professor of Surgery, University of Copenhagen
Chief of Staff, Department of Plastic Surgery and Burns Unit, Hvidovre Hospital, Copenhagen, *Denmark*

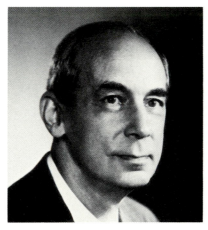

Radford C. Tanzer, M.D.

Clinical Professor of Plastic Surgery Emeritus, Dartmouth Medical School
Consultant in Plastic Surgery, Veterans Administration Hospital, Hanover, New Hampshire

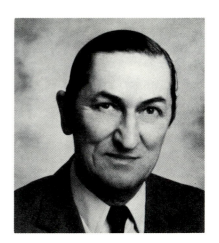

Noel Thompson, M.D., F.R.C.S.

Clinical Tutor, London University
Consultant-Surgeon, Regional Plastic Surgery Centre, Mount Vernon Hospital, London, *England*

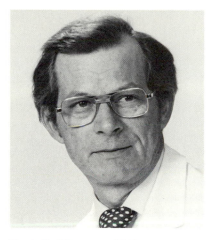

Hugh G. Thomson, M.D.

Associate Professor of Surgery, Faculty of Medicine, University of Toronto
Plastic Surgeon, Hospital for Sick Children
Consultant Surgeon, Ontario Crippled Children's Centre, Toronto, Ontario, *Canada*

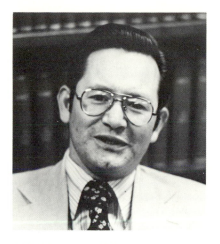

L.O. Vasconez, M.D.

Associate Professor of Surgery (Plastic), Emory University School of Medicine
Attending Surgeon, Emory Affiliated Hospitals
Chief, Hand Rehabilitation, Grady Memorial Hospital, Atlanta, Georgia

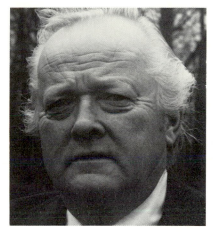

Frederick A. Waara

Waara Optical Laboratories, Ann Arbor, Michigan

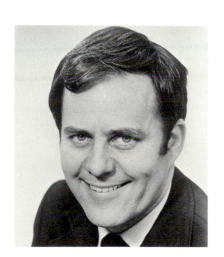

Michael G. Westmore

Professional Makeup Artist, Encino, California

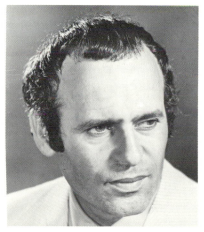

Menachem Ron Wexler, M.D.

Assistant Professor of Plastic Surgery, Hadassah Hebrew University Medical School
Acting Chief, Department of Plastic Surgery, Hadassah University Hospital, Jerusalem, *Israel*

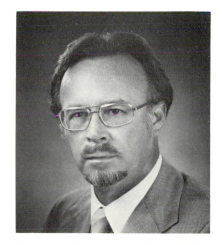

Eugene F. Worthen, M.D., F.A.C.S.

Chief of Plastic Surgery, Chief of Staff, St. Frances Medical Center
Consultant, Plastic Surgery, E.A. Conway Memorial Hospital, Monroe, Louisiana

TABLE OF CONTENTS

Only when we know little do we know anything; doubt grows with knowledge.

Goethe

FOREWORD

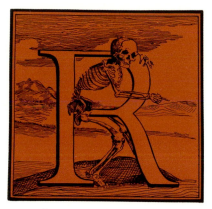

econstruction and Rehabilitation of the Burned Patient, a comprehensive multiauthored treatise, edited by Irving Feller, M.D., and William C. Grabb, M.D., is deservingly dedicated to Reed O. Dingman, M.D., Professor Emeritus of Plastic Surgery, University of Michigan. Many years ago, on a visit to Ann Arbor, I witnessed Dr. Dingman's lonely struggle to provide adequate care to burned patients dispersed in various surgical wards.

Despite the writings by authors who advocated, early in this century, such present-day techniques as the exposure treatment and skin grafting, only since World War II has burn treatment achieved a measure of status in surgery.

During the Battle of Britian the pilots of fighter planes were ordered to land the planes in flames at any cost: the pilots were expendable, the planes were not. Tannic acid, advocated since 1925 as a routine method of treatment, was rapidly abandoned as it was found to retard the application of skin grafts, the prime objective in the therapy of the full-thickness burn.

The full impact of the tragedy of burns was felt in the United States after the Cocoanut Grove and the Hartford fires in which large numbers of victims were trapped in raging infernos.

Today the integument is considered an essential organ of the body, controlling and protecting it from what Claude Bernard referred to as the "milieu exterieur."

Research in burns has provided invaluable information on fluid and electrolyte therapy, improved methods of combating shock and better understanding of the metabolic, nutritional, hematologic, and psychologic aspects of burn care. The problems of infection and the diminution of the burned patient's immunological response have emphasized the urgency of replacing the loss of critical amounts of skin, the final solution in burn therapy.

The reader will find the information he requires in this monumental compendium. The editors and the authors should be justly proud of their accomplishment.

John Marquis Converse M.D.

John Marquis Converse, M.D.

Lawrence D. Bell Professor of Plastic Surgery,
New York University School of Medicine
Director, Institute of Reconstructive Plastic Surgery,
New York University Medical Center, New York

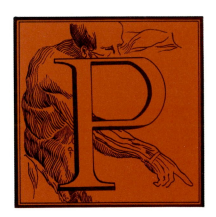

PREFACE

At the Michigan Burn Center we have learned that most burned patients can return to a useful place in society if an organized program of burn care and rehabilitation is followed. This goal is now being attained 90% of the time. These results indicate that an organized team approach works. Successful rehabilitation requires a skilled team, interested in the whole patient, conducting a coordinated program that meshes emotional and physical care and includes inpatient and outpatient follow-up and continued contact with the patient's family and community.

This book has been written to document the state of the art of rehabilitation as it is practiced today. The text has 17 sections, each divided into short chapters. They provide the reader with the principles and practices used by specialists who care for severely burned patients. Each section is introduced by a statement on the principles involved. A summary on the early care of the part of the body is included when anatomic reconstruction is considered. This is intended as a review for the reader who does not practice emergent and acute care.

Rarely can a book of considerable depth be compiled, edited, and readied for publication singlehandedly. Many specialists have contributed unselfishly to this book. They have dedicated years to finding ways of improving their methods and techniques and doing all in their power to make burn patients physically and emotionally whole. Their contributions to medicine and burn care are readily apparent in each of their chapters. There are of course many others who have contributed, and we gratefully acknowledge their involvement:

ACKNOWLEDGEMENTS

Kathryn E. Richards, M.D., Assistant Clinical Professor of Surgery, Division of Burn Surgery, University of Michigan Medical School, Co-Director, Michigan Burn Center; Jai Prasad, M.D., Clinical Instructor in Surgery and Fellow in Burn Medicine, Division of Burn Surgery, University of Michigan Medical School; and Mary E. Haab, R.N., Burn Nurse Specialist, Michigan Burn Center; for clinical coverage while this book was in process.

George H. Koepke, M.D., Director, Physical Medicine and Rehabilitation, St. Mary's Hospital, Saginaw, Michigan and former acting Head and Professor, Department of Physical Medicine and Rehabilitation, University of Michigan Medical School, for his long and enduring interest in and contributions to burn care.

Claudella A. Jones, R.N., Director of Education, National Institute for Burn Medicine, (NIBM), for inspiration and, at times, pointed encouragement, overall efficient organization and management, and good humored persistance as managing editor. Sandra Alexander-Stone, Graphic Artist, NIBM, for design, layout, and encouragement, and for taking time to think about this book on her honeymoon. Connie J. Gill, Graphic Artist, NIBM, for assistance in layout and graphic art. Daniel K. Hill, Photographer, NIBM, for patient photography and business management of color processing and halftones. Patricia C. Masters, Principal Secretary, Department of Burn Surgery, University of Michigan Medical School and Eleanor Dill, Janet S. Karius, Karen Gilson, and Cindy Frez, secretaries, NIBM, for deciphering many manuscripts and revisions, and for meticulous care in typesetting. Susan Marble, Courier, NIBM, for the many go-fors and bring-backs essential to completing the camera-ready copy.

Julia L. Casa, Librarian, NIBM, for efficiency and thoroughness in locating and providing background materials, and for her charm and many kindnesses. Jean L. Barnard, Reference/Rare Book Librarian and Laura B. Hawke, Librarian, University of Michigan Medical Center Library, for their painstaking assistance in locating rare books from the historical collections in the Medical Center Library for use as historical illustrations and citations, and L. Yvonne Wulff, Head Librarian, University of Michigan Medical Center Library, for her support. James E. Haney, for editing the manuscript and editorial suggestions. Harry Shore and Ned Thomson of Thomson-Shore, Inc., for their patient guidance in preparation of the camera-ready manuscript, Professor Gerald P. Hodges, Professor and Director of Medical and Biological Illustration and Professor of Art, Department of Postgraduate Medicine, University of Michigan and Nedra V. Marks, Medical Illustrator, NIBM, for consultation in medical illustration.

Ida Hubbard, Burn Clinic Supervisor, Joanne Helzerman, Secretary, Division of Burn Surgery, University of Michigan Medical School, and Daniel Tholen, Research Statistician, NIBM, for assistance in gathering patient information. Lauralee Lutz, and Anne Van De Walker, secretaries, Section of Plastic Surgery, University of Michigan Medical School, for their assistance in completing the manuscript. J.B. Lyons, M.D., Librarian, Royal College of Surgeons in Ireland, Dublin, and Caroline A. Hutchinson, R.N., Recovery Ward, Queen Victoria Hospital, East Grinstead, Sussex, England, for assistance in obtaining Dr. Barton's photograph. Frank P. Casa, Ph.D., Professor and Chairman, Romance Language and Literature, University of Michigan, for assistance in researching classic binding. Lois C. Withey, Administrative Associate, Department of Physical Medicine and Rehabilitation, University of Michigan Medical Center, formerly of NIBM, and Rita Sheeman, Secretary, Division of Burn Surgery, University of Michigan Medical School, for administrative assistance, early on, in preparation of this text. Cynthia Wojtowicz-Feller, General Administrator, NIBM, for administrative assistance and good-natured support, and Michael H. James, Director of Program Development, NIBM, for moral support.

And finally, an expression of appreciation for financial assistance which contributed to making the book possible; to the W.K. Kellogg Foundation, Great Lakes Regional Burn Care Demonstration Grant, and to the Rehabilitation Services Administration, grant number OHD-13-P-59197/5.

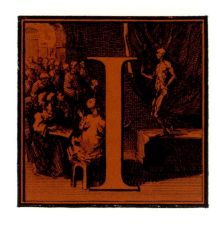NTRODUCTION

Physical and emotional stress mark the long hospitalization for every severely burned patient. For many patients, initial care is followed by a complicated rehabilitative process. Successful care begins at the scene of the accident and ends with returning the patient to a useful place in his community. When the patient is admitted, our immediate concern is survival. During the first few days following the injury, termed the Emergent period, the objective is to resolve problems of fluid balance to stabilize the patient. The second period, the Acute phase, is the longest period during the first hospitalization; all effort is directed to reducing the size of the wound and controlling infections and metabolic complications. Early attention to the basic principles of wound care can minimize functional and cosmetic deformities, and proper management of complications will decrease the residual effect on organ systems. All care during the first two periods provides the foundation for the third phase, Rehabilitation. Rehabilitation for the severely traumatized patient includes correction of functional and cosmetic deformities, management of emotional problems, continued care of organ system complications, and detection and treatment of late complications.

Successful rehabilitation results when all problems are considered simultaneously and resolved according to a plan individualized for each patient. First, correction of functional deformity is usually accomplished by helping the patient to return to normal activity. Cosmetic reconstruction, important to the patient's emotional rehabilitation, should be started as soon as conditions permit. The emotional and social problems that trouble the patient probably constitute the most difficult aspect of the rehabilitation process for the surgeon. Total care requires careful management by members of the Burn Team; surgeon, nurse, social worker, psychiatrist, and therapists working together to provide psychosocial support.

If the emotional needs of the patient are not met during the time when corrective surgery is performed, the patient may not be able to use the physical gain resulting from the operation to his best advantage. For example, the patient with a face burn must be helped to realize that he will never look as he did before the accident, in spite of the many procedures necessary to make it functional and to improve appearance. Simple statements of fact are not enough. The patient requires skilled management for his emotional needs between the hospitalizations for operative repairs. Constant re-evaluation of psychological change is important. If the surgeon does not have these skills, trained therapists should be employed. The surgeon, as head of the Burn Team, has the responsibility to properly select, train, and co-ordinate the personnel who will provide total care during the Emergent, Acute, and Rehabilitation phases. Only through their combined efforts can the patient return to a healthy life, feeling good about himself. This is not easy, nor is it impossible.

During the past 18 years at the Michigan Burn Center we have provided a total program of burn patient care from the time of the accident through rehabilitation. Between 1960 and 1975, of 2,215 patients who survived their burns, 1,616 required no reconstructive procedures. Of the 599 who were reconstructed, 232 required only one corrective operation, but one patient required 34 procedures. Two-hundred-fifty-two required two to five operations, and 114 patients required between six and 27 return admissions for reconstruction. The average age of patients requiring reconstructive procedures was 26. The average area of total burn was 27%, with an average of 16% full-thickness burn. Reconstructive procedures were most often required for the head, including scalp, eyes, nose, lips, face, and ears (644). The upper extremity, including hand, was second, followed by neck, then lower extremity, and last, trunk, including breast and perineum.

Should reconstructive operations be done by a plastic surgeon or a general surgeon? They must be performed by a surgeon who has taken the extra training necessary to manage the specific reconstruction problems. A plastic surgeon who has had only brief exposure to the burned patient during his residency requires additional training before undertaking the full range of care needed by a deformed burn patient. A general surgeon with no training in reconstruction, desiring to do reconstructive operations on the burned patient, should consider where his time is best spent. If he is dedicated to total patient care, he should arrange for training in burn reconstruction. The surgeon must be an expert in choosing the correct operative procedure and carrying it out successfully. He should understand the timing for the initial operation and timing between procedures, as well as knowing that scar tissue maturation and age of the patient, among other variables, will influence outcome of the operation.

The successful total care of the severely burned patient requires a highly trained team, following a well-organized program in a specialized facility. This combination of resources makes it possible for the patient to attain maximum rehabilitation and leaves the members of the Burn Team with a feeling of satisfaction that they have done their work well.

I. Feller, Wm. C. Grabb

I.

RECONSTRUCTION OF THE BURNED PATIENT

PRINCIPLES OF RECONSTRUCTION

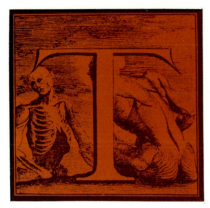

he successful repair of functional and cosmetic deformity is based upon proper diagnosis of the problem, skilled application of the correct reconstructive operation, and meticulous postoperative care. To attain the best possible results all members of the Burn Team must work with the surgeon during this entire period. This introductory section identifies postburn problems and deals with basic approaches to correcting these problems by different specialists on the burn team, including consideration of the patient's age, sex, occupation, and individual needs. Problems and repair methods not included here can be found elsewhere in this book. The basic problems seen in burned patients are these:

- Surface wounds may result in scar contracture and a shortage of tissue, requiring release and closure of the defect with split-thickness autografts, pedicles, or Z-plasty.
- Loss of scalp hair and eyebrows, requiring repair with hair-bearing transplants.
- Hypertrophic scar or keloid formation, which can be corrected with form-fitting elastic stockings, steroid injection, or partially removing the scar and leaving the base for overgrafting.
- Inappropriate skin texture and coloring and thin skin cover, best corrected by dermabrasion and overgrafting.
- Tendon, muscle, bone, and joint deformity or destruction, resulting in fusion of joints or amputation. Repair may require tendon transplants, joint fusion, pedicle graft for full-thickness coverage, bone grafts, or finger transplantation.
- Heterotopic bone formation, requiring close follow-up with excision at the optimal postburn time.
- Squamous cell carcinoma formation (Marjolin's ulcer) resulting from delayed wound healing, necessitating deep and wide excision and grafting or amputation.
- Polyneuropathy which may require medical intervention, casting, splinting, or bracing.

Reconstruction should be planned to obtain the maximum functional, cosmetic, and emotional result. Some problems can be corrected with one operation, while others require long-term planning with staged procedures. Children must be followed through the growth years to reduce the possibility of permanent functional loss from skin graft and the scar tissue not keeping up with the growth. Timing based on scar maturation must be considered, e.g., the child requiring release and graft of hypertrophic scar contracture of the anterior neck. Release and grafting can be done initially and repeated as needed as the child grows, with the cosmetic-or-functional-deforming scar excised during the last reconstructive operation. Time away from work and financial problems have to be considered for the adult. All patients must be closely followed to ensure maximal result of the individual procedure, e.g., special splinting and physical therapy may be necessary to obtain maximum function, and in some cases a special prosthesis should be adapted. The choice of the procedure to correct scar deformity depends upon the defect and the condition of surrounding tissue. Often a combination of several different procedures will be used for optimal outcome. Thought must also be given to the stress resulting from anesthesia, the length of anesthesia time, and the agent used during staged-reconstructive procedures.

Irving Feller

RELEASE OF SCAR CONTRACTURE

Irving Feller

Scar contracture results in a shortage of skin in the affected area, and often the quality of the scar tissue is inadequate for permanent cover. These are two separate problems. The lack of tissue causes loss of joint function, postural changes, and cosmetic deformity. The quality of the scar is a function of the scar type, i.e., hypertrophic scar, atrophic scar, or keloid. Each may or may not have ulcerations.

When possible, both problems can be managed simultaneously. The contracture is released, the inadequate scar excised, and a skin graft is used to cover the defect. However, in many cases the defect is very large when the contracture is released. In these cases, excision of inadequate scars would only make the defect larger and more difficult to graft. The method of choice is to release the contracture first and then determine if the resulting defect should be made larger by excision of the adjacent inadequate scar.

The exception would be the presence of an ulcer within the scar, which would be excised at the time of the release to remove the tissue as a source of infection. When both conditions exist and it is not desirable to both release the contracture and excise the undesirable scar tissue, two procedures are required.

A satisfactory method for releasing scar contracture utilizes the double "Y" incision, the artists' illustration of which is shown in Figure 1. A double "Y" is drawn perpendicular to the line of contracture, Figure 2. A., B., C. This allows for maximum release at the ends of the contracture without increasing the length of the incision. A comparison is made with the conventional length of incision required to obtain the width of release necessary to correct the contracture as is seen in Figure 2. D. and E. Figure 3 demonstrates the procedure on a patient with a severe contracture of the elbow.

Fig. 1. A. Artist's view from above showing a flexion contracture with lines drawn to show the method of release. B. After the incision is made and the flexion contracture release accomplished, the double "Y" lines give way to form a rectangle.

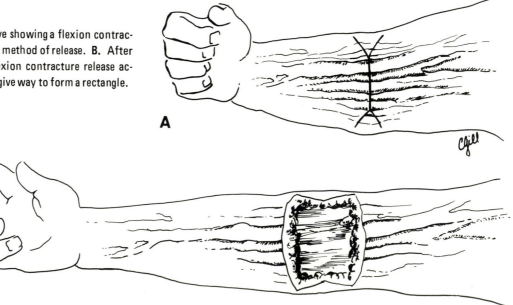

A

B

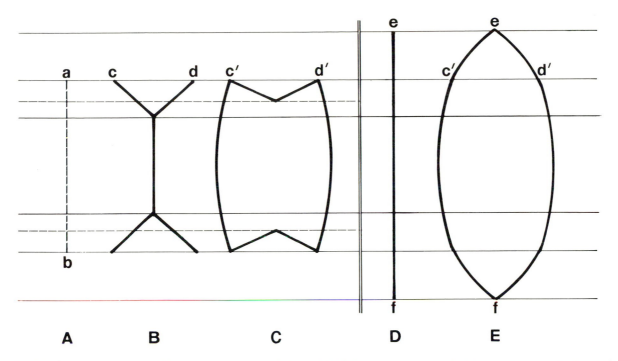

A   **B**   **C**   **D**   **E**

Fig. 2. This figure was prepared to illustrate the principles of the double "Y" release technique. **A.** Line a to b represents the width of the scar. **B.** The double "Y" is drawn to cover the width of the scar. Distance c to d is the minimum width that can be obtained after the incision has been made and the release accomplished. **C.** The full release after the incision has been made (no tissue removed). The distance c' to d' is the maximum width that can be obtained by this technique. **D.** The conventional length of incision, one line e to f, required to obtain the same release that was obtained in C. **E.** The size of the defect that results from incision e to f. The width (c' to d') is the same, but the overall size of the defect is longer than that which results from the double "Y".

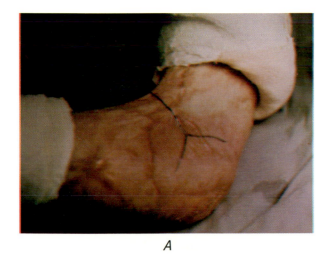

A

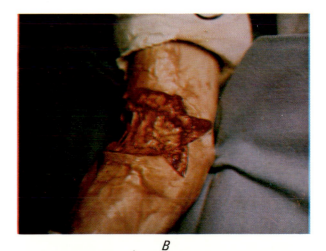

B

Fig. 3. A. A severe antecubital space flexion contracture. Lines have been drawn to mark the location for the releasing incision. **B.** The release has been accomplished by incising the scar along the lines of the double "Y". No tissue has been removed. The defect shows the shortage of tissue in this contracture. **C.** The area is shown after healing. The forearm is in full extension and the elbow now has a full range of motion.

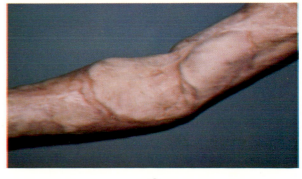

C

3

HETEROTOPIC BONE

E. Burke Evans

Heterotopic bone associated with burns is mainly if not exclusively located around major joints. It has been observed in adults at elbow, shoulder, and hip, in that order of frequency. In children, the elbow and hip are probably affected equally. We have not observed shoulder involvement in children and have observed knee involvement in only one adult. Wrists, ankles, and smaller joints have not been affected in our patients.

The bone lies in the planes of ligaments and muscles. It has been found to incorporate or replace ligaments but not to invade muscle.

In the adult elbow, it most often lies posteriorly in the plane of the medial fibers of the triceps, extending from the olecranon to the medial epicondylar ridge (Figure 1). In children osseous bridging of the elbow is often anterior in the plane of the brachialis, extending from the coranoid or from the radial tuberosity toward the anterior surface of the humerus (Figures 2 and 3).

If adult elbows are bridged anteriorly, there is usually an associated posterior bridge (Figure 4). The radius and ulna are also occasionally joined at the level of the radial tuberosity (Figure 5). This bridge has not been observed in the absence of a posterior bridge.

In the adult shoulder the osseous bridges occur beneath the deltoid, extending from the acromion to the greater tuberosity of the humerus (Figure 6) and in the plane of the subscapularis passing from the lateral border of the scapula to the upper end of the humerus (Figure 7). Occasionally there are shell-like extensions from either osseous mass which cover the head of the humerus in the plane of the capsule.

At the hip in adults and children the bone usually lies in the planes of the iliacus or of the glutei (Figure 8). It is rarely disposed in the horizontal planes of the small rotators.

Although the cause of heterotopic bone is unknown, it is known that severity of burn, length of

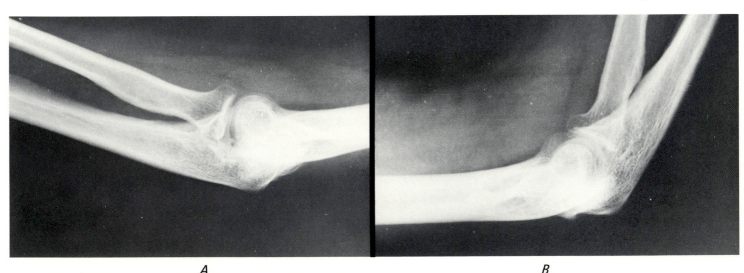

A   B

Fig. 1. Ankylosis due to extra-articular heterotopic bone in elbows in a 32-year-old man six months after 30 percent full-thickness burn involving trunk and both upper extremities. Both forearms could be fully pronated and supinated. **A.** Right elbow. **B.** Left elbow.

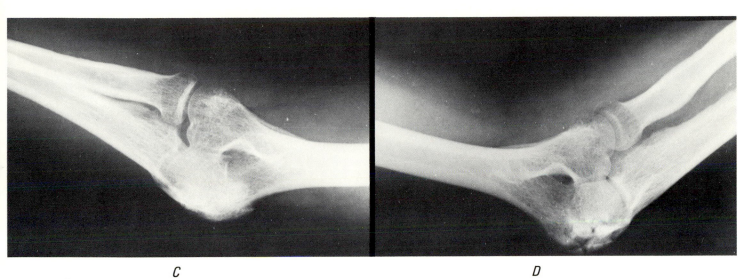

C   D

Fig. 1. (Cont.) Anterior-posterior projections of the elbows show the medial position of the osseous bridges. **C.** Right elbow. **D.** Left elbow.

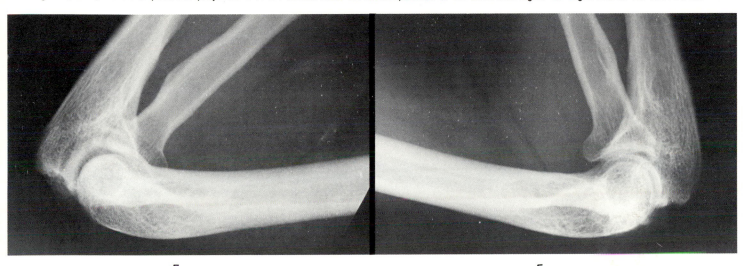

E   F

Fig. 1. (Cont.) Fourteen months after resection of the heterotopic bone both elbows had functional range of motion. Further increase in range was expected. **E.** Right elbow. **F.** Left elbow.

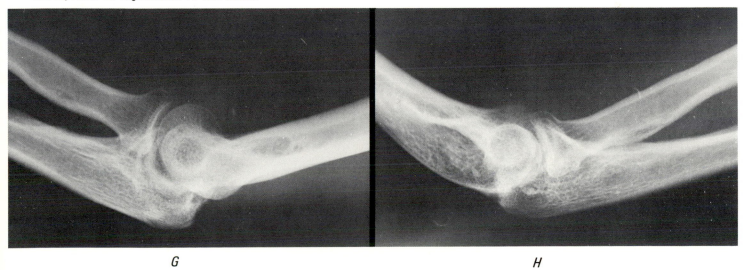

G   H

Fig. 1. (Cont.) Also fourteen months after resection. **G.** Right elbow. **H.** Left elbow.

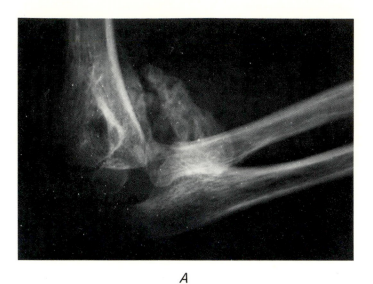
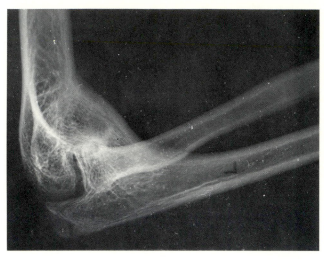

A

B

Fig. 2. A. Immature heterotopic bone bridging the elbow of a 5-year-old girl with 50 percent full-thickness burn. **B.** The bone was resected two months later when it was mature.

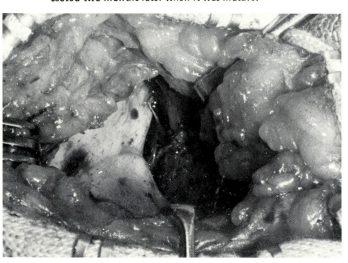
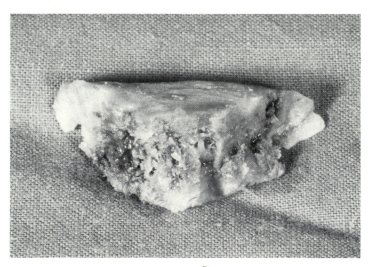

C

D

Fig. 2. C. Operative exposure of the osseous bridge revealed it to have mature cortex. **D.** The resected wedge showed normal medullary bone.

Fig. 2. E. The elbow as it appeared seven years after heterotopic bone excision. The elbow regained full range of motion.

Figure 2. A., B., and D., are reprinted with permission from Journal of the American Medical Association; June 3, 1968; Volume 204; pp. 843-848. Evans, E. Burke; Larsen, Duane L.; Yates, Sam. Copyright 1968, American Medical Association.

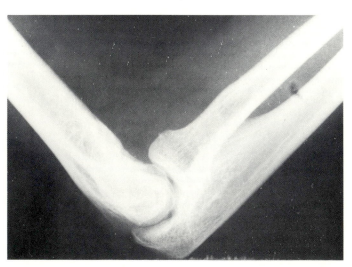

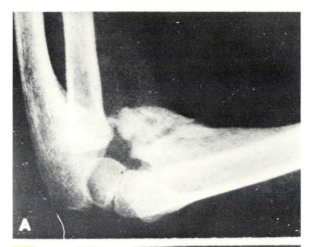

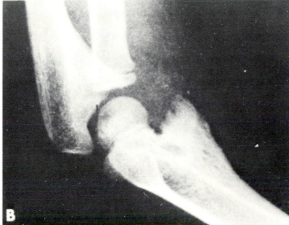

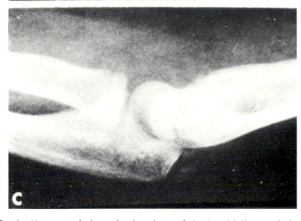

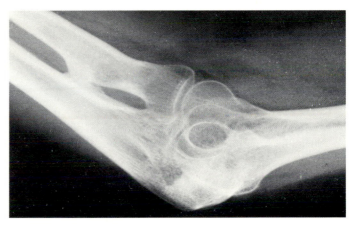

Fig. 4. Heterotopic bone bridges the elbow posteriorly from the olecranon to the medial condylar ridge and anteriorly from the coranoid to the coranoid fossa one year after 40 percent full-thickness burn in a 38-year-old man. (Same patient as Fig. 7.) There was advanced articular destruction. Resection of the bone restored limited motion but intra-articular ankylosis occurred in a short time.

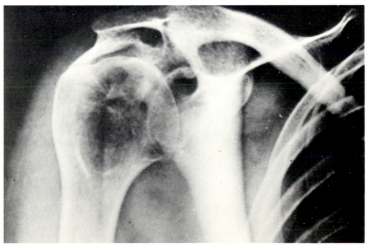

Fig. 5. There is proximal radio-ulnar synostosis and posterior bridging of the elbow in this 33-year-old woman with 20 percent full-thickness burn. The burn involved neck, upper chest and both upper extremities. (Same patient as Fig. 6.)

Fig. 3. **A.** Heterotopic bone in the plane of the brachialis muscle in an 8-year-old girl six weeks after 40 percent full-thickness burn. The affected extremity was only slightly burned. The bone did not bridge the joint. **B.** In three months it had diminished in size. **C.** In one year it had almost disappeared.

Fig. 6. A shell of heterotopic bone extends from the entire acromial border to the greater tuberosity of the humerus. The ectopic bone was resected. Muscles attaching to the tuberosity were intact. Gleno-humeral flexion and extension were restored completely. Abduction and rotation were not. (Same patient as Fig. 5.)

Fig. 7. Large heterotopic exostoses projecting from scapula and humerus in the plane of the subscapularis in a 38-year-old man with 40 percent full-thickness burn. Ankylosis did not take place and it was not necessary to resect the bone. (Same patient as Fig. 4.)

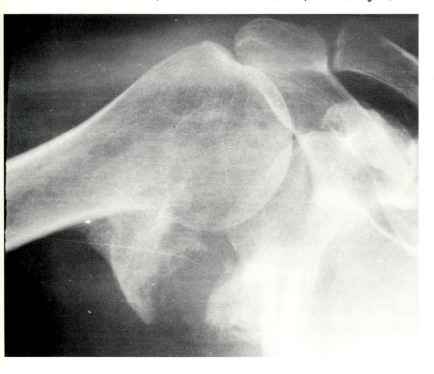

bed confinement, superimposed trauma, and individual idiosyncracy or familial predisposition may favor its formation.

The location of heterotopic bone is not strictly determined by the distribution of the burn. It may occur in a slightly involved or even an uninvolved extremity.

The behavior pattern of the heterotopic bone of burns is similar to that of transient paralysis, in that once the primary disease has resolved the bone no longer forms. However, it is unlike that of post-traumatic myositis ossificans, in which the heterotopic bone commonly reforms after its resection.

Recognition of the following four facts is helpful in planning the treatment of heterotopic bone occurring as a result of burns:

1) Para-articular heterotopic bone will persist and may even increase in dimension as long as there are open granulating areas.

2) As soon as the burn wounds have healed, heterotopic bone which has not bridged a joint may in children disappear, while in adults it will at least diminish in size (Figure 3).

Fig. 8. A. Ankylosis of the left hip due to heterotopic bone extending from pelvis to lesser trochanter in the plane of the iliacus. The slender deposit of bone on the right did not limit motion. The 30 percent full-thickness burn in this 10-year-old girl involved lower trunk, groin, and lower extremities. **B.** After resection of the bone there was partial recurrence but the new bone did not bridge the hip and motion was restored.

A   B

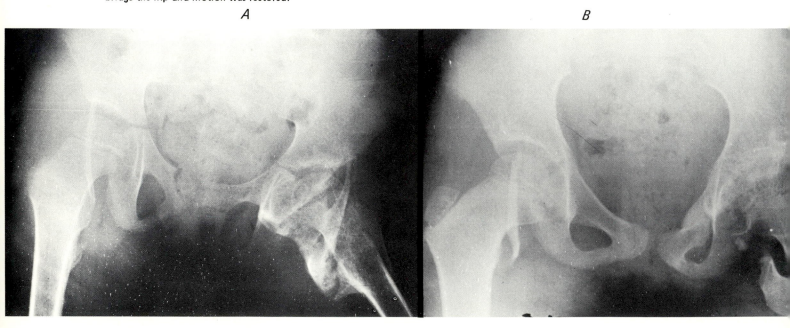

3) Heterotopic bone which bridges a joint in one plane spares the articulation; and thus, as a rule, after it is removed a functional range of joint motion is readily regained.

4) When heterotopic bone bridges a joint in more than one plane, the likelihood of restoring joint motion by surgical resection of the bone is correspondingly decreased regardless of apparent sparing of the articulation (Figures 4 and 5).

It is probably best to postpone surgery until all burn wounds have healed and certainly until the heterotopic bone is well defined and no longer increasing in dimension.

In the surgical approach the skin incision should be generous and accurately placed to minimize the need for retraction and to facilitate deep dissection. The skin often appears to be fragile but if it is managed delicately, it will heal beautifully. Dissection can most always be in tissue planes and thus the knife is not as useful as the closed scissors or hemostat or finger tip. The heterotopic bone is removed with a sharp osteotome after the osteotomy site has been incised and defined with a knife to assure a clean edge and to prevent shredding of soft tissue by the osteotome. The excision site is checked digitally after removal for any remaining ridges. A slight excavation is preferred.

Deposits bridging the shoulder from acromion to greater tuberosity have been approached through a transverse or peri-acromial incision. Deltoid fibers have been detached at origin if necessary and split longitudinally for access to the bone. Deposits below the joint have been approached through a routine delto pectoral incision. This is preferred to the transaxillary approach because of better visualization of the antero-superior aspect of the joint and because of its proximal extensibility.

The anteriorly disposed heterotopic bone at the elbow, whether radial or ulnar in origin, is easily exposed through a double curved incision beginning along the medial border of the brachialis above the elbow and ending along the medial border of the brachio-radialis below. The incision should cross from medial to lateral at the level of the radial tuberosity.

If the bone extends from the coronoid process it is well to remember that the process can be generously trimmed without compromise of elbow or brachialis function.

Osseous bridges between the radius and ulna at and above the tuberosity are best approached posteriorly through a linear incision paralleling the lateral border of the proximal ulna and olecranon.

Through this approach only the anconeus and the upper fibers of the supinator must be dealt with. If the bone extends proximally to the radio-ulnar joint a portion of the anconeus will be lost in the excision.

The approach to heterotopic bone extending from the olecranon to the medial epicondyle is through a double curved incision beginning proximally along the medial border of the triceps, crossing laterally distal to the tip of the olecranon and ending distally at the medial border of the extensor muscle bundle. The incision may be extended distally if there is a bridge of bone between radius and ulna. See Figure 9 for details of this commonly used approach.

At the hip only anterior osseous bridges have required surgical excision. These have been approached through an anterior ilio-femoral incision beginning along the anterior inch or two of the iliac crest and curving distally at the anterior superior spine to extend along the interval between the tensor fasciae latae and the sartorius to about the juncture of the upper and middle one thirds of the femur. The bone may be expected to lie deep to the iliacus or glutei and is reached by reflecting these muscles.

Fortunately, heterotopic bone rarely bridges the hip and if it does not it should be left alone, because a functional range of motion will likely be restored even if resorption of the abnormal bone is incomplete.

Following complete resection of the heterotopic bone, adhesions can usually be broken down by gentle progressive manipulation of the joint. Pericapsular soft tissue can be incised if necessary. An elbow which has been ankylosed in extension should be mobilized to at least 90 degrees of flexion if the ulnar nerve has been transposed forward, but one ankylosed at 90 degrees of flexion should not be forced into

Fig. 9. A. After skin reflection the ulnar nerve (a) is isolated proximal to the elbow where it emerges along the medial border of the triceps (b). Fibers of the triceps tendon attaching to the olecranon are visible (c).

Fig. 9. B. The triceps muscle (b) is retracted laterally; the fibers of attachment being carefully removed by sharp dissection from the olecranon (d). The bridge of heterotopic bone extending from the olecranon to the medial border of the humerus is exposed (e). The ulnar nerve is dissected free of the field and retracted (a).

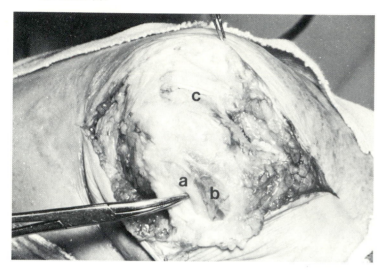

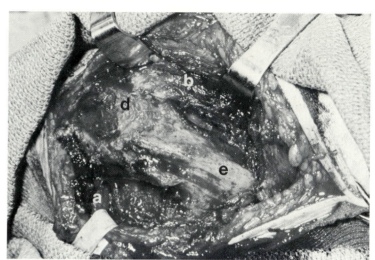

Fig. 9. C. The heterotopic bone is generously excised exposing raw bone of the ulna (d) and humerus (f) and the intact but somewhat irregular cartilaginous surface of the trochlea (g). Following resection of the bone the ulnar nerve (a) is transposed anteriorly and the triceps is sutured back in place. The intact distal attachment of the triceps is shown (c).

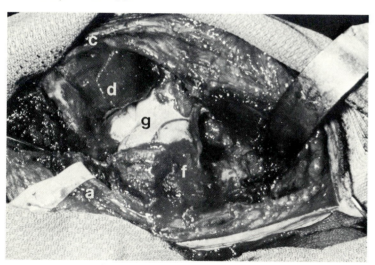

complete extension because of the danger of stress on the anteriorly disposed nerves and vessels.

In general, postoperative positioning of the elbow should favor correction of the previous deformity. The extremity should be immobilized with plaster for three days or so, following which active assistive and isometric exercise should be started. Hips and shoulders are generally positioned at neutral after surgery.

A good range of motion may be gained rather quickly, but I advise patients that if the joint remains free of new bone growth it may take as long as 18 to 24 months to gain maximum benefit from the surgery. If heterotopic bone is going to recur it will do so much sooner than that.

Although I have operated upon joints more than once for recurrent abnormal bone, I shall be reluctant to do it again because none of these operations has been successful.

Happily, heterotopic bone is now so rarely observed as not to be a problem among our own patients. We are convinced that the practice of mobilizing burn patients quickly is largely responsible for this favorable change in incidence.

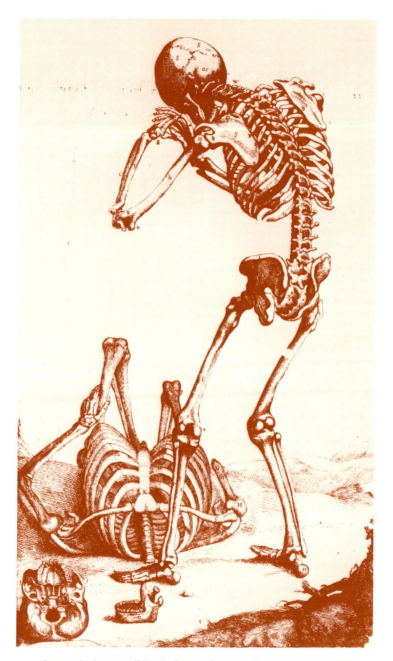

Anatomie der wtterlicke deelen van het menschelick lichaem, 1660.

Life must be lived forwards, but can only be understood backwards.

Kierkegaard

4

HYPERTROPHIC SCARRING AND KELOID: SHAVING AND OVERGRAFTING

Irving Feller

At the extreme ends of the continuum of burn injuries, the healing response of patients is similar, while in the mid-ranges of skin damage and destruction, healing differences among patients are very apparent. Superficial partial-thickness burns heal well in all cases where infection has been avoided. Full-thickness burns also follow a satisfactory and predictable course if they have been properly debrided and autografted. However, the response to the deep partial-thickness burn is not predictable. It is here where the problems of scarring, hypertrophic scarring, and keloid appear. All of these responses make up the spectrum of the human's skin response to the burn injury.

In reviewing the skin's response to various depths of burn, we find that superficial partial-thickness burns, where the damage to the skin is minimal, produce erythema and pain. Healing is complete within a few days, leaving no evidence that injury had occurred. The response to deeper superficial burns is blister formation. At this level of injury, variations among patients become apparent. Some patients heal and show no evidence of injury. Others form enlarged openings to the sweat glands and hair follicles, pigment changes, or flat and mildly contracted scars.

Deep partial-thickness burns result in the greatest variation; they heal in some patients, leaving little or no evidence of injury, as described above, while similar burns in other patients result in severe contracture, massive hypertrophic scars, or keloids. The treatment of these conditions is now limited by our understanding of the skin's physiologic response to burn injury.

Why one patient's injury leaves marked hypertrophic scars while a similar burn on a different patient results in a minimal change in the skin is not known. Conceivably the spectrum of responses to the burn is constant, and a patient's response depends upon his particular physiological reactions to the injury.

HYPERTROPHIC SCAR

There are apparent differences in hypertrophic scar formation in patients. The color, size, hardness, time of onset, duration, and time of involution varies. The hypertrophic scar appears after the epidermis has regenerated. It is as if the reparatory process does not stop, as it does in most patients, but rather continues, resulting in excessive tissue formation. Intense erythema is usually the first sign, followed by the raised lesion. The patient reports parathesia and dysthesias. The most prominent symptom is pruritus. The lesion then continues to increase in thickness and becomes firm, dark red, and almost cartilaginous in consistency. There may or may not be contracture formation, depending upon the location of the hypertrophic scar. Contractures usually become apparent across joints, resulting in loss of motion. After a period of time varying from months to years, the erythema lessens, the scar softens and decreases in size.

Since we know that individual patients vary greatly in their responses, observation is necessary before treatment is prescribed. The contractures that accompany hypertrophic scars over joints can be lessened by splinting. Some physicians advocate pressure dressings while others surgically release the scar and autograft the defect. Most hypertrophic scars involute over a period of time and further treatment is not necessary. Large intensive scars of the face may result in marked disfigurement and should be corrected early. They will respond to temporary measures such as shaving and overgrafting until the involution is complete. Then a definitive procedure can be done.

KELOID

At the far extreme of the process is the keloid, a benign lesion that continues to grow. The difference between the hypertrophic scar and the keloid is that the hypertrophic scar process is self-limiting, while the keloid continues to grow. Both are pathologic processes. Fortunately the keloid is rare; the majority of raised scars that occur are hypertrophic scars.

The keloid can be treated by shaving the defect down to its base and overgrafting. Care should be taken to stay within the border of the keloid and to leave a thin layer of base scar in place before overgrafting.

SHAVING AND OVERGRAFTING

Shaving and overgrafting of massive hypertrophic scars of the face is a method for interim correction of both cosmetic and functional deformity. Definitive

procedures should not be carried out when a hypertrophic scar is active. If an attempt was made to excise the hypertrophic scar early, more harm than good could result because (1) the hypertrophic scar may recede so that excision is not necessary, and (2) early excision of hypertrophic scar often results in additional scarring and increased functional deformity. However, when the hypertrophic scars are very large, i.e., elevated to 0.5cm or more above the surface, they can be shaved down to the level of normal surrounding tissue and overgrafted. Often this procedure will provide a good result until the hypertrophic scar process shows signs of involution, at which time a definitive procedure can be carried out if necessary.

The method is illustrated in Figure 1. The hypertrophic scar is placed under tension by using skin hooks, sutures, or towel clamps (Figure 1 A). Layers of the scar are shaved off to remove excessive tissue, discolored skin, or irregular surfaces, until the hypertrophic scar is removed down to the base (Figure 1 B). A sharp knife is necessary and the blade

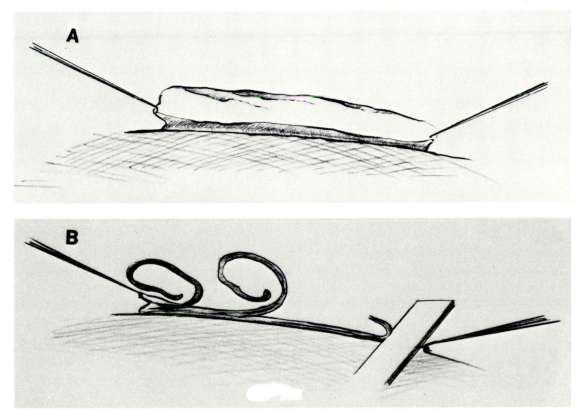

Fig. 1. A. Skin hooks are used to provide traction. **B.** Thin layers of the hypertrophic scar are shaved away. The process continues until only a thin layer of scar remains at the base.

should be changed frequently (Figure 2 A). Care must be taken to leave a thin layer of dermis or scar at the base and at the edge of the lesion with as good a blood supply as possible to avoid regeneration of new hypertrophic scar (Figure 2 B). Sharply curved surfaces are dermabrased to remove epithelium and provide a vascular base for grafts. The circumference of the denuded area is then incised to release any contracture that may exist and provide an edge for securing grafts. A pattern is made of the defect to

mark the donor site and a split-thickness graft is cut. The base is then overgrafted with this autograft. At approximately .020 inch thick, this graft is cut slightly smaller than the defect to apply tension to the base when it is secured in place by suture or metal clips and an appropriate dressing applied. A patient is shown in Figure 3 A with a keloid in the right cheek. This was removed and the defect repaired by the method stated. The appearance of the cheek four years later is seen in Figure 3 B.

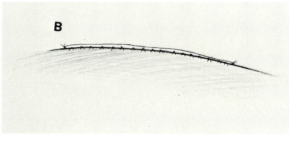

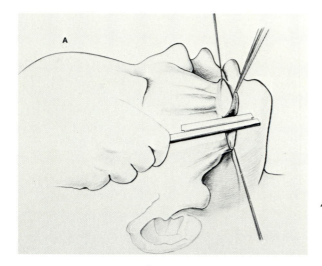

Fig. 2. A. Hypertrophic scars of the face can be shaved using a straight razor. **B.** A split-thickness skin graft is sewn on the defect and a dressing is applied.

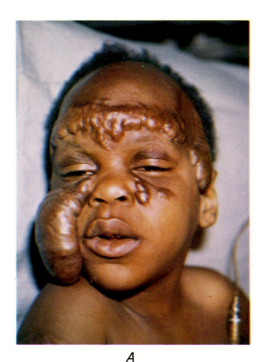

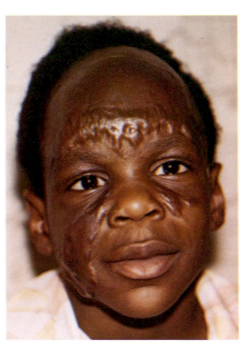

Fig. 3. Keloid. **A.** A patient with a keloid of the right cheek shown preoperatively. **B.** This patient is seen four years after removal of the keloid by the method described.

Figure 4 demonstrates this method as used to remove an active hypertrophic scar. The lesion is shown prior to operation (Figure 4 A). The hypertrophic scar is excised (Figure 4 B) and hemostasis is secured. A split-thickness graft is taken with either a Brown or Padgett dermatome (4 C and D), and 4 E is the artist's conception of the depth of such a graft. Choice of the dermatome is that of the surgeon. The split-thickness graft is applied under slight tension and is held in place using sutures (Figure 4 F). The result is shown one year later (Figure 4 G).

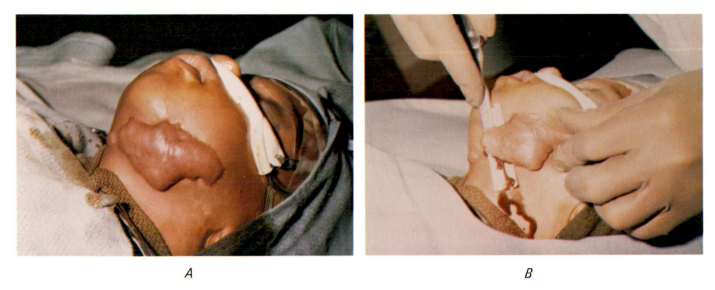

A

B

Fig. 4. Hypertrophic scar. **A.** The hypertrophic lesion prior to surgery. **B.** Excision of the hypertrophic scar.

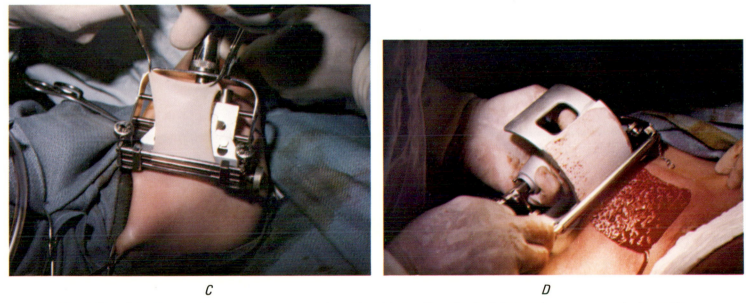

C

D

Fig. 4. (Cont.) C. Use of a Brown dermatome to obtain a split-thickness skin graft. **D.** A Padgett dermatome may also be used by choice of the surgeon.

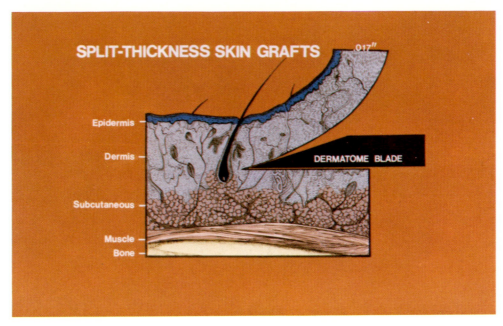

Fig. 4. E. Artist's concept demonstrating the depth of a split-thickness skin graft.

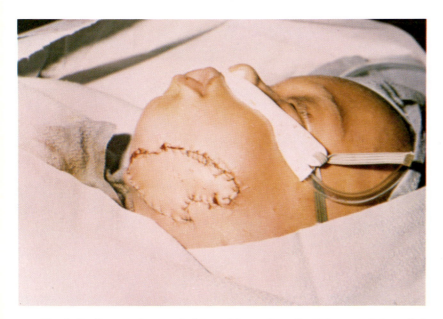

Fig. 4. F. Hemostasis secured after excision and a split-thickness graft is applied and is held in place with sutures.

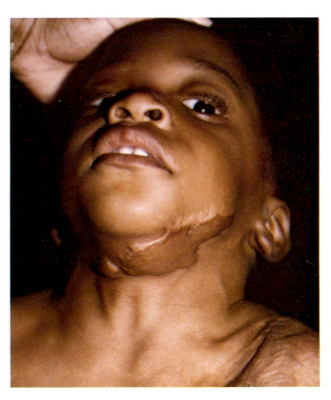

Fig. 4. G. Appearance of patient one year later.

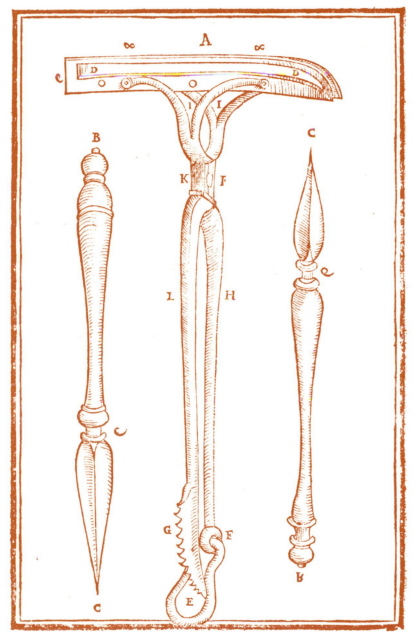

De curtorum chirurgia insitionem, 1597.

5

HYPERTROPHIC SCARRING: PRESSURE DRESSINGS

Donald H. Parks
Duane L. Larson
A.J. de la Houssaye

Hypertrophic scar formation and scar contracture following thermal injury constitute a serious and perplexing problem in the rehabilitation of burned patients. These sequelae are too often accepted as unavoidable, particularly in children.

The use of special nonsurgical techniques based on histopathology has been invaluable in the prevention and correction of hypertrophic scar formation. These techniques include a carefully supervised program of splinting and positioning instituted immediately post-burn, and the simple application of constant and controlled pressure in the post-healing phase, using elastic wraps or garments and custom-molded splints.

HISTOPATHOLOGY OF HYPERTROPHIC SCAR

Hypertrophic scar tissue develops when the deep reticular dermis has been injured, as in deep partial-thickness burns. It usually appears six weeks to three months post-burn and is characteristically raised, firm, red, and blanches with pressure (Figure 1).

Microscopically, the normal, loose tridimensional collagen-fiber arrangement of the dermis is replaced by a disarray of collagen, which twists and turns to ultimately form the compact whorl-like and nodular arrangement typical of a hypertrophic scar (Figure 2). The increased vasculature, collagen, fibroblasts, and the presence of myofibroblasts account for the gross features of hypertrophic scar and contractures.

Constant controlled pressure induces the features of mature scar tissue—grossly, a flat, pale, soft scar, and microscopically, orderly, parallel collagen fibers with fewer vessels, fibroblasts and myofibroblasts (Figure 3). This property of controlled pressure has led to its therapeutic use in the prevention and correction of hypertrophic scar formation.

POSITIONING AND SPLINTING

A comprehensive program to control the healing burn wound and thus to prevent contractures and

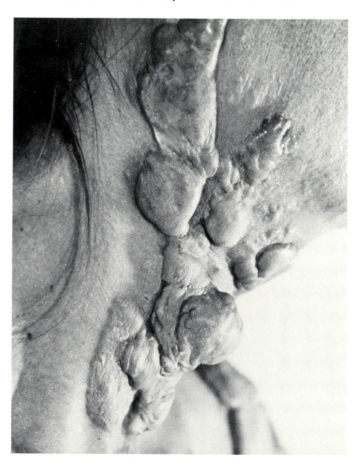

Fig. 1. Raised, firm, red hypertrophic scar on neck.

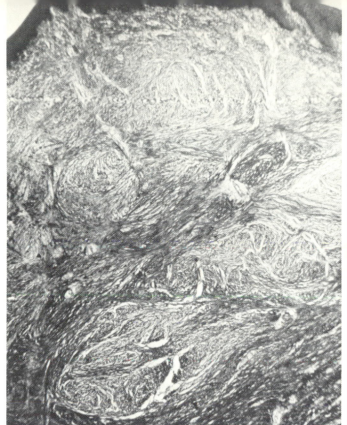

Fig. 2. Hypertrophic scar showing thick whorl-like and nodular arrangement of dermal collagen. (Micrograph courtesy of Dr. H. Linares)

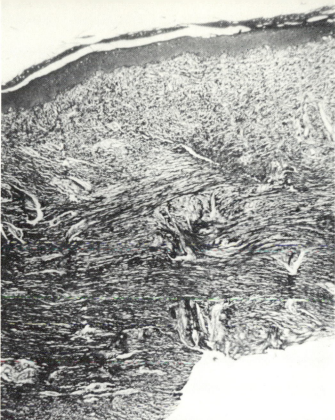

Fig. 3. Hypertrophic scar under pressure. Note parallel orientation of collagen. (Micrograph courtesy of Dr. H. Linares)

hypertrophic scars must begin as soon as possible post-burn. Although the overall management of the burned patient may vary from center to center, the principles of retaining function by proper positioning and splinting remain basically the same.

The physical and occupational therapists are often best qualified to manage the positioning and splinting program and to supervise individually-designed daily exercise programs.

Pre-Healing. Proper positioning and custom splinting are instituted as soon as possible post-burn to avoid the early contractures caused by the patient assuming a position of comfort. Joints must be positioned in the neutral, non-fetal position with simple, static splints (Figures 4A and B). Isoprene provides a convenient malleable material for customized splinting, since it may be cleansed frequently and adjusted easily.

Fig. 4. **A.** Note 3-point extension splints, shoulder abduction and slight flexion. **B.** Note 3-point extension splints, foot-board, hip abduction.

A   *B*

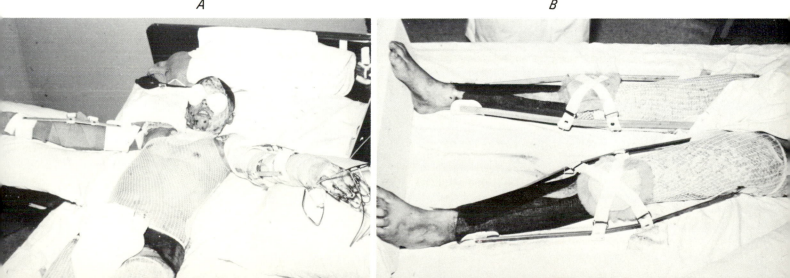

Neck. A custom-made conforming neck splint should be applied over topical dressings as soon as edema subsides. It should be worn 24 hours a day, except when it is removed for cleansing, which should be frequent (Figure 5). The lateral borders of the jaw should be included in the splint and the chin point left open. The chin-neck angle must be definite. On both sides, the molding should extend to, but not beyond, the lateral borders of the trapezius muscle. Two fastening straps are attached: one to fit across the base of the skull, the other at the lower border of the neck.

Axillae. The arms should be abducted 90 degrees and placed in a 15 degree to 20 degree forward plane.

Elbows and Knees. To position the elbows and/or knees three-point extension splints are constructed using ½ inch by 1/8 inch aluminum flat rods, sheepskin pads, and molded isoprene (Figure 4A and B). They must be custom-made, so that the isoprene is shaped to the curvature of the limb. The elbow braces should extend from the deltoid insertion to within one inch of the radial styloid. The knee braces extend from mid-thigh to within 1½ inches of the lateral malleolus. **These splints should be removed only during exercise periods.**

Hips. The hips are maintained in a neutral position in 15 degree abduction from the midline. This can be accomplished with Denis-Brown type braces, or with leg splints which have a spreader bar attached at the knee. Ideally, proper positioning and vigilance by nursing personnel obtains the desired effect without special appliances.

Ankle and Foot. Shortening of the Achilles tendon will occur even in an unburned foot or ankle; therefore, a foot board or positioning splint that maintains the ankle at 90 degrees must be used at all times in bedridden patients.

Wrist and Hand. The wrist is maintained in a neutral position or extended to 35 degrees or less by a splint worn at night and during rest periods (Figure 6).

Fingers. Metacarpophalangeal joints are splinted in slight flexion, IP joints should be straight or in slight flexion, and the thumb should be in ab-

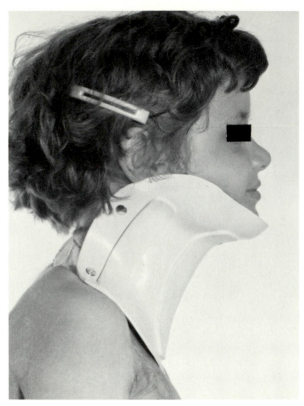

Fig. 5. Neck conformer. Note chin-neck angle and open chin point.

Fig. 6. Basic hand splint. Note neutral wrist, MP flexion thumb index web space preserved with thumb apposed.

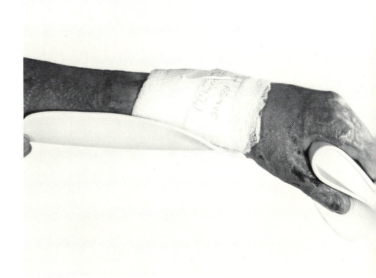

duction and flexion. To avoid damage to the extensor hood mechanism (which is very vulnerable over the PIP joint), only a very cautious range of motion exercises should be carried out. Hand splints are constructed of isoprene and custom molded to each hand. Special emphasis is placed on maintaining the MP joints in moderate flexion and the PIP and DIP joints straight. The thumb-index web must be maintained by placing the thumb in the position of apposition.

Successful early application of these basic principles provides an ideal base for further physical rehabilitation.

Post-Healing. Positioning and splinting must be continued during the grafting phase. As soon as healing permits, constant controlled pressure is used to minimize scar formation and contracture, thus improving both functional and cosmetic prognosis.

The devices and techniques used at the Shriner's Burn Institute in Galveston are summarized.

Neck Conforming Splint. As mentioned above, isoprene neck splints are worn 24 hours a day during the pre-healing phase and discontinued only briefly if skin grafting is required. In the post-healing phase a new splint should be molded directly to the skin and worn 24 hours a day until the scar has been deemed mature.

Elastic Bandage Wraps. During the pre-healing phase, woven fabric and elastic (Ace) wraps are applied to the extremities during ambulation. They are also effective in the proper positioning and maintenance of the hand splints (Figure 7). Each layer provides between 10 and 15mm Hg pressure. Therefore, using more than three layers should be avoided, since the additional pressure may impair circulation.

Post-healing, the wraps are applied over all burn and donor sites and worn 24 hours a day, unless replaced by other pressure garments. To increase or equalize pressure over scars, foam padding may be inserted under the wrap or garment.

Upper Extremity. Arm wraps should be used with a hand splint. The fingertips should be left exposed, and a firm loop should be placed through the thumb-index web to maintain thumb abduction (Figure 7). The wrap is carried up the arm in a spiral fashion except at the elbow, where a figure eight is used.

Thorax. The chest is wrapped in a spiral fashion (Figure 8A and B). Here, more than three layers of wrap may be used, because the greater circumference of the thorax reduces the mechanical advantage of the wraps to only 2 to 5mm Hg pressure.

Axillae. Polyurethane foam pads incorporated under elastic wraps provide controlled pressure in this difficult area. Extreme pressure, which may cause nerve and vessel compression, must be avoided (Figure 8C).

Lower Extremities. Lower extremity wraps should begin at the base of the toes and enclose the heel. Leg wraps are applied according to the method described for the upper extremities.

Fig. 7. Hand splint maintained with Ace wraps.

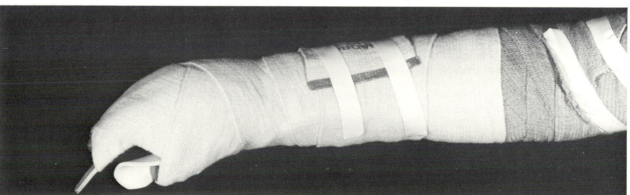

Fig. 8.

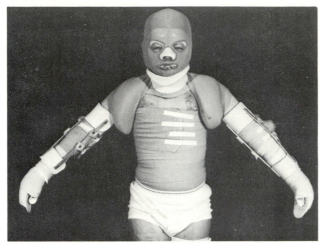

A. Note elastic wraps around trunk, axillary foam pads and wrap.

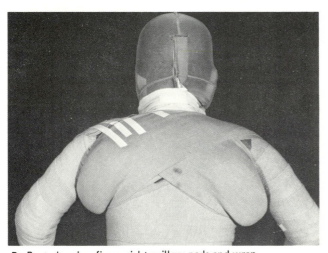

B. Posterior view figure-eight axillary pads and wrap.

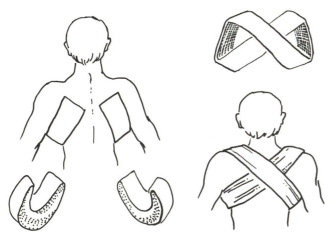

C. Method of applying axillary pads and figure-eight wrap.

JOBST PRESSURE GARMENTS

Jobst* custom-made elastic garments provide a simple and cosmetic means of applying appropriate and constant pressure to the burn scar. Garments are available for virtually any anatomical area, and can be fitted and worn as soon as healing permits. For cleanliness, two sets of garments are usually necessary, and **must be worn constantly except when bathing.** The more commonly used garments will be described (Figure 9).

Gloves. Gloves which leave the fingertips free insure pressure in the web spaces (Figure 10). They should not be incorporated into a body suit or jacket.

Facial Hood. Facial hoods should be used with a silicone facial conformer (Figure 11A and B) or padding, particularly if the scars involve the naso-buccal or nasolabial region. The silicone conformer is made by constructing a plaster cast of the face, then molding a silicone negative conformer on the cast. The silicone is carefully trimmed and augmented to increase the pressure on the nasolabial folds and lips.

To avoid pressure on the ears provide appropriate holes in the hood.

If a neck conformer is used, the facial hood is worn inside its upper edge.

Chin strap. The chin strap exerts pressure along the chin to prevent lower lip eversion.

Jacket, Bodysuit, Panty, Leotard, Hose. Jacket, bodysuit, panty, leotard and hose wraps may be used until the post-burn body weight has stabilized. The jacket would be symmetrically sleeved. If the axilla is involved, Ace wraps and foam pads should be worn over the garment.

High-Top Shoes. Shoes with a well-padded tongue, tip to ankle laces, and metatarsal bar provide effective splinting and pressure (Figure 12A and B). They should be worn over two pairs of socks. To provide a friction surface between socks, the inner sock should be nylon, and the outer sock should be made of heavy cotton.

---

*The Jobst Institute, Inc., Toledo, Ohio 43694.

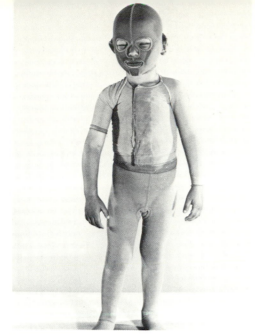

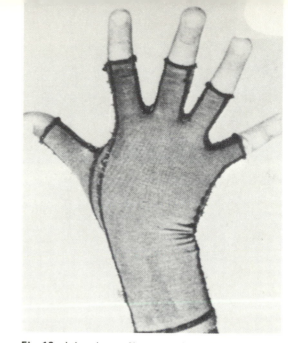

Fig. 9. Child wearing Jobst garments for several body parts.

Fig. 10. Jobst gloves. Note open finger tips.

Fig. 11. A. Child demonstrating molded facial conformer. B. Conformer with Jobst hood. Note nasal obturator and commissure conformer.

A

B

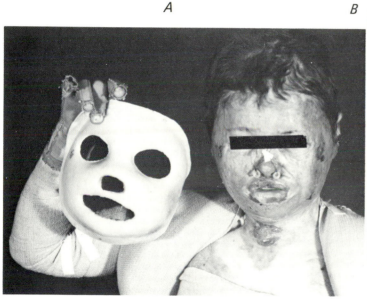

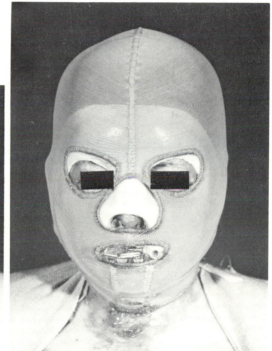

Fig. 12. A. High-top corrective shoe. Note metatarsal bar, Thomas heel and full steel shank. B. One-fourth inch orthopedic padded tongue.

A

B

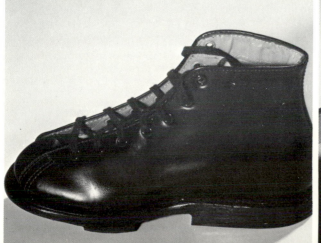

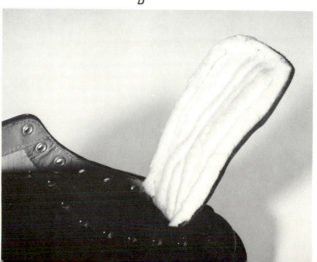

Other Appliances. Oral commissure conformers, nasal obturators, and other special appliances may be constructed by the prosthetist in specific circumstances.

COMPLICATIONS

The most common problem with pressure techniques is skin breakdown due to friction or undue pressure. Careful patient supervision and refitting of splints or garments, when indicated, can eliminate this problem.

Compromising the vascular or nerve supply by the application of extreme pressure must be avoided, particularly in the axillae.

DISCONTINUING PRESSURE

Pressure may be discontinued only after the scar is mature. The time required for the scar to gain maturity, which is characterized by a soft, flat, and pale appearance, may take six to twelve months or longer. Discontinuing pressure for 24 hours is an

excellent initial method of evaluating scar maturity. If the scar becomes hyperemic or raised, pressure must be reinstituted.

CORRECTION OF EXISTING HYPERTROPHIC SCAR CONTRACTURES

Nonsurgical correction of contractures and hypertrophic scars can be accomplished as long as the scar remains active. Once radiological joint changes have been ruled out, serial splinting and sustained stretch techniques may be employed.

Sustained stretch on the hypertrophic scar contracture is accomplished by stabilizing the limb above the joint to be stretched, then suspending a one to two pound weight distal to the joint (Figure 13A and B). When blanching of the scar tissue occurs, an isoprene conformer is applied with elastic wraps. The patient is instructed to attempt extending the limb away from the conformer. Conformers are checked daily and modified as joint extension increases (Figure 14A and B).

Fig. 13. A. Sustained stretch applied to hypertrophic scar contracture of elbow. Five months post-burn. **B.** Fifteen minutes after sustained stretch was begun note increase in extension.

A   *B*

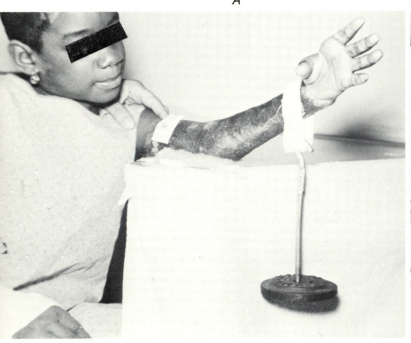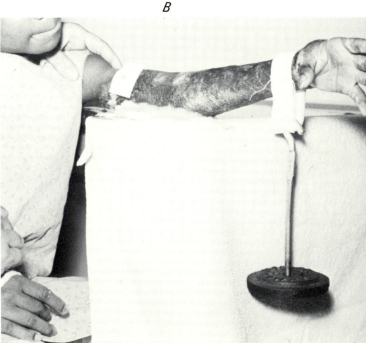

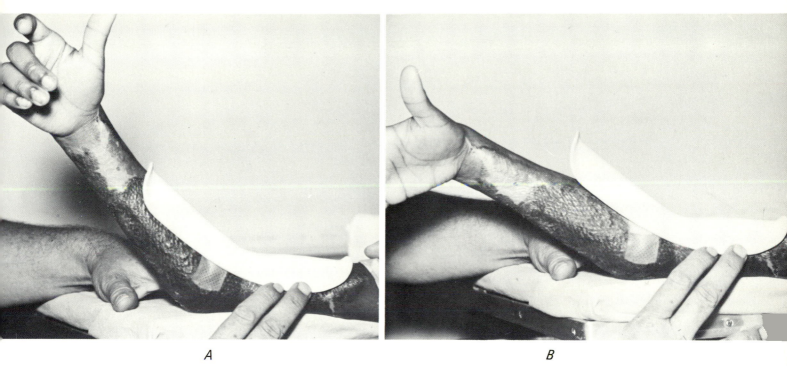

A   *B*

Fig. 14. A. Serial splinting of elbow contracture with isoprene custom conformer. Five months post-burn. **B.** Twenty-four hours later note gain in extension as a result of patient's attempts to extend away from conformer. Conformer will now be modified.

This method works equally well on elbows and knees, but does require strict supervision. Once full range has been achieved, Jobst garments and extension splints may be used.

HOME PROGRAM

Explicit written instructions on wound care, splint and pressure garment application, and exercises must accompany the patient home. Careful follow-up is essential to avoid complications and to gain the best results from the techniques described.

SUMMARY

Significant improvement in cosmetic and functional rehabilitation of the burn patient is possible using special techniques. A carefully planned program of positioning, splinting, exercise, and the application of constant controlled pressure can avoid the dreadful contractures and hypertrophic scar formation so common following burns.

A book is a mirror: if an ass peers into it, you can't expect an apostle to look out.
Lichtenberg

6

HYPERTROPHIC SCARRING: SPONGE FIXATION METHOD

Ryosuke Fujimori

Hypertrophic scarring may form following any burn, trauma, or surgical intervention. In several years, it may regress to some extent without any treatment, but eventually it leaves a functional or cosmetic disability.

Among the causes of hypertrophic scar formation are extensive skin defects, infection, and foreign bodies. All contribute to delay in wound healing and, therefore, a delay in scar tissue maturation. Another important factor is motion (e.g., intermittent tension), which increases contraction and hypertrophy of the scar.

In general, because a scar is unstable and immature in the early stage, it is easily affected by mechanical stimuli. It is my opinion that continuous expansion, pressure, and immobilization of the early, plastic scar might prevent or reduce cicatrical hypertrophy and contraction. Hence, the need for the sponge fixation method (Figures 1 and 2).

SPONGE FIXATION TECHNIQUE

When using the sponge fixation method for the prevention or treatment of hypertrophic scars, a self-adhering sponge has the following advantages: (1) It sticks firmly without rolling and sliding, (2) An open-cellular sponge permits passage of air, perspiration and secretion without irritation or reduction in adhesiveness, and (3) It retains elasticity to produce a constant pressure (Figure 3). An adhesive sponge* is cut into a desired shape and size and is applied directly to the skin area which has been wiped with ether or benzine. For primary wound closure or skin grafting, the adhesive sponge is usually applied one to two weeks after the operation. For hypertrophic scars, it should be applied as early as possible. If there is an ulcer in the hypertrophic scar, the ulcerated area should be excluded from the area of sponge fixation.

When the sponge is applied, is it pressed down firmly with an elastic bandage or other supporter. If the area of sponge fixation is on the neck or in a joint area, a brace is employed to produce expansion and immobilization under constant pressure (Figure 4). On the face, a double-stick adhesive sponge is preferable. One surface is stuck to the skin and the other surface is stuck to a plastic or aluminum plate which has been trimmed and molded into the shape of the affected skin area (Figures 5 and 6). This plate is then pressed down with an adhesive or elastic tape. The molded plate will: (1) Keep the skin area expanded and immobilized, as if a brace were applied, (2) Give sufficient pressure down into a hollow area (e.g., the nasobuccal groove), and (3) Prevent or reduce cicatrical contraction and hypertrophy.

An adhesive sponge may be applied to the inner side of a brace which corresponds to the affected skin area when it is difficult to apply a sponge directly to the skin because of contact dermatitis or irritation. Sometimes it is very convenient to use eye glasses with an adhesive sponge stuck to the nasal or temple frame to press on scars in the interorbital area or the cephalo-auricular sulcus. Also, a modified hand-wrist supporter may be used to prevent or reduce the severity of cicatrical web formation on the hand (Figure 2).

---

* One-sided adhesive sponge (Reston) produced by Medical Products Division, 3-M Company, St. Paul, Minnesota. One-sided or double-stick adhesive sponge (Soft Tape) produced by Nitto Electrical Industrial Company, Sankei Building, Umeda-Machi Kita-ku, Osaka, Japan.

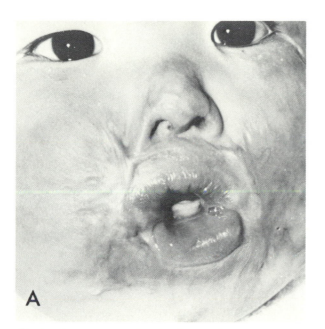

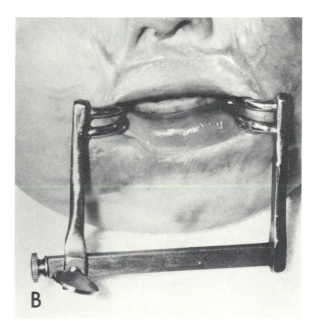

Fig. 1. **A.** This six-month-old baby has a burn scar about the lips and nose of three months duration. He could not suck his mother's milk because of the circumferential scar contraction of his mouth. **B.** Appearance two weeks after initiation of the treatment with a newly designed instrument employed every night and day for about three months to expand the scar.

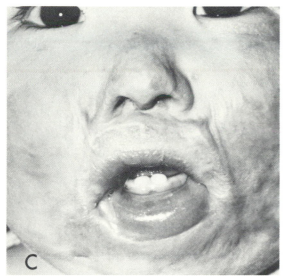

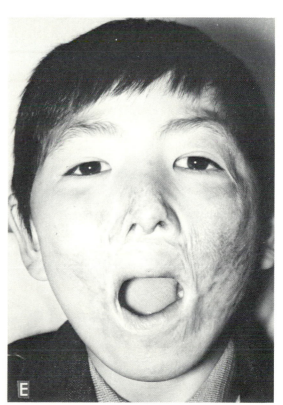

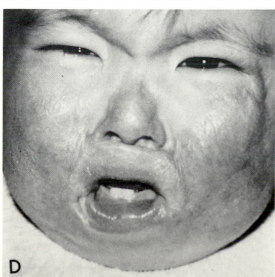

Fig. 1. **C.** Appearance after two months. **D.** Appearance after six months. No recurrence of cicatrical contraction developed later. **E.** Appearance after eight years, and without any operation.

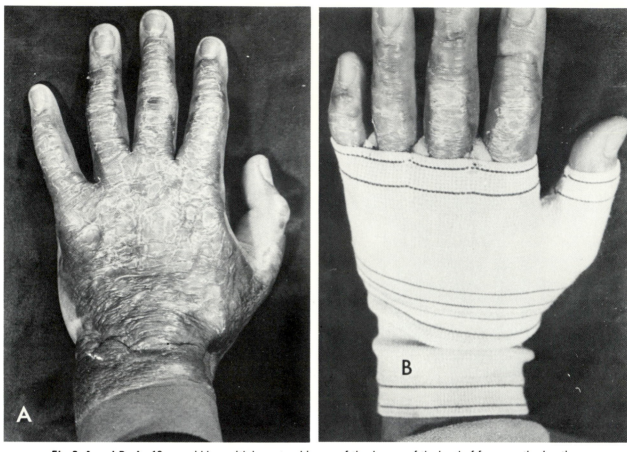

Fig. 2. A. and B. An 18-year-old boy with hypertrophic scar of the dorsum of the hand of four months duration.

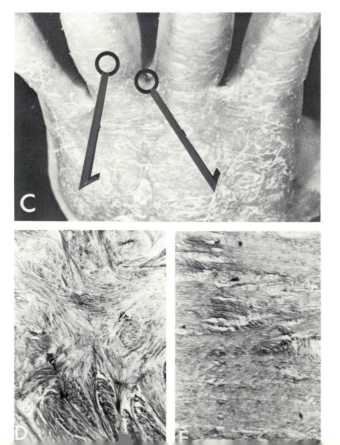

Fig. 2. C. Appearance after two weeks of sponge pressure treatment using appliance shown in **B**. Circle on ring finger indicates site of biopsy depicted microscopically in **D**. Web space biopsy is shown in **E**.

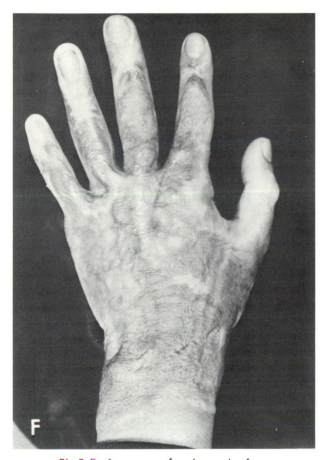

Fig. 2. F. Appearance after six months of sponge pressure treatment.

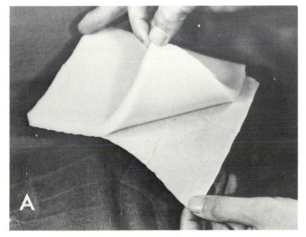

Fig. 3. A. One sided adhesive sponge.

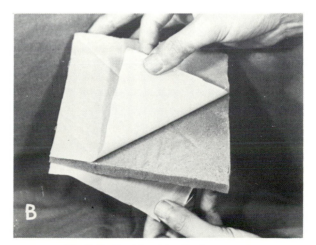

Fig. 3. B. Double-stick adhesive sponge.

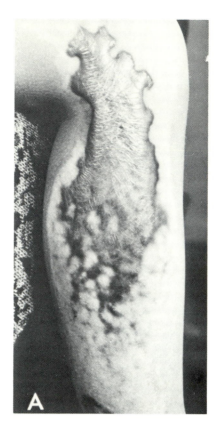

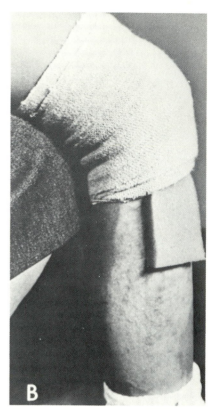

Fig. 4. A. This 10-year-old boy had a hypertrophied burn scar of three months duration. **B. and C.** Details of sponge fixation method. **D.** Appearance after three months of the fixation treatment. **E.** Appearance after final excision of upper part of scar.

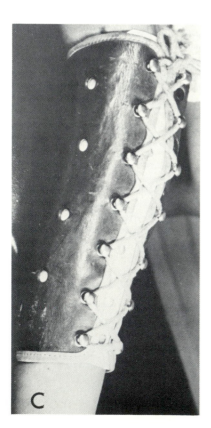

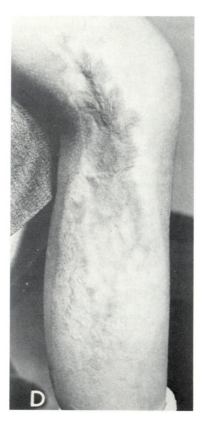

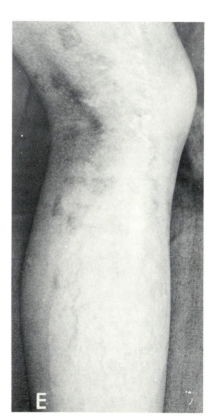

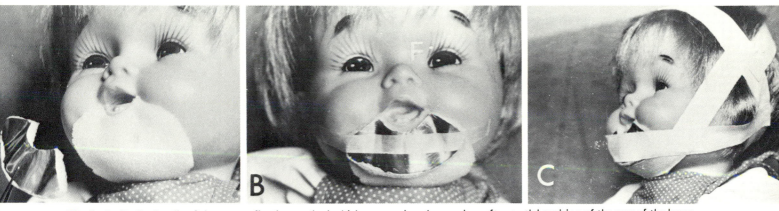

Fig. 5. A., B., C. Details of the sponge fixation method which was employed seven days after partial excision of the scar of the lower lip, using an aluminum plate, adhesive sponge and a specially designed appliance made of elastic tape. Intracicatrical corticosteroid injection accompanied the sponge fixation method.

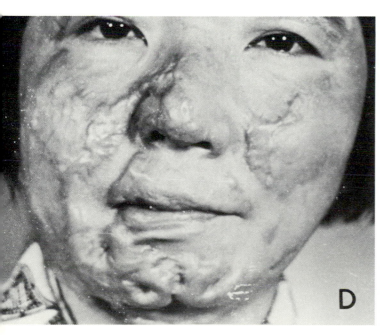

Fig. 5. D. A 35-year-old woman with hypertrophic scar of four months duration.

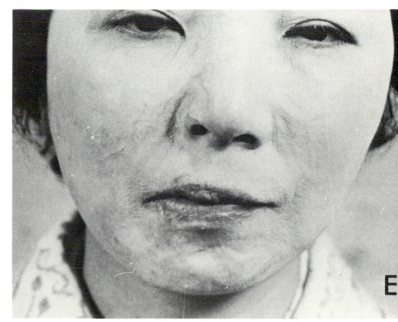

Fig. 5. E. Appearance eight months after the operation and the sponge fixation treatment.

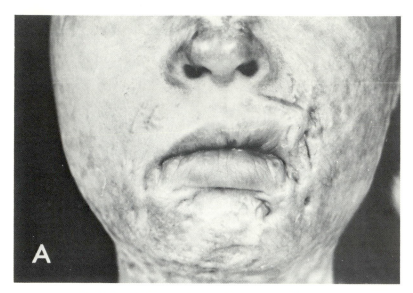

Fig. 6. A. A 16-year-old girl with hypertrophic burn scars.

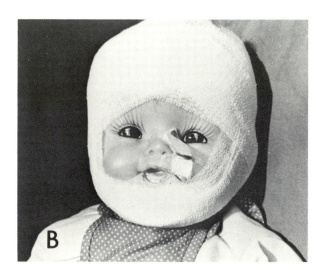

Fig. 6. B. The sponge fixation method was employed seven days after applying split-thickness skin grafts, using an elastic bandage.

Fig. 6. C. Final appearance.

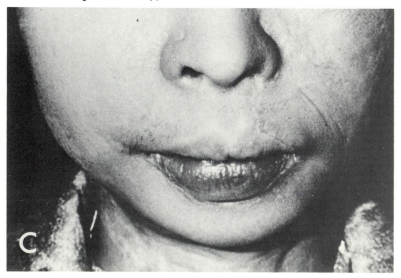

The Figure of Plates to fill or supply the defects of the Palat,

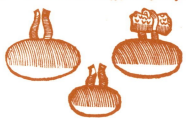

The Figure of another Plate of the Palat, on whose upper side there is a button, which may be turned when it is put into its place, with a small Ravens bill, like this whose Figure is here expressed.

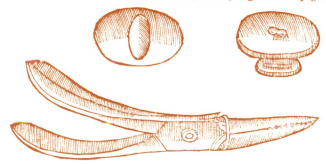

The Works of that Famous Chirurgeon: Ambrose Parey, 1678.

It is easy when we are in prosperity to give advice to the afflicted.

Aeschylus

7

HYPERTROPHIC SCARRING AND KELOID: STEROID INJECTION

Lynn D. Ketchum

The steroid injection of burn scars includes burn scar contractures as well as keloids and hypertrophic scars. Hypertrophic scars are found at the periphery of skin grafts, in areas of healed second degree burns and in skin graft donor sites. Granulation tissue that is covered with a thin sheet of advancing epithelium is most likely to contract, especially in flexion creases, producing burn scar contractures.

PREVENTION OF HYPERTROPHIC SCARS AND SCAR CONTRACTURES

Before going into the treatment of these scars, some thought should be given to the prevention of scars and contractures in conjunction with their treatment, since this is not a static but a dynamic process.

Because partial-thickness burns, especially deep ones, are the most common source of thick, ropey scars, developing during the chronic phase of wound healing, this phase can be modified by the covering of the raw dermis with thin autografts as soon as possible. This accomplishes two things: Firstly, because the stimulus for regeneration and ultimately hyper-regeneration is the loss of a partial thickness of the skin and the greater the loss the greater the stimulus for hyper-regeneration, **coverage with epithelium turns off the stimulus.** Secondly, and also closely related, is the fact that epithelium is essential for remodeling of wounds by its inductive effect on mysenchyme in producing or stimulating production of collagenase very early in the course of wound healing. In many severe burns, autografts cannot be used for this purpose if there are large areas of granulation tissue to be covered; moreover the areas of partial-thickness burns may be the source of split-

thickness autografts themselves, and may even be re-harvested in the 80 percent burn. Even so, the treatment of these areas with homografts has been shown to decrease the amount of hypertrophic scarring.

For the prevention of burn scar contractures, it is helpful to apply moderate split-thickness skin grafts (.020 to .025 inch) across flexion creases or where the area to be covered is small, full-thickness grafts. However, all grafts contract and adequate splinting must be initiated early in the course of a burn, both before grafting and after grafting for several months, until the tendency to contract is overcome (Figure 1).

TECHNIQUE OF STEROID INJECTION OF SCARS

When does one begin thinking about injection of triamcinolone into hypertrophic scars or contractures? Ideally, it would be desirable to accelerate the remodeling of scars with triamcinolone at the first sign of contracture or hypertrophy, since the collagen is relatively immature and most responsive at that time. In limited areas, this is definitely possible. Occasionally, however, the hypertrophy of scars becomes evident while uncovered granulating areas are nearby; this is seen particularly in extensive burns where donor sites are precious few, or where life-saving homografts have been recently rejected. In any event, injection of hypertrophic scars or scar contractures should begin as soon as possible after skin coverage of the burn wounds is achieved. There are guidelines that are helpful regarding the surface area that can be treated and the dosage for a given area relative to the size and age of the patient. A crude dosage schedule for the injection of triamcrinolone into a scar is as follows:

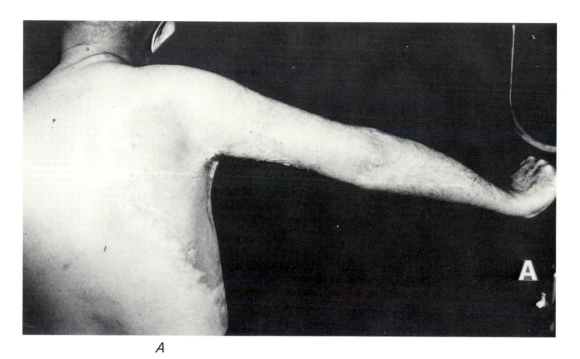

A

Fig. 1. This man had an axillary burn scar contracture which was treated by two injections, four months apart, of 120mg of triamcinolone each, into the area of scarring. **A.** Prior to steroid injection. **B.** At the completion of steroid injection.

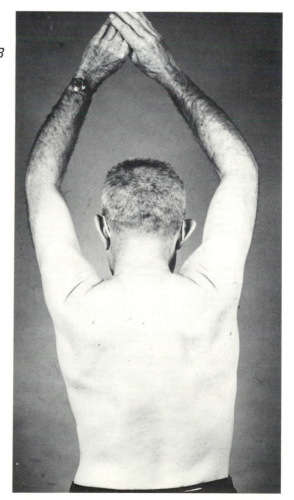

B

Dosage. ADULT: Based upon the surface area of the scar, the following dosage is usually injected at approximately monthly intervals:

1. 1 to 2cm square lesion — 20 to 40mg
2. 2 to 6cm square lesion — 40 to 80 mg
3. 6 to 10cm square lesion — 80 to 120 mg

A maximum dose of 120mg repeated once a month for six months.

CHILDREN: A maximum dose each time is as follows:

1. 1 to 2 years old — 20mg
2. 3 to 5 years old — 40mg
3. 6 to 10 years old — 80 mg

Areas of the Body. In addition to the above dosage schedule, we have developed an approach to scars in different areas of the body as follows:

Scars on trunk and extremities.

1. If the scar is less than $15cm^2$ inject with steroids only — no other treatment is necessary.
2. If the scar is greater than $15cm^2$ excise and resurface the scar with a split-thickness skin graft, injecting the wound edges at the time. It is too time consuming to attempt injection treatments alone for these larger scars.
3. **Scars about the face.** If the direction of the scar is in the line of least tension, excise it, inject the wound margins with triamcinolone, and close it primarily if there is not too much tension; splint the wound for one month. If the scar is not in the line of least tension,

alter the direction of the wound by a Z-or W-plasty and inject the wound edges of these flaps. This has been found to be effective in preventing a trap-door effect from contracture of the flaps in a Z-plasty, and the subsequent need for dermabrasion of these areas to smooth the contour is avoided.

If there is tension on the wound's margins after excision, inject the wound margins and close the wound with a local skin flap or a skin graft.

Multiple hypertrophic scars. Handle one scar at a time by excision, injection of the wound edges with triamcinolone, and primary closure if there is too much tension.

True keloid former with multiple keloids. Do a small test area first to learn the response of the individual to injury, and the ability of triamcinolone to modify the fibroblastic response. Some keloid formers require large doses of triamcinolone for small areas. If a large area is attacked, it will probably be uncontrollable. In addition to triamcinolone injections, continuous pressure over the scar is recommended in these individuals wherever possible, for a minimum of three months.

If a split-thickness skin graft is required, make it very thin (.008 to .010 inch). Deeper grafts may result in a keloid of the donor area. Take the graft from an area where continous pressure can be applied throughout the postoperative period.

Burn scar contractures can be effectively treated, in many instances without grafting, by injecting the maximum dose of triamcinolone for age and weight into the area of scarring at monthly intervals.

Health of body and mind is a great blessing, if we can bear it.
Newman

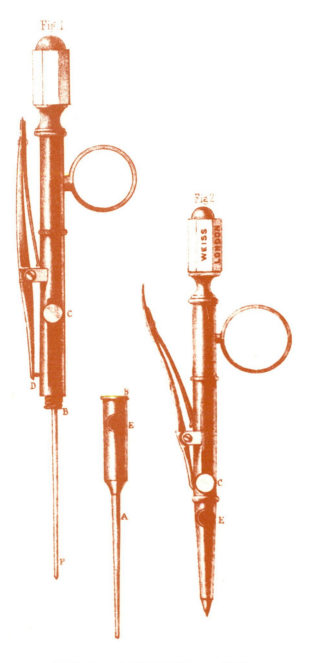

Dublin Journal of Medical Sciences, 1861.

8

MARJOLIN'S ULCER

Irving Feller

Marjolin's ulcer is a descriptive term for squamous cell cancer degeneration of an improperly healed wound. Marjolin first described this phenomenon in 1823 when he noted that cancerous change occurred around the opening of sinus tracts draining long-standing osteomyelitis. It was also noted that the same changes occurred in poorly healed burn wounds. With the advent of the x-ray and radiation therapy, squamous cell cancer was observed to occur in areas of overexposure.

These three situations have several things in common: (1) an initial damage to the skin which cannot be healed completely by the body's reparative process; (2) a long period of attempted repair by the body, the duration of which is approximately 10 to 20 years; (3) the existence of open ulceration for months or years. It appears that metaplasia of highly active squamous cells surrounding the ulceration results in the change to cancer.

The common history obtained from burned patients with cancerous changes in the burned areas is that they were injured about 20 years ago and the wound never healed satisfactorily. Either no grafting was done or inadequate skin cover was provided. The wound broke down, ulcerated intermittently at first, and then remained open for months or years prior to the examination.

After the history and physical examination, three additional steps are necessary to complete the diagnosis. The first is differentiating lower extremity ulcers from those caused by venous insufficiency in circumferential burns. The second diagnostic procedure is biopsy of the wound in several places to obtain a tissue diagnosis. The third is to examine the area for regional lymph node involvement.

The definitive treatment is wide and deep excision of the ulcer with autografting. In many cases the biopsy and excision can be carried out simultaneously. It is always necessary to excise all of the ulceration, which should include a border of normal tissue in all dimensions to assure complete removal. In cases where venous insufficiency and chronic burn ulcers exist together, it is necessary to excise, ligate, and strip away the incompetent veins. When hemostasis is secured, thick autografts should be placed to cover the wound.

Fortunately, the degeneration of burn wounds to cancer is not common, and, when it does occur, metastases are not frequent. In most cases it appears that metastases are rare and slow to spread. Because of this, radical procedures for cure may not be necessary. Each patient should have careful evaluation to determine the best possible treatment.

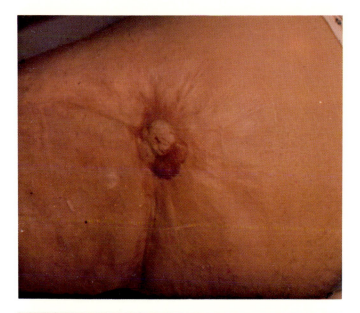

Fig. 1. A. This 60-year-old patient noted the onset of ulceration in the site of burns on his left thigh that occurred 18 years prior. When healing of the ulceration did not take place after six months, he appeared for consultation. Biopsy indicated squamous cell carcinoma with no known metastasis.

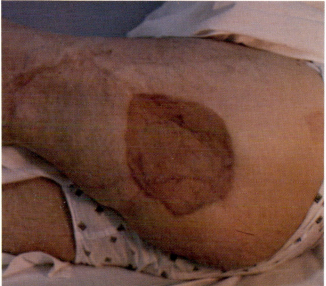

Fig. 1. B. A wide excision and grafting was carried out to remove the lesion. A border approximately three inches around the region was excised and grafted to cover the defect.

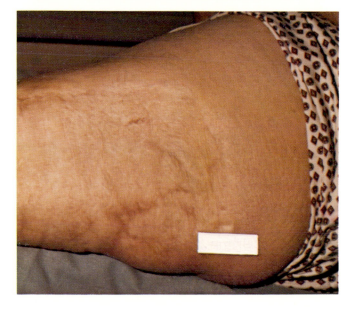

Fig. 1. C. Examination ten years later revealed that the site remained free from recurrence and there was no evidence of metastasis.

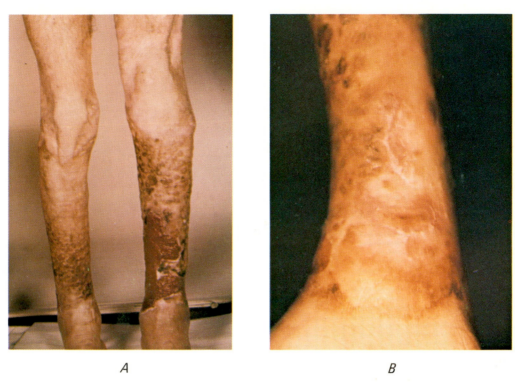

A   B

Fig. 2. A. Patient is a 29-year-old male who appeared for evaluation and treatment of recurrent ulceration of his left lower extremity 18 years following initial burn. The initial burn wound was grafted with pinch grafts and patient survived many months of slow healing before the wound finally covered. **B.** When the patient was first seen, the ulceration was excised and the area grafted after it was determined that he had no evidence of metastasis.

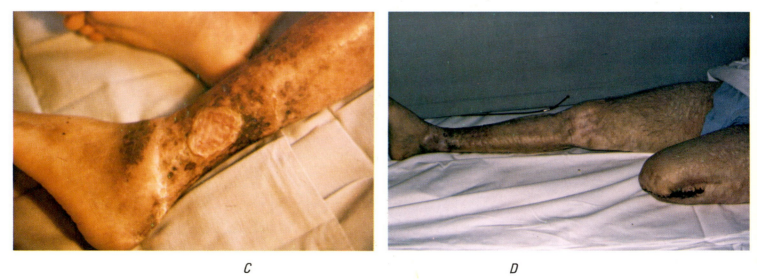

C   D

Fig. 2. C. Patient returned within a year after the grafting and recurrent Marjolin's ulcer was found in the middle of the graft. **D.** Because of the local recurrence after the initial wide-deep excision and grafting, an amputation was advised. The secondary factor in considering amputation, was the marked damage and destruction to the lower extremity that had taken place with the initial burn and the inadequate subsequent healing of most of the leg.

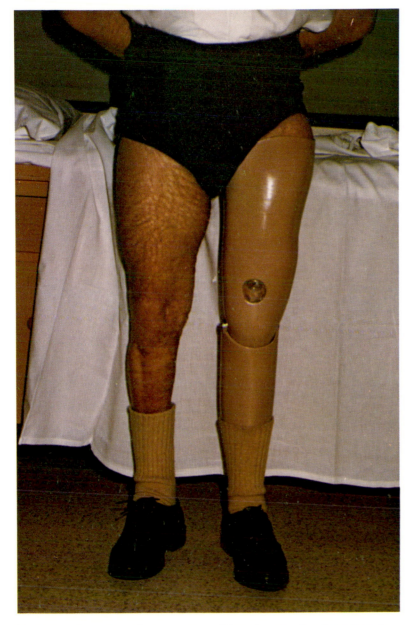

Fig. 2. E.   Shows the patient on a return visit to the outpatient department three years after the amputation.

9

NEUROMUSCULAR AND SKELETAL COMPLICATIONS

George H. Koepke

NEUROMUSCULAR COMPLICATIONS

This discussion is limited to some of the neuromuscular and skeletal problems that are usually associated with burns that cover at least 20 percent of the body surface. Polyneuropathy seems to be the most common neurologic deficit. Its high incidence, however, may be more apparent at the University of Michigan Burn Center because of our interest in this entity. In a study of 249 unrelated admissions to the Burn Unit, 44, or approximately 13 percent, developed electro-diagnostic evidence of a polyneuropathy more than three weeks after their admission. The criterion for neuropathy was evidence of delayed conduction velocities in two or more peripheral motor nerves. Of this number, approximately 15 percent had clinical evidence of neruopathy (e.g., varied amounts of impaired hearing and weakness). A few required drop foot braces and crutches. A follow-up of patients, one to three years later, revealed several with residual severe hearing impairment, peripheral muscle atrophy, and weakness. Three continue to use braces, but none require crutches. Although one single agent could not be implicated, all of the numerous antibiotics administered to the patients are known to be potentially neurotoxic, especially if the blood levels should exceed therapeutic levels.

Peripheral nerve entrapment syndromes that follow burns are usually associated with edema or contractures. They include the median nerve in the carpal tunnel, the ulnar nerve in either the Canal of Guyon or near the medial epicondyle. The peroneal nerve may develop neuropraxia or neurotomesis secondary to pressure on the nerve near the head of the fibula. This is commonly associated with pro-longed bed rest. We have recognized only one case of tarsal tunnel syndrome associated with swelling, hypertrophic scar, and contracture.

Each year at least one patient is seen with the results of a complete stroke. This may be due to acute hypertension or dehydration that developed during the treatment of the burn.

Patients that are burned in explosions often have hidden injuries. In two patients the neurologic manifestations of spinal cord injuries were unrecognized until late in the course of their burn treatment. Further investigation revealed vertebral fractures.

A discussion of late neurologic complications would be incomplete without comment on the depression that is associated with severe burns. In most instances, depression is a natural reaction to the extensive scars and disfigurement that result from the burn. Other factors are: functional impairments, financial impact, and the loss of friends and family. Ordinarily the depression is transient, but a few have required psychotherapy.

Muscle and tendon shortening may form as a response to deep thermal injury, but more often the limited motion is more apparent than attributable to a true muscle contracture. Skin contracture may be considered a normal part of the healing process of a burn. If excised early, muscle, tendon, and joint capsule motion can be easily restored. To obtain good correction, the body segment should be immobilized immediately after surgery in a position opposite the deformity. Fingers and toes are exceptions to this concept and frequently require release of a joint capsule, tendon, and/or joint fusion.

It is common for the burn victim to have associated injuries such as tears of a ligament, tendon, or joint capsule, or a fracture. They are often overlooked because pain associated with early treatment of the thermal injury will make the patient lie immobilized. Later, with activity, a sprain, fracture, or nerve deficit will become apparent. For this reason, burned patients involved in explosions or moving accidents must be examined carefully for other injuries so that appropriate treatment is given early.

HETEROTOPIC BONE

Loss of motion in large joints may not be attributed merely to a change in rheologic properties of muscle, but may result from calcific deposits in soft tissue. A review of more than 1,500 cases seen at the University of Michigan Burn Unit revealed that approximately 2 percent of those who have suffered full-thickness loss of skin from 20 percent or more of the body will develop heterotopic bone. Paraarticular calcification is most common near the elbow, along the posterior aspect of the humerous adjacent to the triceps tendon and superior to the medial epicondyle (Figure 1). It is interesting that burned areas may be remote to the ectopic calcification and that joint spaces may be well preserved. Although the etiology remains unclear, prolonged pressure and inactivity appear to be associated factors. Severe calcium, potassium, and phosphorous levels are usually normal, but alkaline phosphatase levels are elevated during the acute post-burn period. These gradually return to normal, with the onset of joint stiffness. Within a few days after the onset of impaired motion, there is x-ray evidence of a progressive calcium deposit. When it is small and in the early stage, treatment by manipulation under anesthesia is usually successful in restoring normal motion. This can be done at the time that a split-thickness skin graft is obtained, but care must be taken to apply splints promptly that will stress the joint alternately from flexion to extension at four hour intervals. Good motion can often be restored by this conservative treatment. The calcific deposit is evident by x-ray many years later, but the joints retain full range of motion as a response to breaking adhesions between the heterotopic bone and soft tissue. Good motion can usually be restored in those cases that are

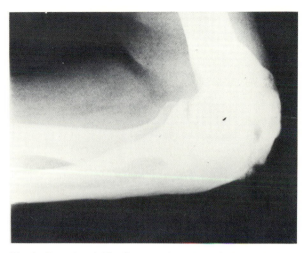

Fig. 1. Ectopic calcification near insertion of triceps tendon.

resistant to conservative treatment by the excision of sufficient calcific material to ensure good passive motion at the time of surgery (Figure 2). It is important to begin an early postoperative program of frequent active and passive exercises.

SKELETAL COMPLICATIONS

Pyarthrosis may recur as the result of a deep burn and the associated infection extending to the joint, or it may develop from a hematogenous infection. The pyarthrosis may result in dislocation of a hip. The customary treatment is prompt incision, drainage, reduction of the dislocation, immobilization, and appropriate antibiotics.

Bone surface exposed by deep burns will usually die and eventually separate from the surrounding healthy bone. The application of appropriate wet dressings will expedite the process and will promote eventual healing. Hematogenous osteomylitis will usually require incision and drainage as well as appropriate wet dressings.

Osteoporosis is a common complication of severe burns and is associated with contracture and prolonged immobilization. It will usually respond to procedures that will restore good range of motion and activity.

Functional or postural scoliosis is a common sequel to hemithoracic and axillary scars. The functional scoliosis of a child may lead to a structural

Fig. 2. Ectopic calcification removed from near triceps tendon.

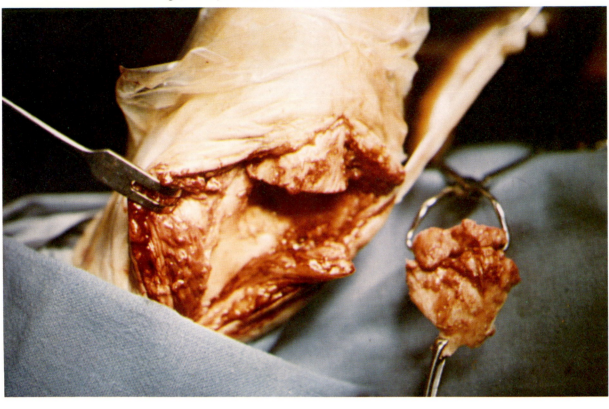

curve unless the scar is excised and split-thickness skin grafts are applied to the area that is devoid of skin. A plaster jacket or removable splints should be applied immediately following surgery to ensure correction of the scoliosis. The child should be held in a corrected position from six weeks to six months, depending on the severity of the spinal curvature.

An uncommon skeletal complication is shown in Figure 3. This resembles a subcapital epiphyseal

separation or dysplasia and may occur unilaterally or bilaterally among severely burned patients. These patients are without history of trauma and the subcapital separation has occurred during the course of the treatment for their burns and before weight bearing. The etiology remains unclear. One wonders if this may be a reaction to burn-induced stress. Of course, weight training must be deferred, and when the patient has recovered sufficiently from his severe burns, the dead femoral head is replaced with an endoprosthesis.

SUMMARY

It is quite clear that the victim of burned skin may undergo local and systematic changes in remote areas. The neuromuscular and skeletal complications may be severe and disabling. For these reasons, prolonged follow-up is important for those patients that have suffered full-thickness loss of skin across joint surfaces or full-thickness loss of skin from more than 20 percent of the body.

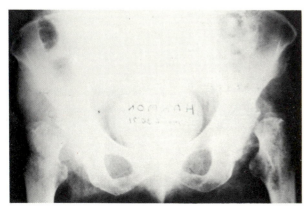

Fig. 3. Spontaneous epiphyseal separation.

The form of an Iron Breſt-plate, to amend the crookedneß of the Body.

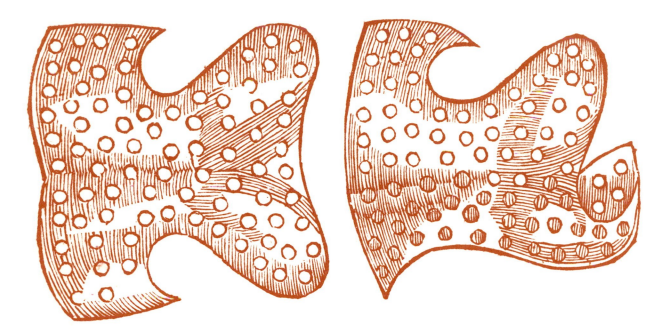

The Works of that Famous Chirurgeon: Ambrose Parey, 1678.

Art is I; Science is We.

Bernard

II.

THE SCALP
AND
SKULL

PRINCIPLES OF TREATMENT

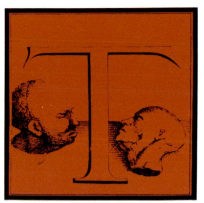

he treatment of localized bone necrosis due to an electrical or thermal burn was greatly advanced by Worthen's technique of early debridement followed by local scalp flap coverage of devitalized bone. Another method is the time-honored technique of removing or drilling through the outer cortex, then applying split-thickness skin grafts to the diploic bone, or to the granulations which form over a period of weeks. This method of maintaining and covering the burned skull is especially suited to the treatment of areas too large to be covered by a local scalp flap, or to the late treatment of the burned skull.

Late reconstruction of full-thickness skull loss in the growing child is best accomplished by the split-rib grafts championed by Longacre. Split-rib grafts, iliac bone grafts, or acrylic can be used successfully in late reconstruction of skull defects in the adult. The use of acrylic for frontal bone reconstruction is now acceptable.

Full-thickness skin loss results in the majority of problems following burns of the scalp. With good wound management, partial-thickness burns of the scalp will heal during the acute phase of treatment and hair will regrow. But full-thickness burns result in permanent hair loss. Split-thickness grafts are generally used to cover these full-thickness areas, and reconstruction during the rehabilitative period concerns reducing the size of the defect.

The multiple excision technique has been the workhorse for reinstituting non-hair-bearing areas. In the adult, these excisions may be of any length and of 8cm wide, while in the child, the width that can be multiply excised is less. If the anterior hairline has been lost, it is usually reconstructed first with local hair-bearing scalp flaps.

Local flaps, used mainly to reconstruct the anterior, temporal, and posterior hairlines, move hair-bearing scalp into a position of higher esthetic importance. Small skin grafted areas away from the anterior hairline can be covered in females by combing the hair over the graft. In a relatively small number of males and females, similar small skin grafts have been rendered hair-bearing by multiple hair transplants.

A hairpiece is indicated for coverage of non-hair-bearing defects too large to be closed by the multiple excision technique. Occasionally we will narrow a large defect by two or three multiple excisions, so that the hairpiece may be of smaller size. We have had difficulty fitting a hairpiece for an isolated non-hair-bearing area in the upper posterior neck. We resolved this problem by moving a hair-bearing scalp flap into the posterior neck defect and then putting the hairpiece over the scalp flap donor site.

Irving Feller

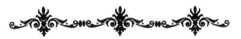

11

EARLY MANAGEMENT OF THE SCALP AND SKULL

Irving Feller
Kathryn E. Richards

Burns of the scalp and skull may be caused by any of the physical or chemical forces; however, many of the deeper burns are caused by electricity. The mechanism of injury is illustrated in Figure 1. The severe burn will have destroyed the outer layers of skin, and may also have destroyed some bone, meninges, and brain tissue. Fortunately most burns of the scalp and skull do not penetrate the skull. Under the layer of dead tissue will be a zone of injured tissue. The eschar is removed to avoid deeper tissue damage and death by infection, and to promote development of good granulation tissue which forms the base for skin grafts.

Burns of the scalp require special attention to wound care. The hair, if not shaved, becomes incorporated in the crusts or eschar, making it difficult to remove dead tissue and drain exudates. Therefore, the scalp should be completely shaved on admission if any part is burned, and a program of daily dressing changes started.

If the injury is only partial-thickness, the hair will continue to grow, necessitating shaving at least once a week. If the scalp is not kept clean by repeated shaving and cleansing, the growing hair will incorporate into crusts, creating an abcess which may then destroy the injured deeper tissues to produce a full-thickness loss.

Dressing changes and repeated shaving will permit complete healing of the partial-thickness burns and removal of the full-thickness eschar. If bone is exposed, it is necessary to keep the wound moist by using physiologic moistened dressings every two to three hours to avoid drying of the periosteum and live bone. The full-thickness burned areas can be autografted when the granulation tissue is mature.

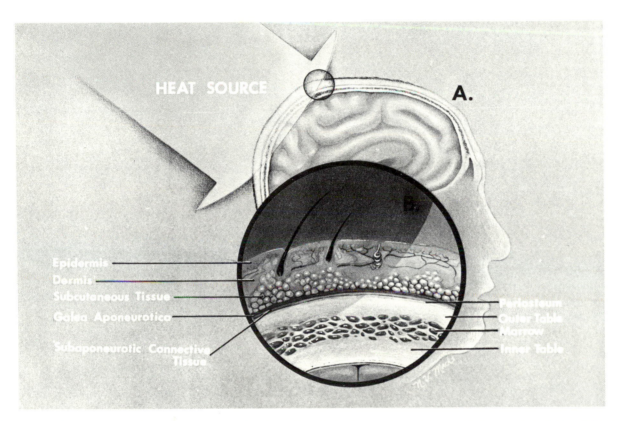

Fig. 1. The Mechanism of Scalp and Skull Burns. **A.** The heat source burns inward from the outside for a period of time. Both the intensity of the heat and the duration of time result in death to the outer layers and damage to the tissues below. **B.** Magnification of one area to demonstrate the layers of scalp and skull as the damage is taking place. The outer layers: epidermis, dermis, subcutaneous tissue, galea aponeurotica, periosteum and outer table of bone are often destroyed. The marrow space, inner table, meninges and brain may also be damaged by the injury. The principles for treatment, therefore, are careful debridement of the dead tissue and protection of the injured tissue during the early treatment process.

12

DRILLING THE OUTER CORTEX

Irving Feller

The principle supporting the practice for this procedure is that granulation tissue forms below the dead bone of the outer table. When holes are drilled through the dead bone, granulation tissue (Figure 1A), will grow through the holes and then coalesce above the dead bone (Figure 1B). The dead bone is then reabsorbed or rejected and the granulation tissue bed becomes the base for the autografts.

The operative procedures can be carried out with minimal or no anesthesia, depending upon the patient. All devitalized scalp tissue is removed, exposing the dead outer cortex. The wound is then cleaned with an antiseptic solution and the field is redraped. The surgeon changes gloves to complete the double preoperative technique.

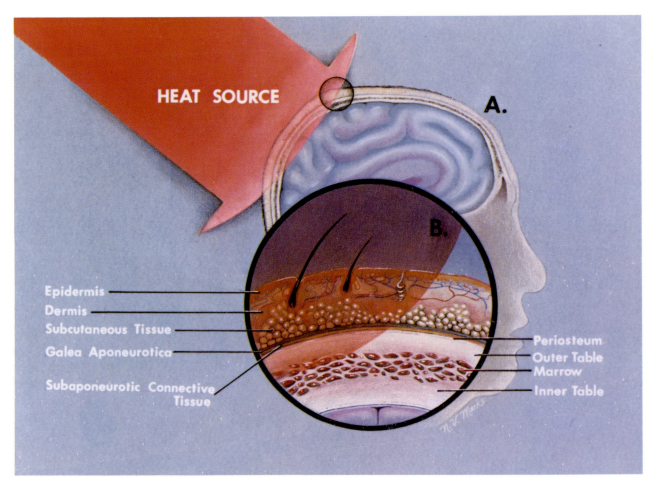

Fig. 1. A. Mechanism of scalp injury. Both tissue damage and tissue death follow the physical or chemical force causing the burn. **B.** The outer layers of tissue will be subject to the burning agent for a longer period of time, and therefore, will be killed. The deeper layers may only be damaged.

The depth of the drill point is set (Figure 1C) using a 1/8 inch bit, and a depth gauge (Figure 1D) is set so that the bit penetrates the outer table and, if necessary, into but not through the inner table.

The friction of drilling causes heat which can burn the surrounding tissue. Therefore, irrigation with a balanced saline solution is necessary. A steady stream of the irrigation fluid directed at the point of penetration of the drill will cool the area and avoid burning. Each hole is drilled until blood flows or the depth gauge stops the penetration. The holes are drilled approximately 4mm (1/8 inch) apart.

When the drilling is complete, the exposed bone is covered with a dressing containing a physiologic saline solution. This dressing is changed at least every eight hours and must be kept moist at all times. If the granulation tissue is allowed to dry, it will die back and the process is retarded. The granulation tissue will appear in the holes and then overgrow the dead bone (Figure 1E).

The dead bone will then be reabsorbed or rejected in whole or in part, and spicules of bone will be seen extruding through the granulations. These can be gently lifted from the granulation as they appear.

When the sequestration ceases and a good granulation tissue has been formed, autografts are applied (Figure 2).

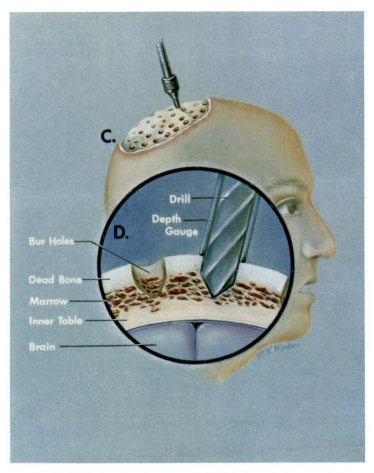

Fig. 1. C. This drawing demonstrates drilling through the outer table of bone into the deeper healthy bone and the appearance of the skull after drilling. D. Illustrates the depth gauge on the drill allowing the bur holes to enter only healthy marrow.

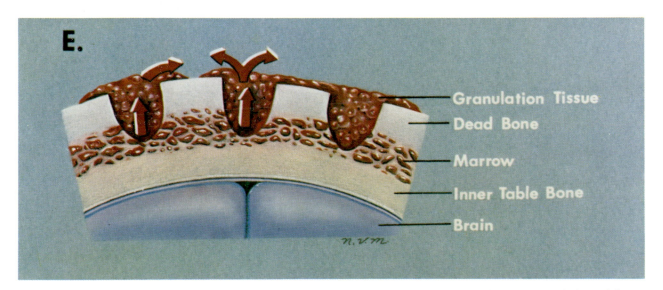

Fig. 1. E. Shows blood clots filling in the holes. The granulation tissue grows through and then coalesces to cover the bone defect.

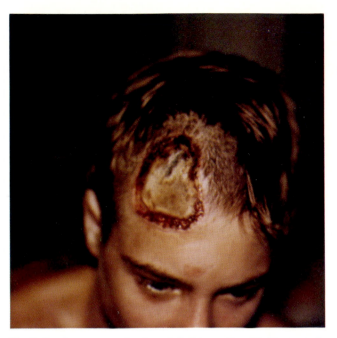

Fig. 2. A. Appearance of scalp and skull burn after debridement of eschar.

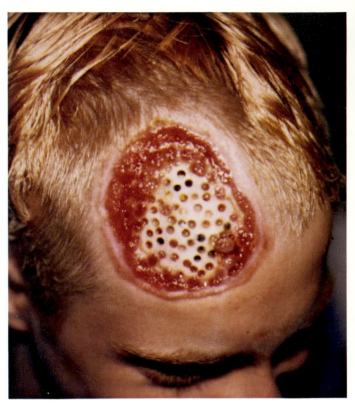

Fig. 2. C. Granulation tissue is seen growing through the holes covering the surface of the dead bone.

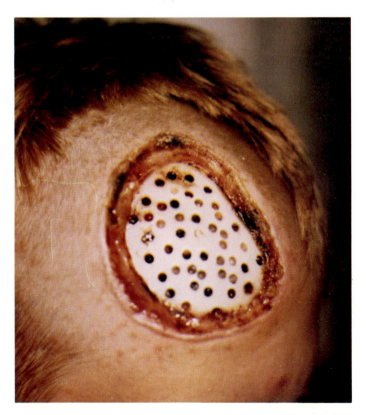

Fig. 2. B. The outer table of bone is dead and holes are drilled to allow granulation tissue to grow through from the deeper healthy bone. The surrounding area will heal spontaneously where it is partial-thickness or the full-thickness area will be autografted.

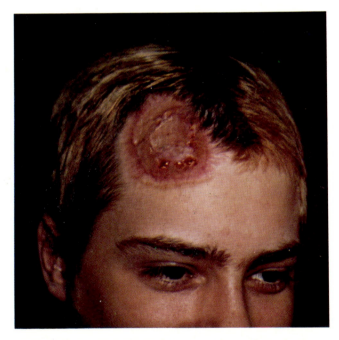

Fig. 2. D. Autografts have been placed on the granulation tissue one month after the holes were drilled. Healing will continue and the scalp defect can then be covered by operation or hair pieces, depending upon the size of the defect.

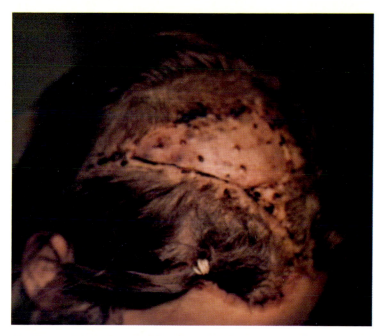

Fig. 2. E. A full-thickness hair-bearing pedicle has been rotated from the middle of the scalp to cover the defect.

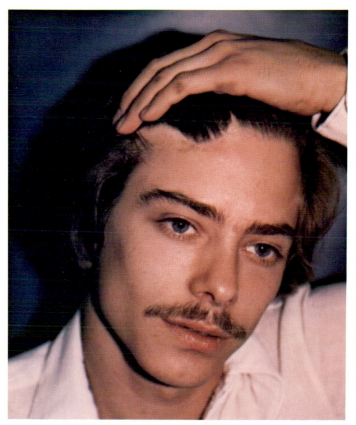

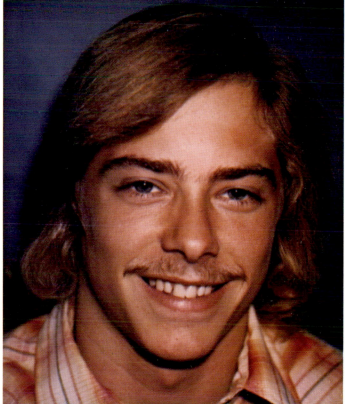

Fig. 2. F. and G. The patient exhibits the hair-bearing flap in place. The defect in the middle of the scalp that was created by rotating the flap anteriorly has been excised by serial excisions and primary closures, gradually stretching the scalp to close the donor defect.

13

REMOVING THE OUTER CORTEX

In Chul Song

Decortication of the outer cortex of the cranium was suggested by Geinitz in 1920 and later reaffirmed and actually performed by Kazanjian in 1946. The procedure is most expedient and effective in restoring a bare cranium. The main advantages are (1) the elimination of a prolonged waiting period until the granulation bed forms, and (2) the applicability of the procedure in the presence of a necrotic outer table. The chisel, osteotome, or neuroosteotome is used for the decortication of the outer table. The exposed cortex is chiselled away until multiple bleeding points in the spongiosa layer of diploe are exposed. The chiselling is carried out from the edges of the wound inward toward the central part, taking care to avoid cutting into the inner table of the cranium. The use of electrical drills or saws will expedite the decortication process. The cortical bone may also be removed by making multiple drill holes and connecting them with a bone rongeur. The diploic bleeding is controlled by electrocautery using a bipolar coagulation unit. The bipolar coagulation unit produces little heat and does not require a dry operative field. Bone wax is not used unless bleeding canals are encountered. Any interposing substances, such as bone wax or a hematoma between the graft and recipient site, will prevent or retard the success of the graft.

Grafting is delayed for 24 to 48 hours if persistent oozing of blood is noted, and the wound is dressed with moist gauze pressure dressings. Judicious use of saline-moistened dressings is mandatory in the preservation of bone viability. A split-thickness autograft (0.014 to 0.020 inches) is immediately placed over the decorticated bone, if there is adequate exposure of the cancellous layer and satisfactory hemostasis has been obtained. Immediate grafting of the decorticated skull will preserve the anatomical integrity of the bone cell and will also forestall infection. The graft is secured with a moist, bulky gauze dressing. This dressing should consist of a layer of nonadherent fine-mesh gauze covered by saline-moistened gauze and bulky fluffed gauze. A stretch gauze bandage applied to the skull both ensures graft fixation and provides graft protection. Antibiotics are added to the saline solution if indicated. When a skin graft is placed on an oozing cancellous surface, the dressing should be changed in 24 to 48 hours. Multiple perforations of the graft may provide additional drainage routes to prevent the ooze from lifting the graft. At the dressing change, saline is used generously to aid in removal. The fine mesh gauze is carefully peeled from the graft, which is held by forceps, to prevent dehiscence from the recipient site. If a hematoma or seroma is found underneath the graft, it is promptly evacuated, and a saline-moistened bulky pressure dressing is reapplied.

A sclerotic decorticated surface should not be grafted immediately. A vascular granulation surface should be encouraged before skin grafting is carried out. This will require two to four weeks. In a burn that involves the entire thickness of skull, it is essential to remove the necrotic bone down to the dura. At the same time split-thickness skin grafts can be placed over the dura. The cranial dura mater is a tough membrane of connective tissue that accepts skin grafts successfully.

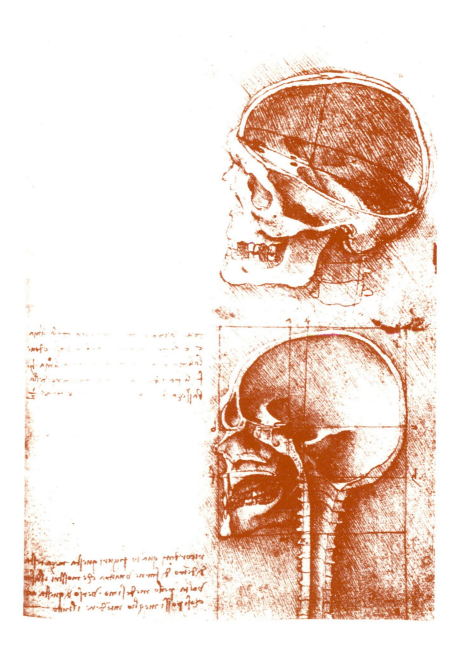

Leonardo da Vinci, 1452 – 1519.

14

MULTIPLE EXCISION AND PRIMARY CLOSURE OF THE SCALP

Thomas M. Hudak

Defects of the scalp resulting from burns as well as other accidents are not rare occurrences. Burns seem to be the major causative factor in partial losses of scalp. Unless the loss is greater than 50 percent, it is possible to minimize, and in some cases completely eliminate, the hairless areas by judicious distribution of the remaining hairy scalp through a series of well planned operations. Small areas can usually be concealed by the surrounding hair, particularly in women patients.

The principle of multiple partial excisions as a gradual reduction of cutaneous deformities was first discussed by Morestin. *The rationale of the procedure is based on the fact that in early and middle life the skin is elastic and rapidly regains normal relaxation and elasticity after marked stretch or tension.* In 1929, in a paper dealing with the gradual partial excision of scars and large disfigurements, Davis reviewed the literature and discussed this consideration. Morestin and Davis excised the maximum amount of tissue that will permit closure without undercutting the bordering skin. Ferris Smith noted that freely undercutting the bordering skin permitted the maximum advancement of normal surrounding skin without distortion of the surrounding structures. This addition to the techniques of Morestin and Davis allowed maximum removal of the lesion and the certainty of exact closure.

The procedure is relatively simple (Figure 1). A precisely determined amount of hairless skin is excised; the surrounding hairy scalp is then freely undermined and advanced as far forward as possible, and the hairy scalp is sutured into the new position. A well planned procedure is necessary to avoid excising such a wide ellipse of tissue that the wound cannot be closed.

The multiple excision technique can be employed in certain larger skin lesions based on the fact that skin which has been placed under tension becomes looser over a period of several months. It has its greatest application in the excision of non-hair-bearing areas of the scalp. This relaxation permits the remaining part of the lesion to be excised in multiple stages. In incising a large burn scar, the initial incision can be made along one side, between the scar and normal tissue. The incision is then carried down to the loose areolar tissue beneath the galea aponeurotica. The scalp can then be undermined extensively at the level of the loose areolar layer and pulled medially over the portion to be excised. The scar is then marked at the level at which the scalp overlaps it and is excised accordingly. Closure of one side of the wound is necessary before the procedure is repeated on the opposite side of the non-hair-bearing portion of the scalp. Several months should be allowed to elapse before any further excision. Multiple operations may be required to remove the non-hair-bearing area from the scalp, depending upon its size.

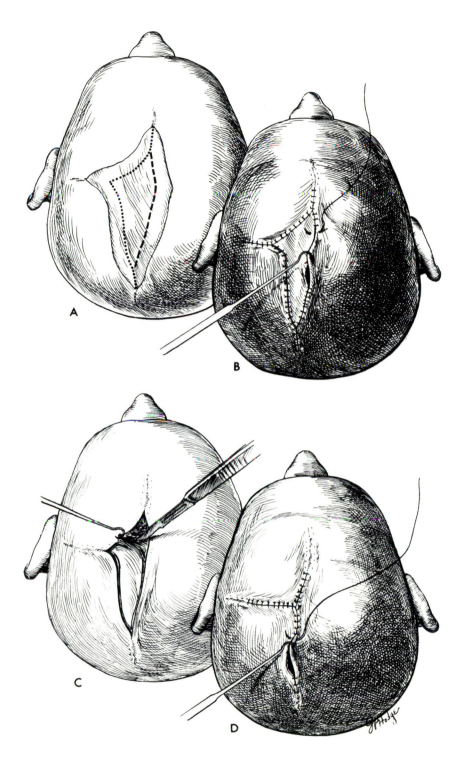

Fig. 1. Multiple excision technique. **A. and B.** The first-stage excision. **C. and D.** The second-stage excision several months later.

15

SCALP ROTATION FLAPS AND SPLIT-RIB GRAFTS

Reed O. Dingman

INITIAL CARE

Severe injuries to the scalp and skull may result from burns caused by electricity. The same destruction of scalp and skull can result from other forms of trauma, including chemical, thermal, and irradiation burns. The final reconstruction required is determined by the defect that results, regardless of the cause.

The following case illustrates the principles of management of the severe electrical burn with full-thickness scalp and skull loss. Early wound treatment consists of debridement of the scalp, skull, and dura and other devitalized tissue, followed by frequent wet dressings for debridement and prevention of infection until granulations appear. A closed wound should be obtained as early as possible by use of split-thickness skin grafts applied directly to the granulation tissues. As a late program of reconstruction, missing bone should be replaced for protection of the underlying brain tissue. This requires full-thickness tissue to sustain the bone grafts. In this particular case, because of the large amount of scalp remaining and the excellent blood supply, it was possible to work out a treatment plan using a full-thickness flap and split-thickness rib grafts for bone reconstruction. Six months after the skin graft placed upon the brain had taken well and a closed wound was established, the anteriorly based scalp flap was then outlined (Figure 1).

Fig. 1. The scalp flap is outlined adjacent to the defect.

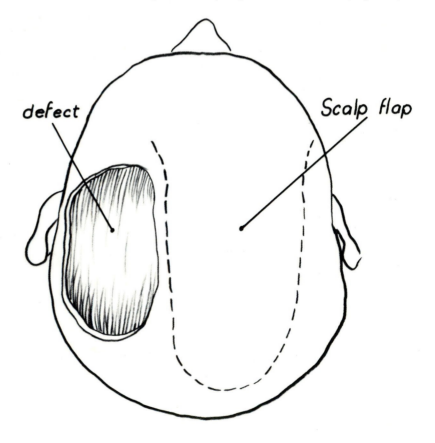

defect

Scalp flap

The flaps should be outlined in such a way that they contain a satisfactory arterial and venous pattern in the long axis of the flaps. This is generally possible most anywhere in the scalp if the flaps are based peripherally. Those based anteriorly depend upon the superorbital and frontal vessels. Lateral flaps depend upon the temporal vascular system and those posteriorly on the occipital and postauricular vessels. The collateral circulation in the scalp is excellent. If delayed, the flaps can be made across the midline for some distance, with the base on the contralateral side with the expectation that the blood supply will be adequate and the flaps will survive. The thickness of the flap should contain skin, subcutaneous tissue, and galea aponeurotica. This will assure a satisfactory

blood supply in the long axis of the flap. In the delay of such a flap, the flap is outlined and carefully measured by use of a pattern of adhesive tape or cloth which can be shifted back and forth over the wound to determine the exact area that the flap will cover. Flaps must be made generously and be designed carefully so that they have an adequate base and adequate length to completely cover the defect.

After a delay of approximately three weeks, the skin graft was removed from over the dura and split rib grafts were utilized to reconstruct the bony cranium, and the flap was transferred over the bone grafts where it was sutured into position (Figure 2A, B, and C).

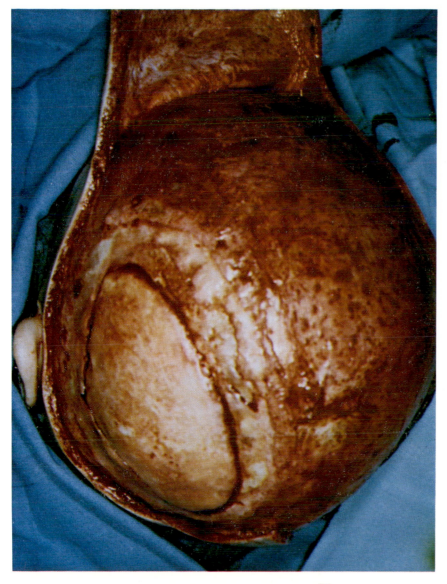

Fig. 2. A. After three weeks the flap is elevated and the split-thickness graft is excised from the dura.

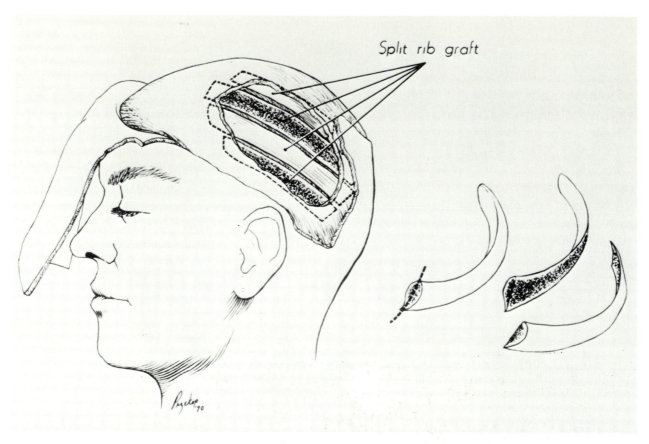

Fig. 2. (cont.) B. Split-rib grafts are placed over the defect.

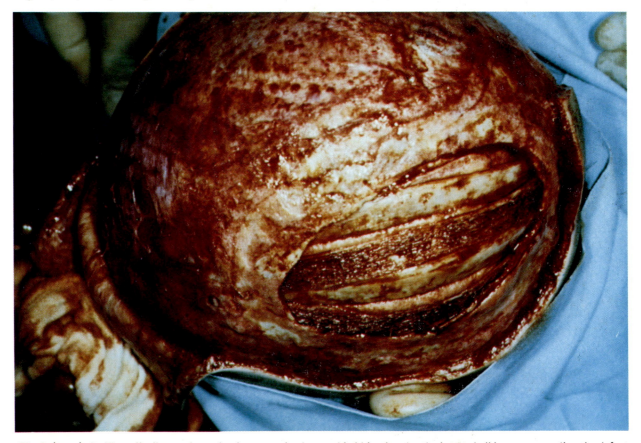

Fig. 2. (cont.) C. The split-ribs are shown in place over the dura and held in place by the intact skull bone surrounding the defect.

The donor site over the pericranium was covered with a split-thickness graft (Figure 3). Grafts will take readily on the pericranium provided it is not damaged during the elevation of the flap which contains the three superficial layers of the scalp.

On large flaps the Y base is rotated. There will be buckling or "dog ear" formation at the base of the flap on the side toward which the flap is rotated (Figure 4). This tissue is vital to the nourishment of the flap and should not be removed until after the flap has become adequately established in its new location and has picked up a blood supply from its periphery. After four to six months, if the "dog ear" has not flattened out, it can be removed surgically (Figure 5). In this instance healing was uncomplicated. There was complete survival of the rib grafts and the hair-bearing pedicle flap worked out very well from the standpoint of coverage and appearance. The split-thickness skin-grafted area over the flap donor site was well covered by the remaining scalp hair.

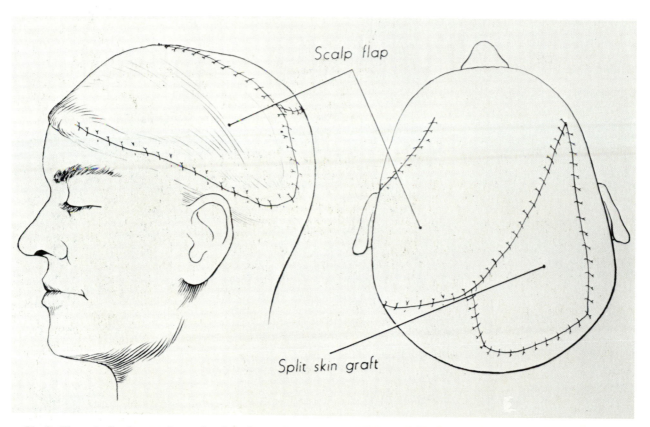

Fig. 3. The scalp flap is rotated over the rib grafts and the previous bed of the scalp flap is covered with a split-thickness graft.

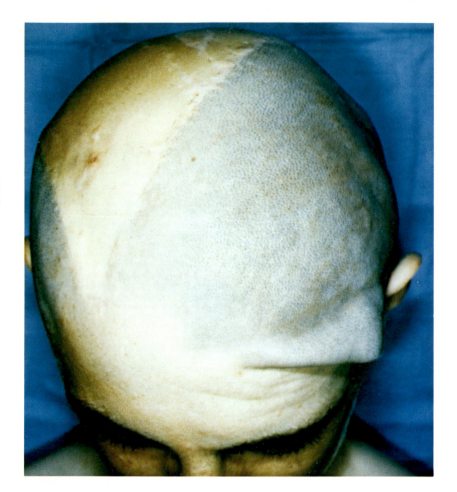

Fig. 4. A "dog ear" fold of scalp is the result of the flap rotation and is shown several months after the flap transfer.

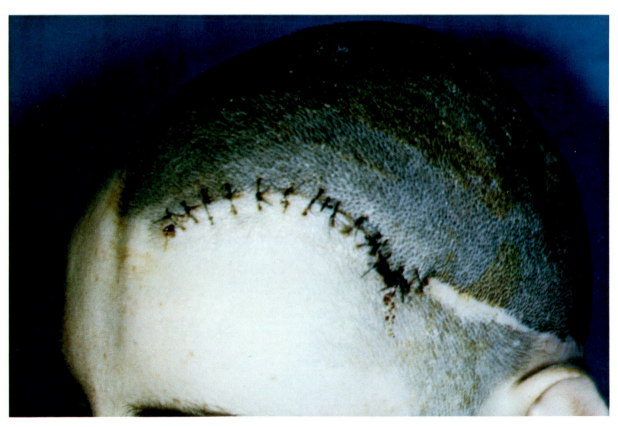

Fig. 5. The "dog ear" is excised and repaired to restore normal scalp appearance.

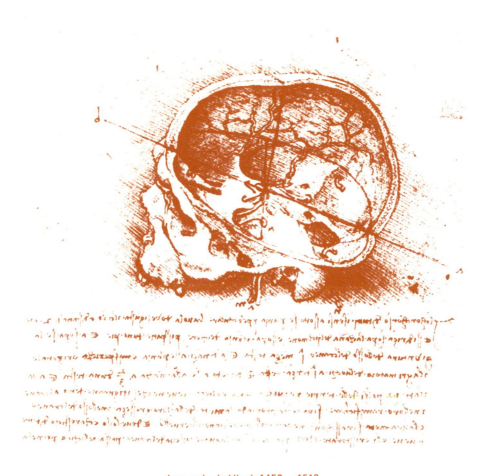

Leonardo da Vinci, 1452 – 1519.

Do not give to your friends the most agreeable counsels, but the most advantageous.

Tuckerman

16

REGENERATION OF THE DEVITALIZED SKULL

Eugene F. Worthen

Management of full-thickness devitalization of the skull has long posed one of the more difficult challenges to reconstructive surgery. When devitalization remains limited to the outer table, a variety of surgical approaches may be used successfully. Surgical removal of the outer cortex, drilling of the outer cortex, or spontaneous sequestration will permit a satisfactory end result because a viable foundation of inner cortex remains with an intact calvarium.

When devitalization of the skull includes the inner table, however, one is faced with the loss of the protective barrier provided by the skull, whether by aggressive surgical excision or conservative spontaneous deterioration. Surgical debridement is not only technically difficult but is also often precluded by location over a major vascular sinus. Spontaneous sequestration is accompanied by a high incidence of epidural abscess formation. Both require subsequent restoration of the intact shield of the calvarium. Covering the bony defect with a prosthesis presents the potential of reaction and ulceration. Bone graft replacement requires the most meticulous attention to contour and mortise if a successful result is to be achieved. Any combination of the foregoing requires many months of hazardous disability. Study of the nature of the electrical burn injury offers yet another approach.

THE ELECTRICAL INJURY

The problem of devitalized skull is encountered most often in the electrical burn. Thermal injury may denude bone of overlying soft tissue, but will rarely generate sufficient heat to produce devitalization of the bone. The depth and extent of a thermal burn of the scalp is initially apparent, because its

greatest damage is at the surface, with diminishing effects in the deeper layers. Electrical current, however, will seek the path of least resistance in the vascular diploe of the skull, with resulting thrombosis and bone death. This may be severe enough to devitalize large segments of full-thickness skull, with minimal apparent superficial change in the initial stage (Figure 1). In such cases, even the entire hair distribution may be intact and appear normal.

Even though bone is the only body tissue with greater electrical resistance than skin, the skull is unique. The broad flat surface and vascular diploe

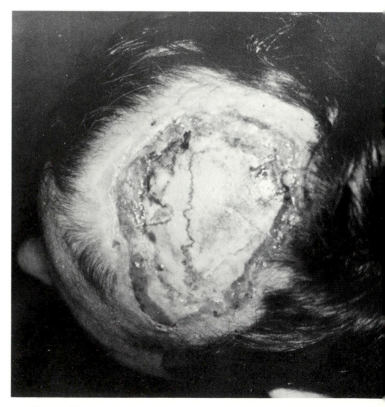

Fig. 1. Electrical burn of scalp with full-thickness devitalization of skull.

allow large amounts of current to flow through un-impeded. It is important to note that this mechanism of devitalization does not involve destruction of the bone or its architecture, but mere isolation from the vascular tree by thrombosis. It is now apparent that in the past a perfectly contoured and mortised graft has been sacrificed in this type of injury. Actual bone deterioration will not commence for several weeks, and it is during this time that the segment of devitalized bone may be salvaged. Once sequestration or infection has interrupted the continuity of bone, the potential of regeneration disappears.

POTENTIAL FOR REGENERATION

The potential of bone regeneration has been confirmed in experimental work by Gage and his colleagues. By freezing with liquid nitrogen, they effected complete devitalization in segments of dog femur. (This mechanism of bone death is comparable to that observed with electrical injury.) After complete devitalization of the bone and periosteum (confirmed by microscopic study), the wounds were closed primarily, enveloping the dead bone with normal soft tissues. After three weeks, new periosteal bone was observed extending across the devitalized segment from the upper and lower margins. Within eight weeks, segments as long as 10cm were covered with new bone. Vascularized tissue then entered the haversian and Volkmann's canals. The canals en-larged as non-vital bone was absorbed, then new bone appeared on the walls of the canals. Complete replacement was noted within six months in some cases.

When the regeneration potential of the devita-lized skull is recognized, its treatment evolves into immediate management of the devitalized scalp. Determination of bone viability becomes a matter of academic interest only.

SURGICAL MANAGEMENT

When the electrical burn has been sufficient to devitalize bone, the overlying scalp will gradually become a dry hard plaque of tissue. Hair distribution may remain undisturbed. **It is at this time that plans for reconstruction should be formulated.** The head is shaved and an exploratory incision made in the center of the demarcated plaque. This incision, which re-quires no anesthesia, should extend down to the underlying bone. Absence of pain and bleeding confirms at least full-thickness soft tissue destruction. Exploration and biopsy of the underlying skull will be of documentary interest only, since it has no bearing on the subsequent course of surgery.

If the island of devitalized scalp has a diameter of less than 6cm, an adjacent flap of viable scalp is outlined for rotation in a manner that will permit primary closure of the secondary defect. Under endotracheal anesthesia, the eschar is excised com-pletely and the flap mobilized. In these smaller defects, periosteum may be transferred with the flap to hasten regeneration of the bone, but this is not a necessary adjunct. The scalp flap is sutured into position without tension over the devitalized skull. The secondary defect is revised and closed primarily.

When the devitalized scalp presents a diameter of 6cm or more, plans must be made to skin graft the secondary defect. After the plaque is excised, the flap is elevated without periosteum and transferred. The periosteum on the base of the secondary defect provides an excellent bed for immediate application of a split-thickness skin graft. This method is appli-cable to any defect exposing less than half of the calvarium. Due to radial orientation of the vascular system of the scalp, flaps unlimited in size may be transferred. Flaps may be rotated from any direction so long as a peripheral base is maintained with a suitable base-to-length ratio (Figure 2). Subsequent excision of the split-thickness graft in stages offers an optional refinement (Figures 3 and 4).

In massive defects involving 50 percent or more of the scalp, preliminary development of a distant skin flap is completed before excising the eschar. When the flap is ready for transfer, the soft tissue debridement is performed, the flap is sutured into position, and the donor site is treated in the appro-priate manner.

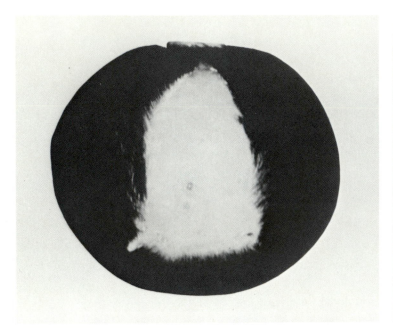

Fig. 2. Two months following coverage of burn with local scalp flap with split-thickness skin graft of the flap donor site.

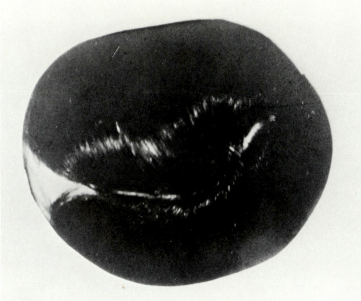

Fig. 3. Appearance of the scalp after excision of the split-thickness skin by the multiple-excision technique.

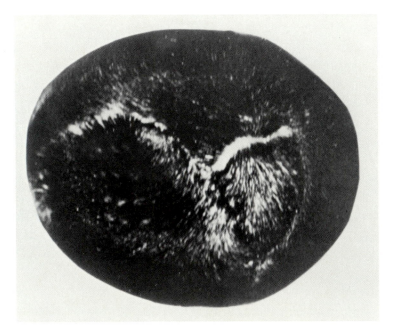

Fig. 4. Appearance of the scalp three years after electrical burn.

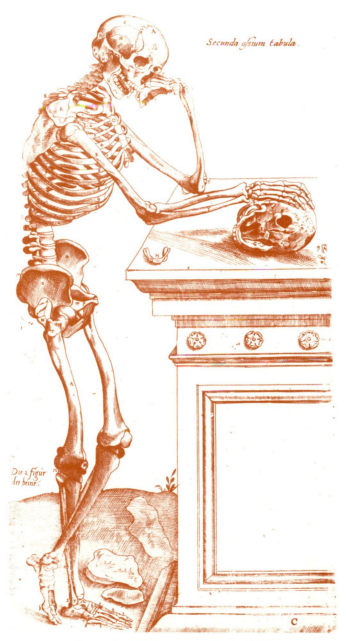

Secunda ossium tabula.

Die 2 figur der beine.

Anatomia viri in hoc genere princip, 1617.

_____

To have doubted one's own first principles is the mark of a civilized man.

Holmes

17

SPLIT-RIB BONE GRAFTS

Jacob J. Longacre

Large defects of the skull present a problem. Rarely does the calvarium regenerate and then only in very young children after a portion has been removed for craniosynostosis or osteomyelitis. Ossification of a linear fracture of the skull requires a much longer period than a fracture through the base. This is because the calvarium originates as membranous bone while the base is chondral bone.

BONE GRAFTS

Severe burns, such as those suffered by a child or an epileptic who has fallen into an open fire, often terminate in exposure and later sequestration of the cranial bones. In addition, electrical burns may result in destruction of the cranium and facial skeleton. Should the adjacent scalp be insufficient to be used for rotation flap coverage, a new blood supply can be brought in by using a jump flap from the abdomen, with the arm as the intermediate carrier. Direct microvascular anastomosis of omental vessels to the *in situ* artery and vein and then skin graft on the omentum is another choice. Once vascular cover is attained, the defect can be reconstructed with autogenous bone grafts. These may be obtained from adjacent bone, but this creates an additional defect. In growing children the iliac crest should never be used because of the disturbances in growth. The use of the tibia similarly creates an unsightly defect. The use of homologous banked bone grafts has proved disappointing.

The literature is filled with preliminary reports of bone grafts and so-called follow-ups of a mere two to three years. Results which first appear to be excellent may not be as good when observed over a longer period. **Only careful long-term follow-up will yield the basic data necessary to provide a secure foundation upon which to build our specialty.** This is particularly true when the growth factor must be taken into consideration in the reconstruction of extensive defects of the cranial bones and facial skeleton in the developing child.

SPLIT-RIB GRAFTS

We have carried out more than 1,000 operations on humans using split-rib grafts during the past 20 years. Figures 1 through 4 illustrate such a long-term result. In addition, several long-range experiments have been carried out on several large series of Rhesus monkeys. Our findings in humans closely parallel our more detailed observation in monkeys.

Clinically, we have noted that the skulls in these children have developed at a normal rate. This is further confirmed by our observations in young monkeys. After a follow-up of 2½ years (equivalent to 7½ years in man) the split-rib grafts can still be identified in the developing skull. This is counter to the old theory that the calvarium develops by absorption from the inner table and replacement by onlay on the outer table. Though we have utilized split-rib grafts to repair very extensive defects (six patients had a loss of 75 to 90 percent of the cranial vault) and have followed these from 15 to 20 years, *in no instance has there been any sign of epileptic seizures following the insertion of the split-rib grafts.* This is in sharp contradistinction to the incidence of seizures following the use of tantalum and other alloplastic substances.

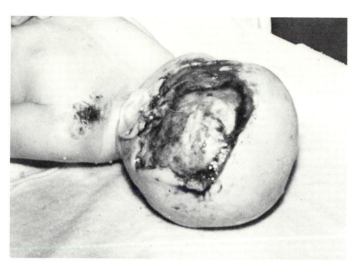

Fig. 1. Extensive traumatic defect of 40 percent of the calvarium, soft tissues, and coverings of the brain.

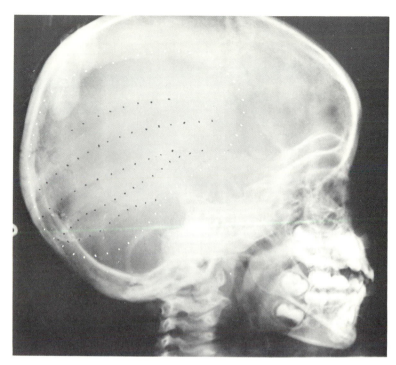

Fig. 3. Note regeneration of skull with remnants of the split-rib grafts still evident eight years following reconstruction. No bone grafts were placed in the occipital region. The original defect and the rib grafts are outlined to improve orientation.

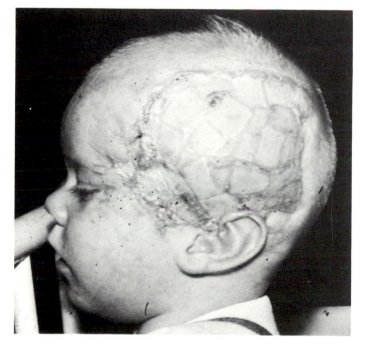

Fig. 2. Following control of infection the exposed dura was covered with split grafts to provide physiologic cover. The child was provided with a protective helmet which he refused to wear.

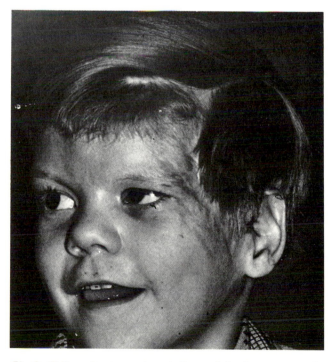

Fig. 4. Oblique view two and one-half years following reconstruction. Child is very alert.

The rib cage will constantly and repeatedly replenish itself to provide a bank of fresh autogenous bone. Large amounts of bone can be taken, provided alternate ribs are taken and the rib bed is carefully closed with a running catgut suture. Children are able to get out of bed the day after the operation, and the degree of morbidity is low compared to that following removal of a similar amount of bone from the tibia or iliac crest should never be removed from a developing child.

18

SKULL IMPLANTATION MATERIALS

Glenn W. Kindt

Closure of cranial defects by cranioplasty has a long history. Trephination has been practiced among civilizations diverse both in time and location. Evidence recovered among archeological findings attests to the frequent success of such operations, although the reasons for this practice remain a mystery. In most instances of trephination the defect was not covered. However, there is evidence that practitioners in the South Pacific attempted cranioplasty with coconut shells, and South American Incas occasionally employed gold plates.

The first recorded successful cranioplasty was performed in 1670 when J. van Meekren implanted a bone from a dog into the skull defect of a man. His success was of short duration because violent church opposition prompted him to remove the graft. The modern era of cranioplasty began approximately 200 years later when a number of physicians reported results of cranioplasty in collected series of patients.

CRANIOPLASTY MATERIALS

Autogenous bone grafts from almost any available site have been used successfully for covering skull defects. Rib grafts, once popular, are still occasionally employed in children. Grafts can be taken from the ileum that closely approximate both the thickness and the curvature of the skull. A most ingenious method, in which advantage is taken of adjacent intact pericranium and skull, was advanced by Müller and König. An autogenous flap is made by cutting a mirror image of the cranial defect from the outer table and pericranium of the adjacent skull. The split-bone flap with attached pericranium is then rotated into the defect. Prolonged operating time and improved artificial substances, however, have led

to the gradual abandonment of this excellent method. Preserved cadaver bones, also used for cranioplasty, have lost popularity because of frequent absorption after implantation.

In more recent years, metallic implantable materials have been used extensively. Gold can be easily molded, but is soft and certainly expensive. Silver and aluminum, as most metals, conduct temperature fluctuations to the underlying brain and perhaps occasionally cause headaches. Tantalum was the metal most commonly employed for repair during World War II. The metal is tough and nonreactive and can be easily cut and molded in the Operating Room.

Plastic materials are most popular among surgeons performing cranioplasties today. Acrylic was apparently first used for cranioplasty by Zander in 1940. The simplicity of molding the plate in the Operating Room in a one-stage operation allows a short operating time. Plastic surgeons have found multiple applications for Silastic, an inert plastic which can be obtained in several variations of hardness. In recent years medical-grade silicone has been employed in skull defects, particularly those involving the forehead.

CAUSES OF SKULL DEFECTS

There are multiple causes of skull defects which require cranioplasty. The majority are produced surgically in the process of therapy for open skull fractures. Common treatment for a compound skull wound with loose and contaminated bone fragments consists of removing the fragments and allowing primary wound healing without infection. It is sometimes safe, however, to replace bone fragments, particularly in relatively clean wounds in children. Bone fragment replacement was first employed by Macewen in 1885 and should be considered in civilian cranial trauma. Skull defects are also produced during removal of brain tumors, such as meningiomas, which involve the cranium. Part of the standard therapy for any infected craniotomy wound is excision of the bone flap which serves as a nidus for infection. The bone flap excision results in a prominent skull defect requiring cranioplasty. Congenital skull defects, such as patent biparietal foramina, occasionally require cranioplasty. Skull defects due to thermal burns are not common. A defect can occur, though, when the scalp wound is deep and extensive, such as an electrical burn. **The full-thickness of the skull may also be lost in any scalp burn or avulsion if the exposed skull is not kept moist during the healing stage.**

INDICATIONS FOR CRANIOPLASTY

The indications for cranioplasty can be divided into three main categories: (1) protection from external trauma; (2) cosmetic; and (3) reduction of pulsations which may be associated with seizures or with thinning of the cortical mantle.

Skull defects, even of a small size, should be repaired in children who must weather the hazards of the sandlot. However, we have rarely seen brain damage produced through an open skull defect. Frontal skull defects may produce an unsightly facial appearance, which may be markedly improved by cranioplasty. The closure of skull defects in order to prevent seizures or thinning of the cortical mantle is somewhat controversial.

Seizures are a common sequela of open skull fractures, particularly when the dura has been torn and the brain lacerated. Follow-up of war injuries in which the dura was torn revealed a seizure incidence of 43 percent in veterans of World War I and World War II, and 42 percent in veterans of the Korean War. Closing the skull defect is thought to be beneficial for preventing post-trauma seizures. However, some observers do not believe closure of the skull defect reduces seizure incidence.

Pneumoencephalography performed on a patient with a skull defect often shows a thin cortical mantle over the site of the defect. Thinning of the cortical mantle has been described as a migration of the ventricle toward the cortical surface. This may occur because of pulsations of the choroid plexus, also described as the etiology for ventricular dilation in hydrocephalus. The ventricular wall toward the skull defect may gradually dilate due to these pulsations. Conversely, thinning of the cortical mantle may be secondary simply to scarring and atrophy from brain damage occurring at the time of trauma. Thus, it is probable that brain pulsations through an open skull defect are harmful, at least in some instances. Preventing these pulsations can be cited as one indication for cranioplasty until more definitive information is available.

TIME FOR CRANIOPLASTY

Proper timing for performance of the cranioplasty is an important consideration. If craniotomy and bone removal are elective, cranioplasty should usually be performed at the primary operation. In some cases of extensive tumor removal, the skull defect can be closed later, after brain edema has subsided. The customary time for closing a skull defect due to an open skull fracture is six months following the injury, to allow any infection to resolve. This waiting period need not be rigid; less time is required for a relatively clean open skull fracture and probably more time is allowed if osteomyelitis is present.

TECHNIQUE OF ACRYLIC CRANIOPLASTY

The procedure is a major operation performed under general anesthesia. A complete head prep is preferred. Of considerable concern is the scalp incision, which must expose the entire skull defect and be designed so that it does not interfere with the blood supply of the scalp flap. Blood supply across an old scar is minimal and not dependable. It is therefore essential that the incision is not made across the remaining blood supply of a scalp segment. The skin incision should also be planned so it does not cross the implant (Figure 1). If a plastic or metal plate is located beneath a fresh scalp incision there is a tendency for the healing scar to be thin and expose the plate.

Separating the galea from the scarred dura can be the most difficult part of the operation and requires care. The dura must be separated from the scalp throughout the entire extent of the bony defect, as well as approximately one centimeter beneath the bone margin. Small bleeding sites from the dura and the scar can be annoying; peroxide irrigation of the area will aid in obtaining a dry operative field. Accidental incision of the dura requires a water-tight re-approximation. If the frontal

sinus is inadvertently entered during dissection, the mucosa should be removed and the cranioplasty delayed to another date. Any exposure of the cranioplasty plate to the sinus cavity will likely result in chronic infection requiring later removal of the plate.

The presterilized, packaged methyl methacrylate polymer and reagent are mixed according to directions to produce a workable molding material. Polymerization, an exothermic reaction, starts when the acrylic increases in temperature, which is readily discernible to touch. The material is then molded into the approximate dimensions of the cranial defect. The dura must be protected from heat con-

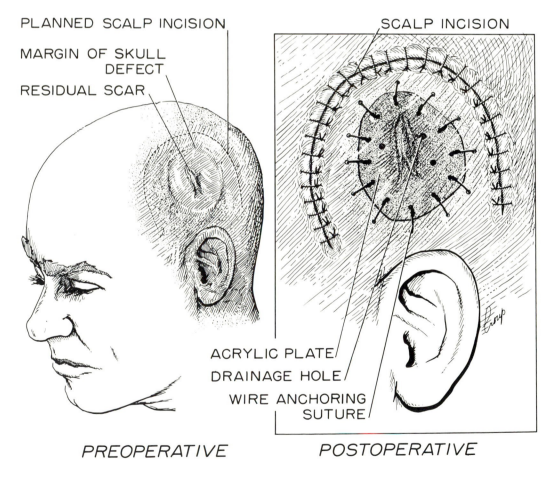

Fig. 1. Schematic drawing of skull defect and cranioplasty. Preoperative diagram demonstrates the planned incision and underlying skull defect. Postoperative diagram shows the acrylic plate anchored in place with the overlying scalp sutured.

duction with wet cotton pledgets and a thin sheet of plastic. The acrylic material is inserted into the defect and allowed to harden during frequent saline irrigations.

A number of small holes are placed in the central area of the plate for drainage of fluids from beneath the plate during the postoperative period. Fibrous union occurs later between the dura and the scalp through these holes and serves to anchor the scalp. Holes in the plate for wiring are placed approximately 1cm apart and one half to 1cm from the edge (Figure 1). Opposing holes are then made in the skull near the edge of the defect. A flat metal retractor is placed between the bone and the dura during drilling to prevent perforation of the dura and the brain. Number 2-0 or 3-0 wire sutures are then used to solidly anchor the acrylic plate to the skull edge (Figure 1). It is essential that the plate be in place in the manner described or it will loosen with time, even if it is solid at the time of the operation. The wound is irrigated and the scalp incision closed with wire sutures. A head dressing is applied.

POSTOPERATIVE CARE

Preoperative anticonvulsant medications should be resumed postoperatively. The initial brain trauma dictates the need for the anticonvulsants, not the cranioplasty itself because the cortex of the brain should not have been disturbed. A prophylactic antibiotic is usually given for a week following the insertion of the foreign body although the efficacy of antibiotic use may be disputed. During the initial few days of the postoperative period, the head dressing should be removed to check for fluid collection under the scalp incision. A small amount of fluid will usually reabsorb without difficulty, but if the skin flap is bulging this may compromise the suture line and sterile needle aspiration may be necessary. Sutures are removed after adequate healing takes place and the patient discharged in seven to ten days.

SUMMARY

The history of use of implantation materials in the skull is long and colorful. The type of material used for cranioplasty has changed periodically and undoubtedly will continue to evolve. The most popular material used at present is an acrylic resin, methyl methacrylate. This material is as strong as the normal skull and can be easily molded in the Operating Room. If the procedure is performed properly to avoid certain pitfalls, there should be no complications and the cranioplasty plate should be permanent.

Medicine is the only profession that labors incessantly to destroy the reason for its existence.
Bryce

19

HAIR TRANSPLANTS

Thomas D. Cronin

Free hair transplants have been used in two forms. Small punch grafts of the scalp were first described by Orentreich in 1959. While using the punch grafts, Vallis also advocated strip grafts to establish the frontal hairline in 1964, 1967, and 1969.

Punch scalp grafts are of value when local excision of scars cannot be closed by undermining or by the use of local flaps. Strip scalp grafts 3 to 4mm wide are useful in establishing a hairline, especially if no flap tissue is available. **A limited donor area or too-extensive loss of hair precludes the use of hair transplants.**

The scalp consists of the following layers: skin, superficial fascia, galea aponeurotica, loose areolar tissue, and pericranium. The most favorable situation for the use of hair transplants occurs when there is a loss of the skin only. Transplants are still possible with losses down to the areolar tissue, assuming that split-thickness skin grafting has been performed. If the residual cover of the skull with scarred epithelium or a skin graft is of sufficient thickness to be movable, hair transplants are possible. However, if the scar or split-thickness graft is thin and tightly adherent to the skull successful transplantation of hair is unlikely.

OPERATIVE TECHNIQUE

The technique for punch scalp grafts is the same as that used to treat cases of male baldness. A 3½mm or 4mm punch may be used for both donor and recipient sites. Preferably, the 4mm punch is used to take the graft, while the 3½mm punch is used at the recipient site. Because the hole expands and the graft shrinks a little, the fit is better with this combination.

The operation is performed under local anesthesia (Xylocaine 1 percent with 1:100,000 adrenalin) or general anesthesia. But even if general anesthesia is used, infiltration with Xylocaine and adrenalin should be used to minimize blood loss.

DONOR SITE

Punch Graft. The occipital area is the most common donor site, followed by the parietal areas, because these areas are the least likely to become bald in later life. The hair is clipped with electric clippers, leaving it just long enough to determine the direction of growth. The punch is inserted parallel to the hair so that the roots are not cut off. From 30 to 100 punches may be taken at one sitting.

The punch goes into the fatty superficial fascia layer. The graft is lifted up with Adson tissue forceps and cut off with small eye scissors. The excess fat is trimmed off, exposing but not damaging the hair roots. The grafts are deposited on moist saline sponges until the recipient site is ready or, if two teams are working, the recipient site may be simultaneously prepared and planted. The hole should be deep enough to fully receive the graft. The cylinders from the donor site are discarded.

Many authors, especially dermatologists, leave the donor sites open. However, I close the holes with one suture, being careful to insert the sutures at different angles to avoid undue tension in any one direction, which might cause loss of hair. Suturing seems to lessen discomfort for the patient, healing is quicker, and scarring is less (Figure 1).

The grafts should be inserted with the hair directed in the normal direction for the particular location. Suturing the grafts is not always essential,

Fig. 1. Donor sites in occipital scalp have been closed with single sutures taken at varied angles to avoid tension in any one line. Grafts are sutured by taking a bite through opposite sides of the recipient sites, going over the top of the graft rather than through the graft, and continuing from one graft to the next.

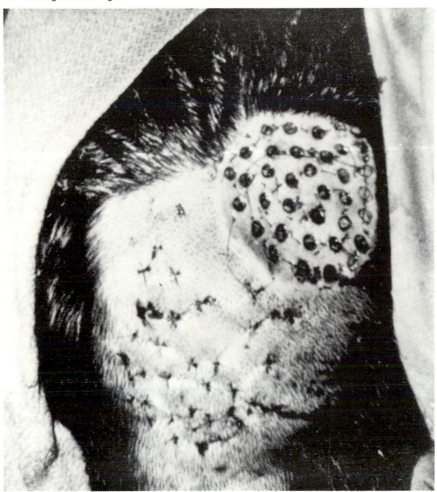

if a nonadherent dressing, such as telfa, is applied carefully so as not to disrupt them. On the other hand, in scarred or skin-grafted areas where the depth of the recipient site may be limited, I use a continuous suture of 4-0 monofilament. Taking a bite through opposite sides of the recipient punch site and going over the top of the graft rather than through the graft, I suture continuously from one graft to the next one to ensure that the graft does not protrude.

Strip Graft. The strip graft is useful for establishing a frontal or temporal hairline (and, or course, eyebrows) if a flap is not available. Vallis points out that the strip should be taken in a transverse direction from the occipital region, since vertical scars are visible. The incisions should be made 3 to 4mm apart, parallel to the direction of the hair shafts. The

frontal or temporal hairline should be carefully sketched in to resemble the normal hairline. Then a single incision is made down through the galea, which allows the skin edges to spread and receive the graft. Hemostasis should be thorough. The hair should be directed in the normal direction, which, in the frontal region, is towards the brow.

Figure 2 illustrates repair of a hairline defect using a combination of transposition flaps, multiple partial excisions, and punch scalp grafting. The use of punch scalp grafts may be somewhat disappointing due to the sparsity of hair. The result is definitely inferior to that obtainable when a flap can be used. Yet punch grafts are of definite value to the plastic surgeon, both alone and in combination with flaps.

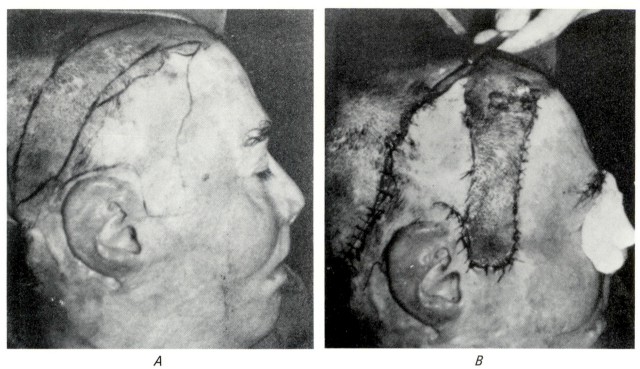

A   *B*

Fig. 2. A. A severe burn with complete loss of hair in temporal area. Outline of a scalp flap to restore anterior hair line. **B.** The bald anterior area and the hair-bearing scalp flap have been transposed, as flaps. As the scalp stretched, it was possible later to excise part of the non-hair bearing area; punch scalp grafts were then put in the remaining area of alopecia.

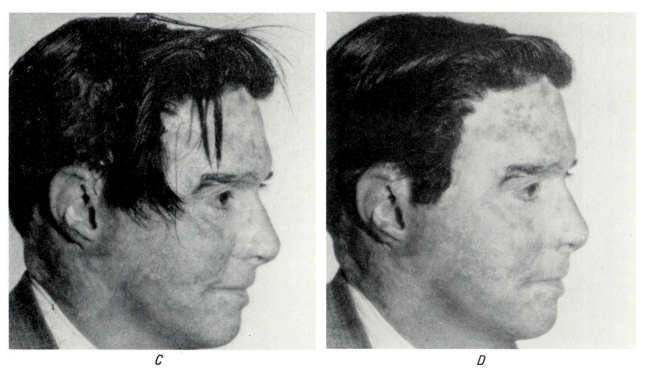

C   *D*

Fig. 2. C. Anterior hair pulled aside to show area of hair-bearing punch grafts (performed in three operations; 16, 12, and 4 months before). **D.** Appearance with grafted area reinforced by combing anterior hair over it.

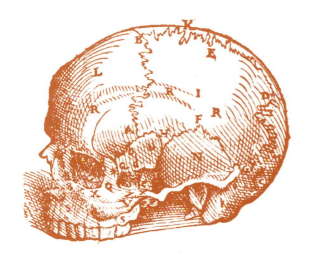 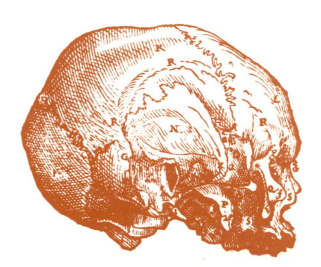

CHARACTERVM TERTIAE, ET QVARTAE
figurarum Index.

Jan Stephen van Calcar, *Anatomia,* 1575.

Advice is like snow; the softer it falls the longer it dwells upon, and the deeper it sinks into the mind.
Coleridge

20

THE CUSTOM-MADE HAIRPIECE

Joseph Paderewski

Extensive burns of the scalp, resulting in the permanent loss of a great amount of hair, when not corrected surgically through scalp rotation, require that the patient be supplied with a partial or complete hairpiece. In instances where the hair is shaved for surgical purposes or to promote healing of the burned areas, the patients may want to be supplied with a temporary hairpiece.

Hairpieces for women or young girls present little problem. They can be purchased as stock items and are readily available with both human and/or synthetic hair. The greater problem lies in properly fitting men and boys. Stock hairpieces are rarely, if ever, useful in these cases and custom-made hairpieces, whether they be partial or full, must be obtained to achieve optimal results.

In larger cities, where the services of wigmakers are readily available, patients are easily accommodated. However, for those medical centers located in smaller cities, arrangements for satisfactory hairpiece fittings can be accomplished through the mails if the wigmaker is furnished with the following information:

1) An impression or casting of the affected area.
2) A measurement around the head, taken behind the ears (Figure 1). This measurement will determine the size of the form upon which the wig is made.
3) A lock of hair, for color match, at least 1/8 inch in diameter secured by a piece of string or scotch tape. (A few hairs are of no value for an accurate match.) Hair color may also be matched through the use of numbered shade guides (Figure 2), which the wigmaker may be able to supply.
4) Photos of the patient (4 x 5's in black and

Fig. 1.

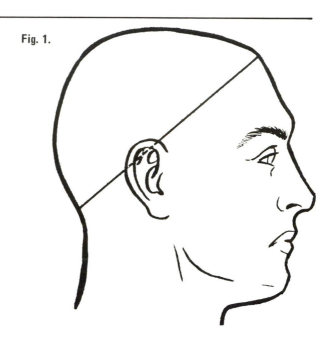

Fig. 2. Numbered hair shade guide.

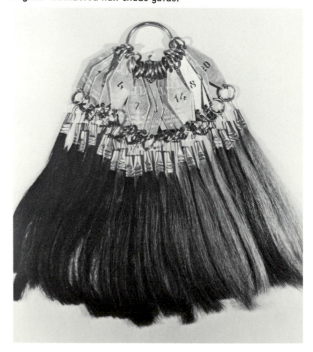

white will do very well) showing the front, both sides, and the back of the head.

5) Additional information required by the wigmaker may be: the amount (thickness) of hair which could vary from very light, if the patient's own hair is sparse, to heavy, if patient's hair is very thick and stands out; the amount of wave in the hair from very tight curl to semi-straight or straight, etc.

IMPRESSIONS FOR FULL HAIRPIECE

Apply a thin coating of Vaseline to the scalp and especially to the remaining hair. With a soft eyebrow pencil draw the proposed hair outline, including the part, onto the scalp. It will seem at first that the eyebrow pencil is merely gliding on the greasy surface. However, after a few repeated strokes the markings begin to "take" (the Vaseline actually dissolves the pencil material). The line should be well-pronounced and quite dark.

A length of strong thread or silk suture is placed lengthwise along the middle of the scalp and fastened with Scotch tape near the eyebrows in front and well below the hairline on the back of the neck. Strips of quick-setting plaster bandage are then dipped in warm water and set into place along both sides of the thread so that the thread will not be covered by the plaster bandage. Continue the application of the plaster bandage to the scalp, overlapping the lines drawn by the eyebrow pencil. At least three layers of plaster bandage should be used, worked well onto the contour of the involved area, and then allowed to set.

A batch of plaster is mixed and applied carefully over the thread, overlapping the plaster bandage about two inches on either side of the midline. The plaster application should be at least 3/8 inch thick.

When the plaster is about to set, remove the Scotch tape and, grasping both ends of the thread firmly, pull upwards. The thread will cut through the partially set plaster, dividing the mold in half. Because this is the most critical part of the procedure, it might be well to practice the "thread-cut" technique on some inanimate object to determine the "feel" of the material. Pulling the thread too early will cause the unset plaster to bond together. If the thread is pulled too late, the plaster will be too hard for the thread to cut through. After the cut has been made, allow the plaster to set and then gently remove the halves of the mold.

The halves of the mold are carefully assembled and fresh plaster is applied over the "join" on the outside of the mold and allowed to set. Upon examining the interior it will be noticed that the hairline marking has been transferred to the mold. Darken this line with an eyebrow pencil, and carefully apply a plaster separator. A layer of plaster about ½ inch thick is then built up inside the mold and permitted to firmly set. The mold is then removed or broken away. The hairline which has been transferred to the cast should be darkened with an indelible pencil, crayon, or felt-tipped marker, and the patient's name plainly marked.

While a full hairpiece can be made from measurements, greater accuracy can be obtained through the use of this technique.

PARTIAL HAIRPIECE

The same basic impression technique is used in making the mold for a partial hairpiece, except that the thread is not employed since a one-piece mold is required. The markings on the scalp are made on the affected area where it meets the remaining hair, keeping the outline simple. Markings on the final cast should include an arrow pointing to the front of the impressions and lines showing the direction of the hair growth.

FITTING THE HAIRPIECE

When the hairpiece arrives from the wigmaker, the hair is usually a bit long or shaggy. Corrections can easily be made by any barber. Partial hairpieces are made so that the hair can be combed into the patient's own hair to hide the join line. The hairpiece is fastened to the scalp with spirit gum or, more popularly, double adhesive tape. Adhesives, hairpiece forms, and hair grooming creams can be ordered from

Fig. 4. Putting on the hairpiece.

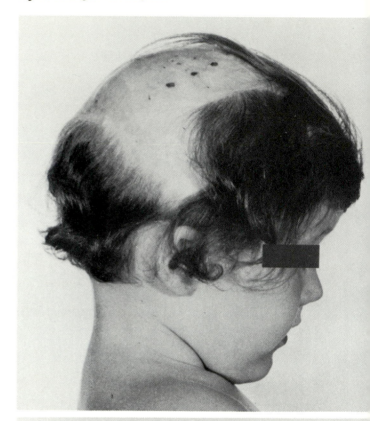

the wigmaker. A generous supply of tape should always be kept on hand.

The patient can easily master properly fitting the hairpiece by following these simple steps:

1) Peel the protective layer off the tape.
2) Cut strips of tape to fit the spot.
3) Place pieces of tape near the edge of the wig (Figure 3).
4) Put the wig on carefully, pull the edges taut, then press down on the tape.
5) Comb the wig with a large-toothed comb and style slightly.
6) Dampen the comb, if necessary, to put unruly hair in place (Figure 4).

SUMMARY

The hairpiece, as well as other prostheses, is very important to the psychological well-being of the patient, and every effort should be made to see that the patient is supplied with items of first-class design and craftsmanship. **Mediocrity will only serve to add ridicule to tragedy.**

Fig. 3.

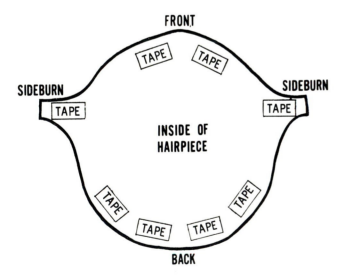

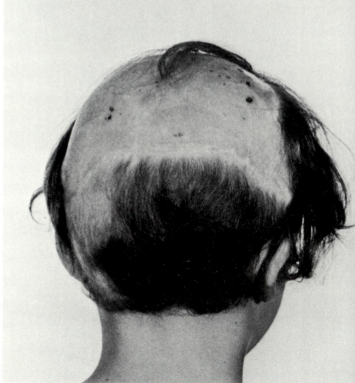

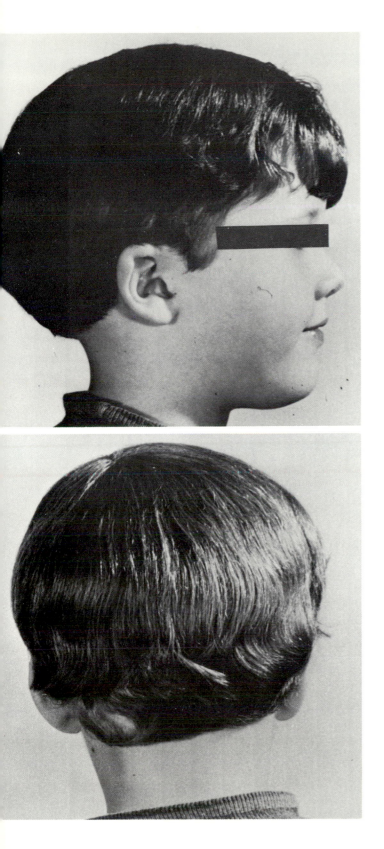

III.

THE EAR

PRINCIPLES OF TREATMENT

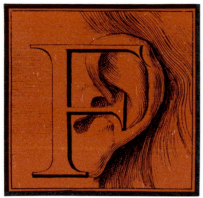

ull-thickness burns of the external ear are common following flame burns. The external ear frequently suffers full-thickness loss, including the cartilage. Reconstruction by pedicles or composite grafts is required. In some cases the patient may prefer to use a prosthesis.

Excessive tissue such as hypertrophic scars and keloids may follow partial-thickness burns of the external ear. These may require excision, which should be carried out at the proper time. Stenosis of the external canal is rare. It can be corrected by using a combination of a pedicle and a thick graft after the defect is opened.

Injury to the tympanic membranes and middle ear requires careful evaluation for proper treatment. Consultation with an otologist is often advisable when middle ear or eighth nerve damage is present. The loss of hearing in most cases of severe burns is due to eighth nerve damage. This damage is often caused by medications. Potentially ototoxic antibiotics are often required when treating severe burns. These may result in partial or permanent hearing loss. Unfortunately, hearing aids are not effective for this problem.

Irving Feller

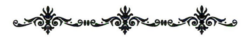

22

EARLY MANAGEMENT OF
THE EAR

Irving Feller
Kathryn E. Richards

The primary hazard to the ear following a burn is loss of cartilage by infection. The skin covering the cartilage is thin and the blood supply to the external ear is easily disrupted.

It is difficult to diagnose the depth of burn of the ear immediately following the accident. However, early treatment is similar for both partial and full-thickness burns. The basic treatment is the use of a topical antimicrobial agent, frequent dressing changes, and daily examination for pain and swelling. If the ear remains normal in size and is pain free, treatment is successful. On the other hand, if the external ear swells and becomes tender, a chondritis is usually present. This condition requires incision, drainage, and excision of all infected cartilage. Systemic antibiotics are also indicated to contain the infection. Early debriding of dead tissue and autografting can often decrease the incidence of chondritis (Figure 1).

Another major problem for many seriously burned patients is loss of hearing. The primary cause for the decrease in or a complete hearing loss is the antibiotics necessary to manage infections in severe burns. The antibiotics may be ototoxic and/or nephrotoxic. If the patient develops renal impairment, the incidence of ototoxicity increases. The paradox is that often the only effective antibiotics are nephrotoxic. When a choice does exist, the nephrotoxic medications should be discontinued when either renal damage is diagnosed or audiograms indicate eighth nerve damage.

Burns of the external canal and middle ear are rare. However, the canal and tympanic membranes should be examined when the patient is admitted and frequently during hospital course for injury and for removal of debris from the canal. Moist dressings and debris can cause maceration of the external canal and tympanic membrane, leading to pain and tissue loss (i.e., perforated tympanic membrane). If injury to the canal or middle ear has occurred, an otologist should be consulted and a program started to keep the area clean. An audiogram should be taken as soon after admission as possible and should be repeated every week.

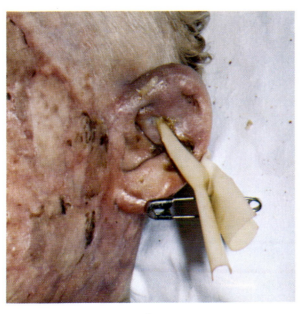

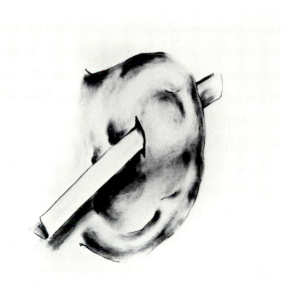

A   B

Fig. 1. When it becomes apparent that part of the external ear has been damaged beyond repair, excision should be complete to remove all dead tissue. Care should be taken to avoid the spread of chondritis to the exposed cartilage. When abscess formation surrounds an area of chondritis, a through and through incision at the point of greatest swelling and purulence provides adequate drainage and avoids excessive loss of earlobe (**A**). The site is kept open with a soft rubber drain. This procedure causes less deformity than bivalving the ear for acute supportive chondritis. **B.** Artist's conception of the procedure.

23

TYMPANIC MEMBRANE AND MIDDLE EAR

Roger Boles

PERSISTENT PERFORATIONS OF THE TYMPANIC MEMBRANE

The vast majority of perforations of the tympanic membrane from mechanical trauma or from acute suppurative otitis media heal and close spontaneously. Those resulting from burn injuries often persist, apparently because of the necrotizing nature of the injury and the associated profound damage to the remaining tissues. This intense scar tissue reaction makes the outcome of conventional surgical repair uncertain. There is little or no hope for closure of such perforations by simple chemical cautery of the margins of the perforation, with or without patching material, a technique which is often very successful in closing persistent tympanic membrane perforations following traumatic rupture or acute suppurative middle ear disease. Such chemical cautery will only add further necrosis and fibrosis to the burned tympanic membrane, and will not generally reduce the size of the opening.

Only operative myringoplasty, utilizing substitute tissue grafts such as temporalis fascia or vein, will have any significant chance of success (Figures 1 and 2). Even then, if the injury has been diffuse and severe, the remaining blood supply of the tympanic membrane remnant and adjacent external canal may not be sufficient to nourish the graft material. Generally, in cases in which the skin of the external auditory canal has been badly burned, it should not be used as a graft material, and it certainly should not be used as a free graft. Only if the burn of the external canal is partial or mild should the skin of the canal be used as a pedicle flap. Recent grafting techniques using homograft tympanic membranes and middle ear ossicles may hold some promise for restoration of badly burned ears. Under no circumstances should tympanoplasty procedures be attempted in the presence of infection in the ear. If all attempts to repair a tympanic membrane perforation fail, the patient should be instructed to avoid water and other solutions in the ear and should be checked periodically to be sure that no complications, such as cholesteatoma and infection, are occurring.

RECONSTRUCTION OF MIDDLE EAR BURN INJURIES

The extent of a middle ear burn injury will determine, to a great degree, the surgical reparability. If there is diffuse coagulation necrosis of most of the epithelial lining of the middle ear, there will be little hope of success in surgically restoring a safe and functional middle ear. This also pertains if the middle ear cannot be kept free of infection for extended periods of time. If only mild or moderate damage is done to the middle ear epithelium, a successful tympanoplasty result is much more likely. One of the more common middle ear ossicular injuries is necrosis of the long process of the incus, which constitutes a disruption in the sound-transmitting ossicular chain and usually results in a moderate, conductive-type hearing loss. Depending upon the nature of the middle ear or ossicular injury, the appropriate type of tympanoplastic technique will have to be used, all of which are premised upon absence of infection and good eustachian tube function. Should neither ear be surgically reparable, the patient should be given hearing rehabilitation by the use of an appropriate hearing aid.

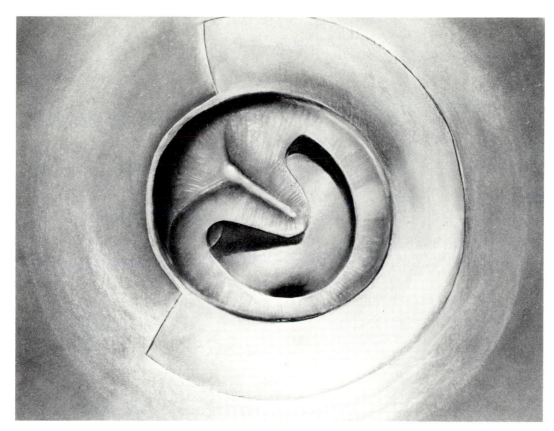

Fig. 1. Surgical dissection of the outer squamous epithelium from the tympanic membrane and adjacent external auditory canal. (from M.M. Fletcher, M.D.; Artist, G.S. Lashbrook.)

Fig. 2. Temporalis fascia graft placed against the surgically desquamated tympanic membrane remnant. (from M. M. Fletcher, M.D.; Artist, G.S. Lashbrook.)

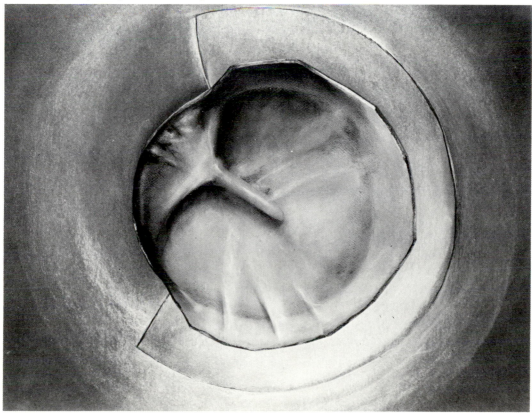

24

EXTERNAL CANAL

John E. Magielski
Irving Feller

The problem of stenosis of the external auditory canal can be a particularly troublesome dilemma for the surgeon. Many methods have been devised in attempts to reconstruct the meatus of the external auditory canal as well as the canal itself. The method described here is certainly not the definitive solution to this problem but illustrates an effective method which may be used.

In Figure 1 the external meatus is shown obliterated by burn scar with complete overgrowth of scar tissue and epithelium externally. This requires correction in order to restore hearing to normal levels, provided that the middle ear structures and the auditory nerve are functioning properly. In addition, it is necessary to re-establish the patency of the canal in order to avoid the trapping of squamous debris from the skin-lined bony auditory canal wall. The dotted line illustrates the line of the incision which is made at the attachment of the anterior crus of the helix and parallels the spina helicus of that structure, extending into the scar tissue of the meatus and approximately finishing where the cavum conchum of auricle lies.

The next figures (2 and 3) demonstrate the undermining of the flaps of skin posteriorly and anteriorly to the incision. Then scar tissue is removed by sharp dissection, Figures 4 and 5, to the level of the bony external auditory canal where the epithelium lining the canal is noted and preserved. At this point, incisions are made inferiorly off the anteriorly and posteriorly undermined skin about the proposed meatus, and the pedicles are rotated medially to the level of the epithelium of the external auditory canal (Figure 6) and fixed with 5-0 nylon sutures. At this point it is obvious that there will be deficient skin over the auricular cartilage inferiorly and the soft

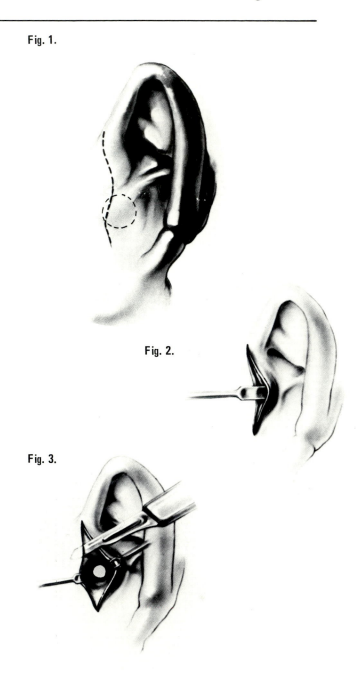

Fig. 1.

Fig. 2.

Fig. 3.

Fig. 4.

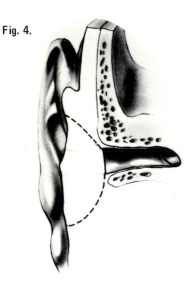

Fig. 5.

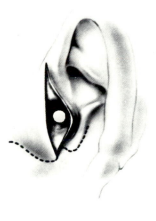

Fig. 6.

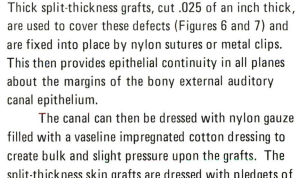

Fig. 7.

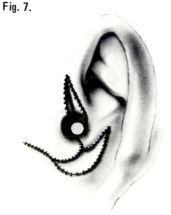

tissue overlying the temporalis muscle superiorly. Thick split-thickness grafts, cut .025 of an inch thick, are used to cover these defects (Figures 6 and 7) and are fixed into place by nylon sutures or metal clips. This then provides epithelial continuity in all planes about the margins of the bony external auditory canal epithelium.

The canal can then be dressed with nylon gauze filled with a vaseline impregnated cotton dressing to create bulk and slight pressure upon the grafts. The split-thickness skin grafts are dressed with pledgets of cotton soaked in sterile physiologic solution. These are placed into position to develop contour and pressure for proper adherence of the graft to the underlying tissues. An external dressing is then applied and allowed to remain in place for approximately one week. Care is taken with the dressing that it is not of a highly compressive nor abrasive nature. This is to avoid abrading any of the skin over the auricle itself.

Figure 8 A and B shows the result in a patient with this particular problem. Restoration of the meatus and external auditory canal communication to the ear drum have been accomplished although some hypertrophic scarring remains.

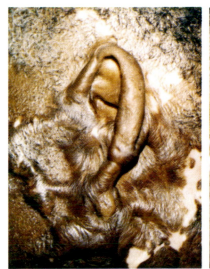
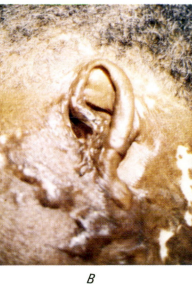

A   B

Fig. 8. A. Appearance of ear prior to reconstruction. The meatus and external canal are obliterated due to hypertrophic scarring. **B.** Removal of scar tissue restoring communication to the ear drum.

25

PARTIALLY BURNED AURICLE

PATHOLOGY AND DEFORMITY OF THE AURICLE

The residual defects of the burned auricle consist primarily of scar-contracted cartilage, healed skin or grafted skin over the cartilage, and hypertrophic keloid scar tissue. The amount of tissue damage depends upon exposure time, secondary infection, and residual circulation of the skin and cartilage. In partial loss of the ear, the helix rim and roll, the most delicate and thinnest parts of the ear, are damaged first. Next is the upper part of the auricle and the lobe, and last is the concha. Damage is greatest when the anterior and posterior surfaces of the auricle are involved. In severe segmental burns, scar contracture may close off the auditory canal.

EVALUATION AND TIMING OF THE RECONSTRUCTION

Several steps are helpful prior to the onset of the reconstructive surgery of the partially burned ear. It is important to first consider the part the ear plays in the total burn problem. Evaluation of the local problem must include consideration of the extent of the correction to be undertaken, the procedures which will obtain that effect, and the endpoint.

The reconstruction should be undertaken only when the skin is stable and cartilage shrinkage has ceased. Most reconstructive procedures will appear better when accomplished with the lowest surgical steps. Certain reconstructive plastic surgery, such as tubed pedicle formation, of necessity will require staging. **The patient should be made aware of these steps. Write down the stages along with their costs for physician, hospital, anesthesia, and any lost wages; it may encourage less surgery.**

RECONSTRUCTION OF THE SCAPHA AND SUPERIOR HELIX

If the major loss is of the scapha and superior helix, the cartilage expansion principle will add between 1 and 1.5cm to the height of the ear in one stage. In this technique the existing cartilage of the scapha is used as part of a composite pedicle based on the postauricular skin (Figure 1). The top of the existing ear is used along with the cartilage and skin of the helix. The anterior skin-cartilage pedicle should contain cartilage at least 1cm wide at its base, and should be long enough to complete the ear contour. Thus, the incision may have to extend into the concha. The scapha incision is made only through the anterior skin and cartilage. The postauricular skin on the concha is dissected away, and will act as the pedicle and carrier. Undermining may have to extend to the mastoid and scalp to give the pedicle enough mobility to be moved up and back. A tangential incision in the temple may be necessary to facilitate this movement.

The defect of the concha-helix donor site may be closed primarily or filled with a preauricular rotation flap. The latter is recommended, since this anchors the free end of the composite flap and molds the anterior contour (Figure 2). The scapha defect of postauricular skin-adipose pedicle is covered with a thick split-thickness graft, full-thickness graft, or a free full-thickness-skin-cartilage graft from the opposite ear, which is held in place with a tieover bolster. The circulation of the anterior helix pedicle is always in jeopardy because of the large ratio of the pedicle length to the width at the base, which may be as great as 4:1. Therefore, the pedicle may be quite blue at the completion of the operation. Tissue loss is rare and minimal.

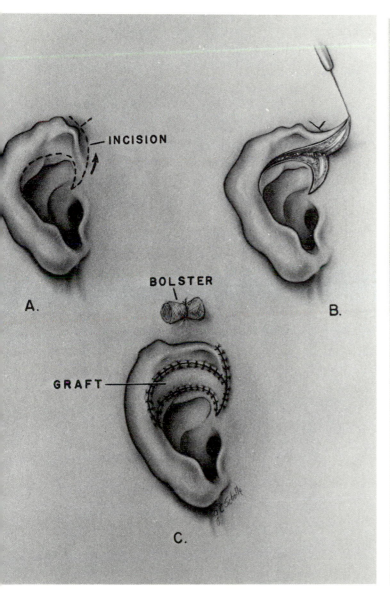

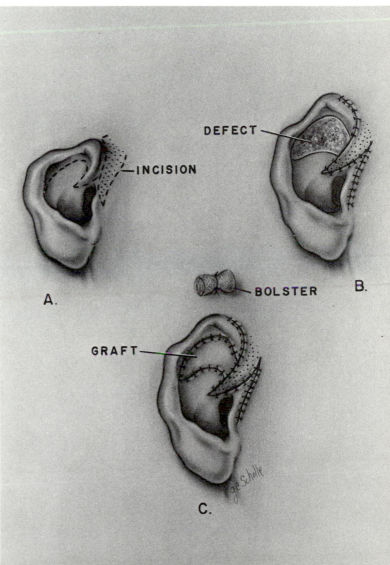

Fig. 1. Cartilage expansion principle for reconstruction of scapha and superior helix. The cartilage composite pedicle flap is moved up and back to give the ear elevation and the desired posterior tilt of the long axis of the ear.

Fig. 2. Variation of the one-stage ear expansion, using a composite skin cartilage flap carried on a postauricular skin pedicle and an anterior rotation flap to mold and hold the composite skin-pedicle. The bolster on the scalp helps to hold the superior tip of the ear in its new position.

Another method of reconstructing the scapha when there is a partial loss or almost a complete loss is a multi-stage method using the spliced autogenous conchal cartilage from the opposite ear al la Drs. Gorney, Murphy and Falces. In this method, the unusable and scarred tissues are discarded and replaced with a full-thickness graft large enough to allow for the formation and convolutions of the framework. The full-thickness graft is made approximately one third larger than the anticipated reconstruction. The skin graft should be placed in the correct topographical angle, namely parallel to the axis of the nose about 20 to 30 degrees from the vertical axis of the head (Figure 3).

The second stage is contemplated once the skin is soft, pliable and can be pinched and elevated between the finger tips. In this stage the anterior parameters are marked on the donor ear and the cartilage is marked with a through-and-through hypodermic needle and ink technique. A postauricular incision is made and the cartilage is cut and, if necessary, a segment is spliced on inferiorly, as shown in the diagram. The donor site ear is closed and also accurately packed for one week to ten days so as to give contour to the ear. A planned postauricular sulcus type of incision about 3 to 5cm long is made along the graft edge of the recipient ear. The cartilage is implanted and, if necessary, sutured to any residual cartilage left from the injured ear. This now softened graft is then carefully elevated with some fatty tissue so as to allow an adequate amount of circulation. The skin graft is secured over the underlying cartilage with bolsters or packings that may be sutured in place to secure the accurate detail of the cartilage. Once healed, this should give adequate framework for the reconstructed ear. When the skin cover is pliable, the ear can be elevated. A sling flap is designed on the scalp to fill in the defect in the postauricular ear where the carti-

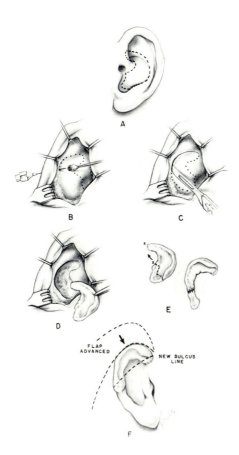

Fig. 3. Reconstruction of the partially burned auricle. **A.** Donor cartilage marked off on anterior surface of donor ear. **B.** Transfer of outline of cartilage graft to posterior surface with ink stained intravenous needle. **C.** Incision of cartilage is carefully done to preserve the anterior skin. **D.** Cartilage removed including part of the antihelix roll. **E.** Enlarging the ear using a cartilage splicing technique and suturing them together. The cartilage graft is rotated 180 degrees with the convolutions toward the anterior surface. **F.** Elevation of top of ear—an incision is made about ½cm beyond the cartilage graft edge inferiorly contiguous with hairline over the mastoid to the dotted sulcus line. The scalp flap is designed and advanced in to the new sulcus. The posterior surface of the ear is grafted.

lage graft is to be elevated with the overlying skin graft. A sling flap is elevated and rotated to form a new postauricular groove and the scalp is advanced to fill the defect created by the sling flap. A split-thickness or a full-thickness graft is placed on the posterior surface of the elevated ear. A tieover dressing to keep compression on the graft may be necessary. The discrepancy between the two ears is now much less and the donor ear is somewhat more flattened and very much like the reconstructed burned ear.

RECONSTRUCTION OF SEGMENTAL AURICULAR LOSS

Segmental loss of the ear or ear rim can be reconstructed by local tissue flaps with or without cartilage. Of value are postauricular transposition flaps, rolled or partially tubed. Again these may have

a strip of borrowed cartilage to hold the contour. Preauricular or postauricular bipedicle tubed flaps with pancake expansions in the middle or end also have merit.

RECONSTRUCTION OF EARLOBE

If both ears are involved and the lobes appear equal, reconstruction may not be required. If only one ear is injured, the noninvolved ear lobe may have to be reduced to match the smaller lobe.

If a lobe is desired, it may be reconstructed using either local flaps or distant tissue. Local tissue flaps can be devised on the postauricular skin, unfolded with the hinge in the dependent position (Figure 4). The newly made flap is surfaced with a facial flap based toward the mastoid, folded on itself and sutured to the earlobe flap. These flaps are almost at right angles to each other.

Fig. 4. Ear lobe reconstruction by the double-flap technique using a postauricular and a facial skin flap.

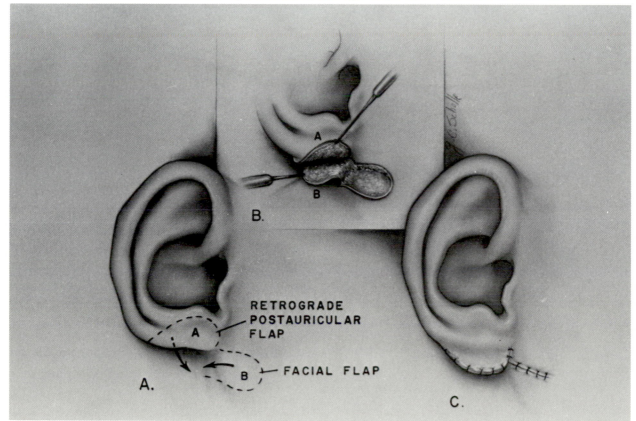

Another method of earlobe reconstruction uses a wide mastoid flap based inferiorly and attached widely to part of the remaining turned down earlobe rim. The defect of the neck is closed primarily or grafted. The flap is divided in stages inferiorly and rolled upon itself to form the lobe. A primary skin graft on the exposed pedicle is desirable to keep the wound covered. Homo- or heterografts will have melted away in time for the folding of the lobe. Permanent grafts on the lobe will shrink and curl the edge. They are less desirable since they make the lobe too thin, unless the original pedicle from the neck was quite thick.

The lobe constructed in conjunction with a tubed neck pedicle will give a pleasing effect (Figure 5). The anticipated lobe will be on the defect side. Plan the tube 2cm longer than its ultimate length, e.g., 15 to 17cm long. Since shrinkage occurs, if it is too short it will not reach the lobe site. The lobe is preformed and will be part of the pancake end. It appears like stunted rabbit ears and will require about 4 by 4cm of skin. The pancake is folded upon itself, the straight part is fastened to the face, the other free edge is sutured to the freshened lobe edge.

RELEASE OF THE CONSTRICTED EXTERNAL AUDITORY CANAL

Canal obstruction occurs when damage to the ear has been great. Chondritis of the tragus, concha, or canal with late healing can close the canal. A skin graft used to cover an adjacent granulating surface can occlude it as it contracts. In each of these cases, preventive measures can be taken by inserting a bougie into the canal for several months. A rubber or polyethelene tube of adequate size can be shaped by notching so it will stay in the canal (Figure 6). Employing an open tube rather than a sponge will permit irrigation and will allow sounds to be transmitted.

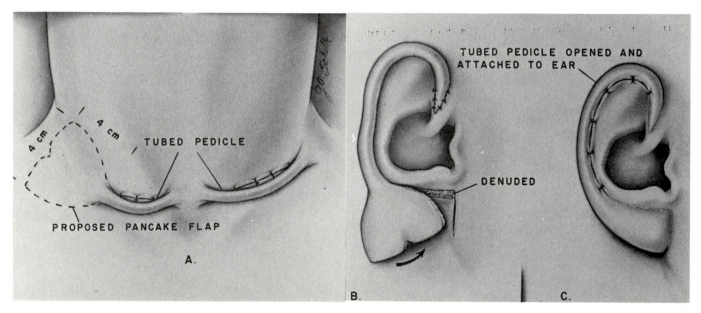

Fig. 5. Helical rim and ear lobe reconstruction with a tubed neck-skin flap involves multiple stages. **A.** This 15 to 17cm long tubed neck-skin flap should have an island attachment in the center. The pancake at the proximal end of the flap can be undermined and the lateral cuts made; the proximal end of this pedicle is the base of this flap and must remain attached. The central island is divided, but requires additional width to prevent pinching of the central tube. The end of the flap on the patient's left neck is delayed, divided from the neck and attached to the right anterior upper helix. The pancake is delayed and later divided, attaching the pancake to the prepared lobe site. **B. and C.** At the first stage the tube is opened and attached to the ear rim, carefully suturing the posterior surface, but barely attaching it anteriorly. This allows scar contracture to form a groove beneath the anterior helical rim.

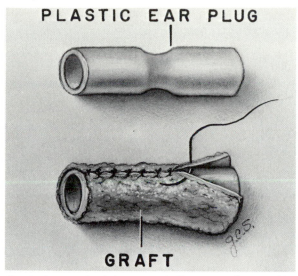

Fig. 6. In stenosis of the ear canal, the raw area is covered by a skin graft with the dermis side out and sutured over a notched tube. This tube permits cleaning deep in the canal and prevents a build-up of secretions. The tube should be left in place for several months.

For the late healed ear, the scar occlusion of the canal has to be resected. Interdigitating flaps are a picture book solution considered technically cumbersome and of limited success. One or more rotation or transposition flaps from the concha are rotated into the ear canal; the defect is covered with a split-thickness skin graft (Figure 7). Maintenance of the ostium is important and is accomplished with a temporary sponge, or more permanent tube or catheter. These should be kept in for several months. Total circumferential skin grafts are to be avoided. If the defect is large, a local skin flap should be placed in the canal. The rest of the canal is then grafted by suturing the graft dermal-side-out around a tube tampon (Figure 8). The skin-covered tampon is placed into the canal to fill the defect. The part of the graft placed over the flap will die off and can be debrided away postoperatively. The tampon is removed after approximately 10 days and replaced with

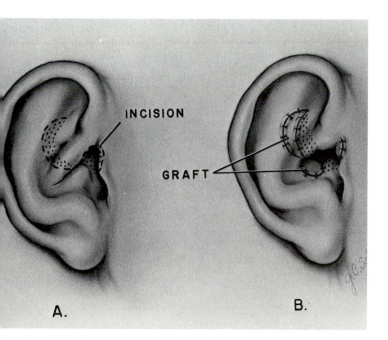

Fig. 7. A double rotation flap is used to open a severely stenosed ear canal. This flap lines the canal on two sides.

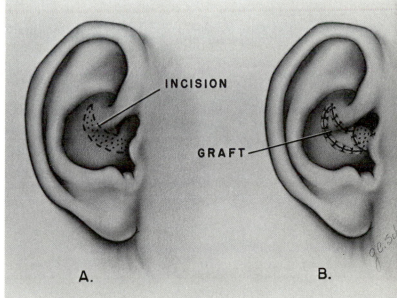

Fig. 8. Stenosis of the canal is best overcome by a local skin flap from the concha. The remaining defect is covered with a full or split-thickness skin graft.

a tube which acts to prevent contracture during the several months of postoperative healing.

HELIXICAL RIM RECONSTRUCTION

Segmental or total ear rim restoration can be accomplished using either tubed pedicles or composite grafts. The tubed pedicles can be made from preauricular facial, postauricular, or neck skin. The composite grafts comprise skin and cartilage from the opposite ear.

TUBED SKIN FLAP

The preauricular tube can be very thin and has the advantage of not requiring an additional delay. It is excellent for segmental rim replacement and partial lobe reconstruction.

The postauricular tube has advantages similar to those of the anterior tube, but it is not as easily

moved and the donor skin is usually damaged by the burn scar. But, it does have a place in the central rim reconstruction.

COMPOSITE GRAFT

This concept of using a composite graft to construct the helical rim is relatively new. The total rim is borrowed from the opposite ear as a free graft (Figure 9). The total rim, including skin 4 to 5mm wide plus cartilage 3mm wide, is excised. This is inset in reverse fashion into the opposite ear rim. If the recipient site is scarred and has poor circulation, the recipient ear is incised a week prior to the transfer. When the incision is again opened, it has a rich granulation tissue base to nurture the composite graft. I have used this technique several times and have been pleased with it when I desired only a minimum of rim definition. The reduction in the donor ear rim helps balance the burned ear.

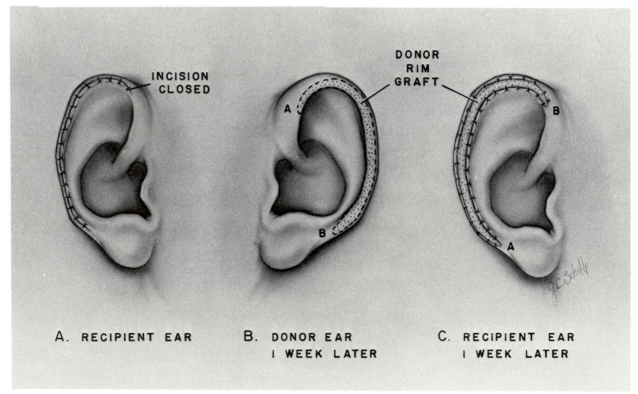

A. RECIPIENT EAR   B. DONOR EAR   C. RECIPIENT EAR
                       I WEEK LATER   I WEEK LATER

Fig. 9. Ear rim reconstruction by a free composite graft of skin and cartilage from the non-injured ear. A two stage procedure is shown in which the first stage is to provide a granulating blood-rich recipient site by incising the recipient ear rim and then closing it. At the second stage, the rim is excised in the normal ear and sutured into the reopened, previously prepared ear incision.

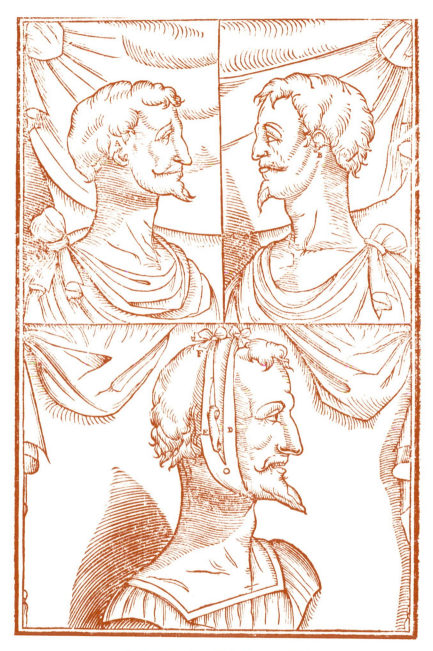

De curtorum chirurgia insitionem, 1597.

26

AURICLE REPAIR WITH CARTILAGE FRAMEWORK

Radford C. Tanzer

The total reconstruction of the auricle may be complicated by several associated deformities that must be corrected before, during, or after the restoration. The potential skin cover in the mastoid region may be supplanted by scar, the hairline may have disappeared, or the external auditory meatus may have become so constricted that hearing is impaired. One feature which distinguishes the plan of repair from that employed in the more severe forms of congenital microtia is the almost consistent preservation of the conchal cavity, although its size may have been reduced considerably, and the integument may have been so badly damaged that replacement is necessary (Figure 1).

One must first evaluate the advantages of surgical repair versus prosthetic replacement. A surgical replacement in a patient over forty years of age should be viewed circumspectly, particularly since rib cartilage itself becomes less suitable for use after this age. Simons has demonstrated the feasibility of an artificial device, but many surgeons would disagree with its use in the younger age group unless dictated by overriding circumstances. It may be necessary to replace scarred skin before a prosthesis can be applied, a step which would be taken in any case prior to a surgical reconstruction. Hence, a prosthetic auricle can be readily tried in the older age group, with resort to surgery later in special instances.

OPERATIVE TECHNIQUE

Preliminary Steps. Considerations must first be given to the integument which is available for furnishing the lateral surface of the new auricle. A burn that has been severe enough to destroy most of the ear has almost certainly rendered the adjacent skin unusable. Therefore, the first step comprises tracing the normal ear (or, in case of bilateral damage, an average ear) on transparent film and transferring this outline to its proposed position on the damaged side of the head. Then the scarred skin of this entire area, together with any other unstable or unsightly skin in the vicinity, should be replaced by a thick split-thickness skin graft from the upper thigh (Figure 2). At the same time, any significant stenosis of the ear canal should be corrected. Less severe forms of stenosis can be improved by introducing the same free graft that is used to resurface the mastoid region. A more complete stenosis requires either a full-thickness free skin graft or a rotated pedicle flap. The latter is feasible if suitable skin is available in the preauricular or conchal region. If necessary, a segment of contracted cartilage may be excised from the region of the meatus, and the defect covered with a free skin graft, creating considerable expansion of the orifice. In any case, an acrylic stent should be worn in the canal for at least three months, or until contracture of the free skin graft has ceased.

At least a portion of lobule usually remains, and should be preserved for use in the reconstruction. Frequently it will have been pulled superiorly by scar contracture, in which case it should be rotated on an inferiorly based pedicle into a transverse position, so that it lies along the margin of the proposed outline of the new ear. This rotation, of course, should be done only after the preliminary resurfacing procedure has been completed. The lobule then can be set properly onto the new skin graft that will comprise the outer surface of the ear. In the event that the lobule has been completely obliterated, provision should be made when constructing the cartilage framework for sufficient cartilage to give proper contour of the lobule.

Fig. 1. Virtually complete loss of auricle due to prolonged contact with hot metal plate.

Fig. 2. After resurfacing of site of future cartilage embedment, and adjacent areas, with thick split-thickness graft.

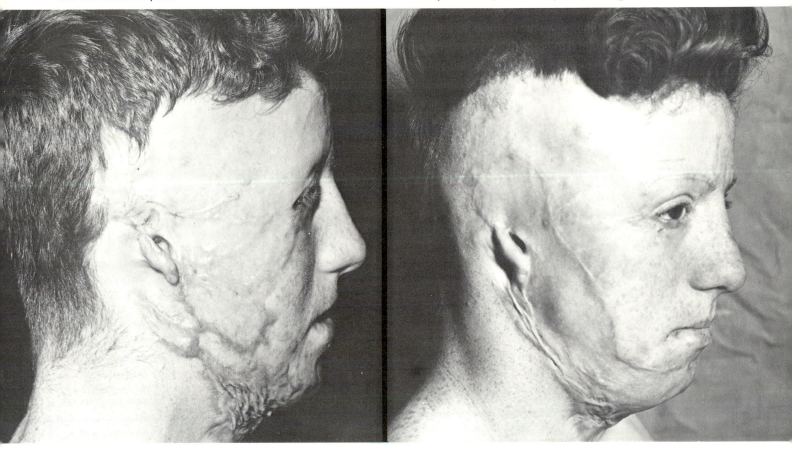

Construction of the Auricle. A minimum of four months should elapse between the time of skin resurfacing and the introduction of an ear framework. At the end of that time, a basic choice must be made between an inorganic material and autogenous cartilage. There is sufficient evidence to preclude the use of allografts, either fresh or preserved. Silicone frameworks have shown a propensity for extrusion, particularly in the presence of scar tissue. For this reason, rib cartilage is recommended as a material which is available in adequate amount and which has demonstrated a marked resistance to extrusion or absorption, even in the presence of scar tissue.

After the preliminary measures have been concluded, a reasonably satisfactory reconstruction can be carried out in two stages.

Stage I starts with the construction of a contour pattern of the opposite normal ear, cutting it out of a piece of transparent x-ray film. (If both ears are in-

volved, a suitable size and shape are selected for the individual case.) A second contour pattern is made from the ear tracing, outlining the shape of the proposed cartilage graft. At the beginning of the operation, the ear pattern, which has been previously gas-sterilized, is traced in proper relationship to the existing ear canal, being careful to keep the long axis of the proposed ear parallel to the bridge of the nose. Next, the cartilaginous portions of the sixth, seventh, and eighth ribs, on the side opposite the involved ear, are exposed through a transverse incision over the sixth interspace, dividing the rectus muscle transversely. The cartilage pattern is then placed on the sixth and seventh ribs, overlying the synchondrosis, to determine the amount of rib cartilage that must be removed to provide the base block for the auricular reconstruction. This block is then removed subperichondrially, leaving the synchondrosis intact. The eighth rib is removed separately. The base block, consisting of the sixth and seventh ribs, is carved to the configuration of the previously prepared cartilage pattern. The concavities of the scapha and fossa triangularis are produced with wood-carving chisels. The eighth rib is carved in the shape of a helix and is attached to the rim of the base block with several mattress sutures of stainless steel wire swaged on straight cutting needles.

Through a small incision beneath the lobule, or in its vicinity, the skin within the markings of the proposed auricle is thinly undermined, and the cartilage framework is slid into position. If the lobule has been lost, a sufficient amount of cartilage should be incorporated in the framework to produce a reasonable simulation of a lobule. The skin overlying the helical sulcus is snugged into the concavity by a series of mattress sutures. These pierce the ear between the helix and the base block and are tied over gauze pledgets, holding the skin in close apposition to the cartilage framework. The entire ear is then packed with fluffed gauze and a voluminous head cap used to avoid undue pressure during sleep. After the sutures have been removed on the tenth postoperative day, an ear guard, something akin to a hockey helmet, is worn nightly, up to the time of the next operation, to avoid pressure on the cartilaginous helix while it is consolidating (Figure 3).

Stage II can be carried out four months or more after the implantation of the cartilage framework. The ear is elevated extensively from the side of the head, carrying the dissection under the conchal cartilage, and lining the defect with a thick split-thickness skin graft taken from the upper thigh. Meticulous hemostasis must be observed to avoid even the slightest loss of skin graft, which might produce exposure of the implant. The skin graft is carefully packed with fluffed gauze, and tie-over sutures are used to maintain firm, even pressure. On removal of the dressing and sutures, the same ear guard is employed at night, until the graft has become quite stable (Figure 4).

The thick split-thickness skin graft has a marked propensity to contract, pulling the newly constructed ear back against the side of the head. In order to counteract this deleterious occurrence, a foam rubber wedge may be used to hold the ear out at the opti-

mum angle to the side of the head. Even with the employment of such a splint, the ear may eventually lie closer to the side of the head than the opposite normal ear. Hence, it may be expedient to set in the opposite ear, in order to place the two ears at the same angle to the side of the head. Other devices for maintaining a proper ear angle are under trial by several plastic surgeons.

SECONDARY REVISION

It is almost impossible to obtain, in the presence of scar tissue the delicate outline that is expected in the primary reconstruction of the auricle in cases of congenital microtia. Secondary revisions are often indicated for the improvement of the basic two-stage reconstruction.

A shallow helical sulcus may be improved by reexcavating a helical trough in the cartilage, using wood-carving chisels through a series of interrupted incisions along the sulcus, then snugging the undermined skin into the sulcus again with mattress sutures tied over gauze pledgets. A more prominent helical lip may also be obtained by the Matthews-Cronin procedure. The skin of the helical rim is advanced laterally, and the resultant raw undersurface covered with a split-thickness skin graft. The latter method is most useful when the defect is recognized early and the revision is executed before the new ear has been elevated from the side of the head. A thin tubed skin flap may also be used to build up a more prominent helix, using preauricular skin if available, otherwise elevating an arteriovenous pedicle of superficial temporal scalp vessels, lining the cylinder of tissue with a free graft, and eventually transferring it to the helical rim, as described by C. Dufourmentel. Cervical tubes should be used only as a last resort since they produce wide scars which create another source of dissatisfaction.

Contracture of the auriculocephalic skin graft may produce so much flattening against the side of the head that a correction is indicated. Usually, a second auriculocephalic graft will produce a satisfactory angle. Minor degrees of flattening may be corrected by implanting a block of costal cartilage in the retroauricular region. Extra cartilage from the initial

Fig. 3. After embedment of cartilage framework. Eyebrow has been restored by free scalp graft and eyelids by full-thickness grafts.

Fig. 4. Ear has been elevated from side of head and defect lined with thick split-thickness graft. Contour of lobule has been restored by the cartilage framework. Hairline has been lowered by rotation of scalp flap. (Conspicuousness of meatus could be diminished by enlarging the tragus with a cartilage disc.)

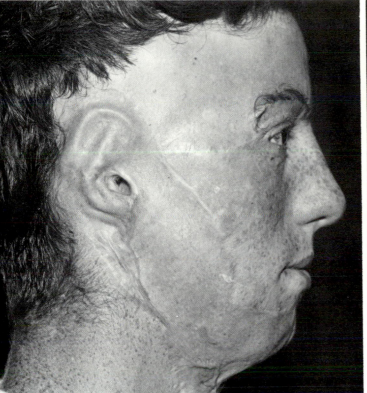

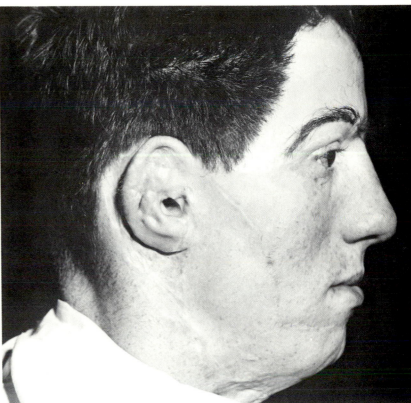

operation is usually banked in the subcutaneous tissues of the abdominal wall for this eventuality.

A diminutive tragus can be improved by implanting a disc of autogenous cartilage, if some banked material is available, or by using a small silicone block, which will plump out the tragus and serve to make the external auditory meatus less conspicuous.

A deformed lobule is best corrected by initially carving the contour of the cartilage implant to build up missing portions. In the event that this maneuver has not been completely successful, any secondary repair will have to be individualized, taking into consideration the nature of the defect and the quality of skin which is available in the vicinity for repair. When reconstructing a burned ear, the usual source of tissue for filling out a lobular defect is the skin immediately subjacent to the existing lobule. This tissue, whether it be native or grafted skin, is elevated as a rotated flap, based anteriorly or posteriorly, and folded into the defect to produce a roll. An alternative method embodies the lifting of a skin flap inferior

to, and in continuity with, the lower border of the dwarfed lobule, then resurfacing its medial surface with another skin flap, rotated from an adjacent area. In either of these basic procedures it may be necessary to introduce some structural support to produce proper contour. Occasionally it is necessary to transfer a tubed pedicle flap from the lower cervical region to furnish usable skin.

SUMMARY

Massive scarring and loss of the auricle should not induce the plastic surgeon to adopt a defeatist attitude toward the problem. Heavy scars can be excised, a usable skin graft can be furnished as cover for a reconstruction, and a framework can be implanted. These will not produce the delicate contours obtainable in unscarred tissue, but will create a serviceable auricle, capable of instilling confidence in the patient suffering the disfigurement of a severe burn.

27

HYPERTROPHIC SCARRING AND KELOID OF THE PINA

Irving Feller

In contrast to the usual loss of tissue of the external ear, there are two conditions that lead to excessive tissue on the external ear; they are hypertrophic scars and keloid formation. Fortunately the keloid is rare; most of the lesions are massive hypertrophic scars.

The treatment for both of these lesions is similar. The operative procedure should not be undertaken until the hypertrophic scar shows signs of involution. In cases when the diagnosis is keloid, the appropriate time for operation is when the growth of the mass slows.

The amount of tissue to be removed is illustrated in Figure 1A and B. The lines for excision should leave a border of hypertrophic scar or keloid to avoid or diminish recurrence if the process is still active. The excision is then completed by removing a wedge of tissue, leaving enough to reconstruct a normal pina (Figure 1C). Figure 1D illustrates the completed procedure, and Figure 2A and B the patient's appearance pre- and postoperatively.

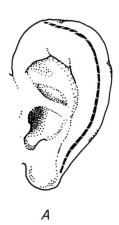
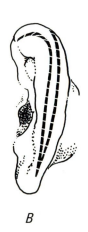
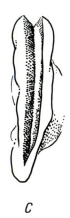
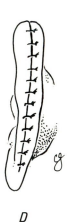

A   B   C   D

Fig. 1. A. and B. The dotted lines depict the amount of hypertrophic scar tissue to be removed. **C.** A wedge of scar tissue has been removed leaving a thin margin of scar to diminish recurrence. **D.** Sutures close the defect approximating a normal ear size.

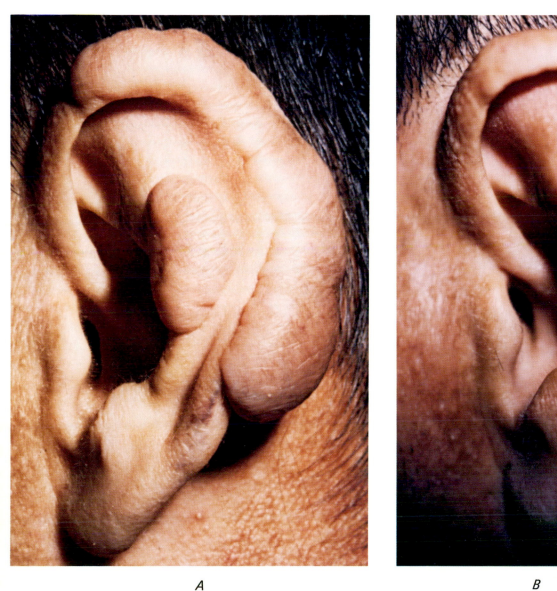

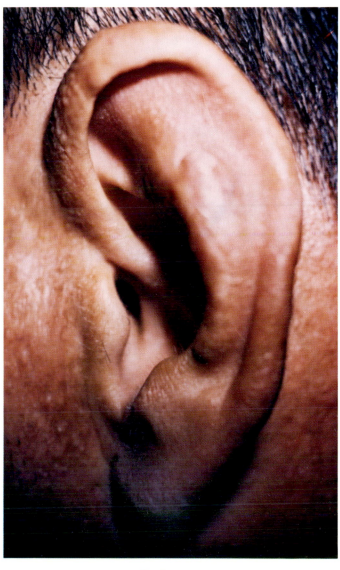

A   B

Fig. 2. **A.** Approximately one year after the patient was burned, the hypertrophic scarring on the ear showed signs of involution. It is noted that there is not only hypertrophic scarring along the edges of the external ear, but one small mass in the middle. Both were treated by the method described. **B.** Appearance of the external ear in the patient, two years after the operation.

28

PROSTHETIC REPLACEMENT
OF THE EAR

Denis C. Lee

A great deal of help is available to the burn patient through the use of cosmetic prosthesis. With recent advances in prosthetic materials and coloring techniques, simple, effective prostheses can easily be prepared for burn patients suffering from damage to the ear, nose, hand, and other areas of the body.

EAR PROSTHESIS

Partial or complete loss of the ear is the most common problem dealt with by the Department of Medical Sculpture (University of Michigan Medical Center). The most difficult prosthesis to prepare is one which covers the upper portion of the ear or the helix, scapha, and triangular fossa. Usually there is some portion of the anthelix left which lends good support for the prosthesis.

An impression is taken of both ears with a hydrocolloid, and a cast is made in stone plaster (Figure 1). The ear or ears are reconstructed in clay. If only one ear is damaged, a cast of the other ear may be used as a model for reconstruction. The edge of the prosthesis that fits over the remaining ear is feathered to blend in with and overlap the remaining portion of the ear so that the prosthesis will fit securely yet not interrupt the natural contours of the ear (Figure 2). For the best cosmetic appearance and prosthesis durability, the entire ear is covered whenever possible.

A two-piece stone mold is then prepared around the reconstructed ear by first pouring the portion under the helix, then covering the rest of the ear (Figure 3). The result including the original cast of the ear is a three piece mold (Figure 4).

The mold is then separated, cleaned, and coated with a separator. The material for this type of prosthesis must be very strong because of the thin edges. I have found a mixture of RTV silicones most satisfactory. Silastic 399 is used for strength and translucency and Silastic 382 is used for a white coloring base. Texture can be controlled by adding small amounts of Silastic 386 foam elastomer. The silicone mixture is catalyzed and colored with pigments to match the patient's lightest skin color. Then the mixture is catalyzed again, quickly brushed into the mold and tightly clamped (Figure 5).

When the silicone has vulcanized completely, the mold is separated and prosthesis removed; the flashing is trimmed, and the rough spots sanded (Figure 6). The prosthesis is now ready to fit on the patient (Figure 7). If the prosthesis is satisfactory, it is glued lightly in place and tinted to match the patient's normal coloring (Figure 8). The tinting is done with premixed colors of silicone and pigment. When the coloring process is completed, the entire ear is sprayed with catalyst to lock in the color. The shine is then removed with a special matting spray which gives the prosthesis a dull, life-like surface. The skin surface of the prosthesis is coated with a thin layer of Silastic 399 and nylon for additional strength. The prosthesis is applied to the patient with medical adhesive B. A small puddle is sprayed on a pad of paper and quickly applied to the prosthesis. The adhesive is allowed to dry for a minute and then pressed firmly into place. The prosthesis should be removed at night to allow moisture in the skin to evaporate. Our ear prostheses last from 12 to 18 months, depending on care and use, and are inexpensively replaced.

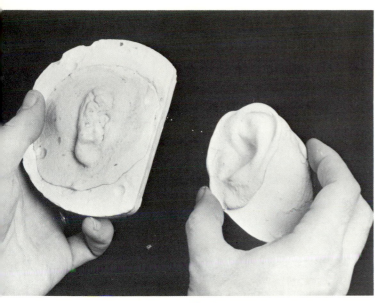

Fig. 1.

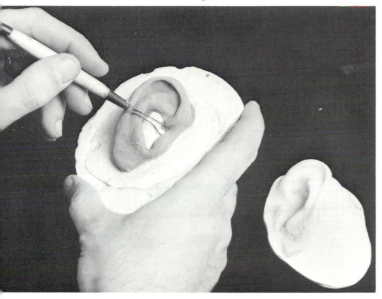

Fig. 2.

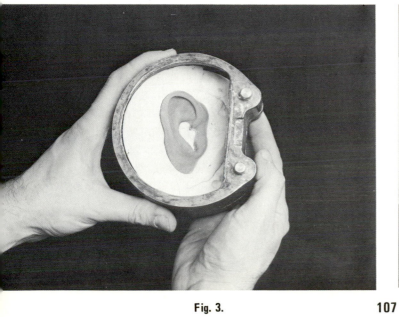

Fig. 3.

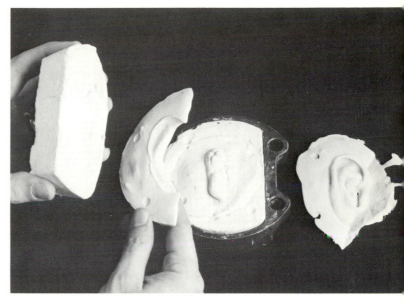

Fig. 4.

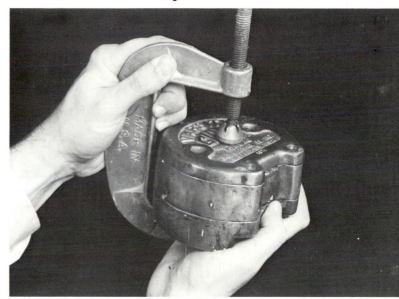

Fig. 5.

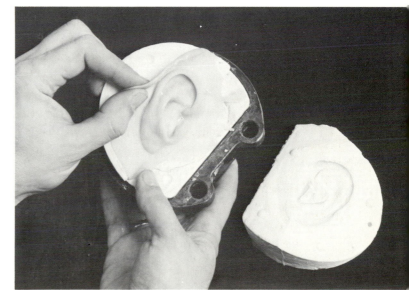

Fig. 6.

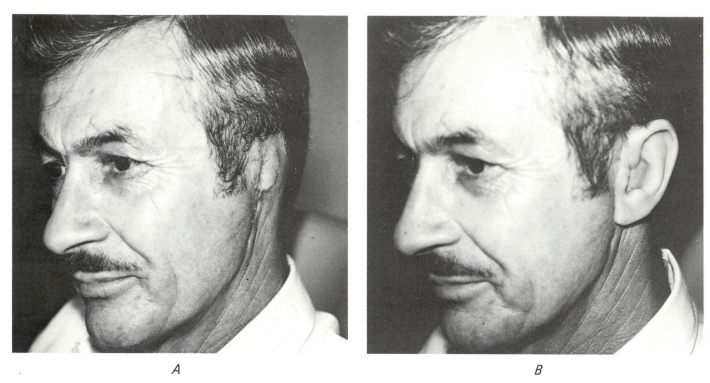

A   *B*

Fig. 7. A. Patient with complete loss of ear. **B.** Appearance after prosthetic replacement.

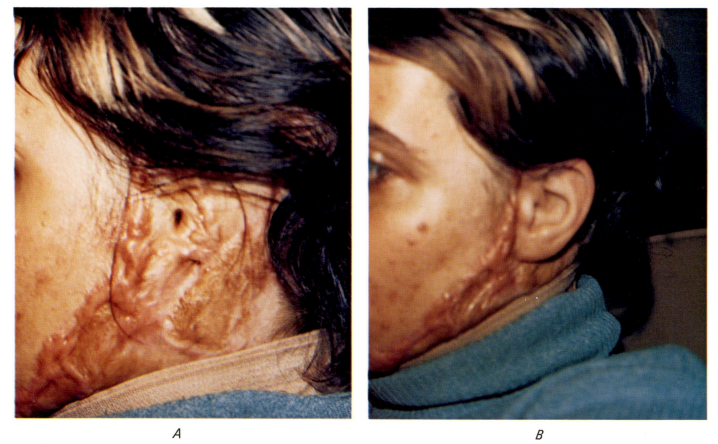

A   *B*

Fig. 8. A. Patient with complete loss of ear and scarred surface. **B.** Placement of prosthesis, tinted to match surrounding tissue.

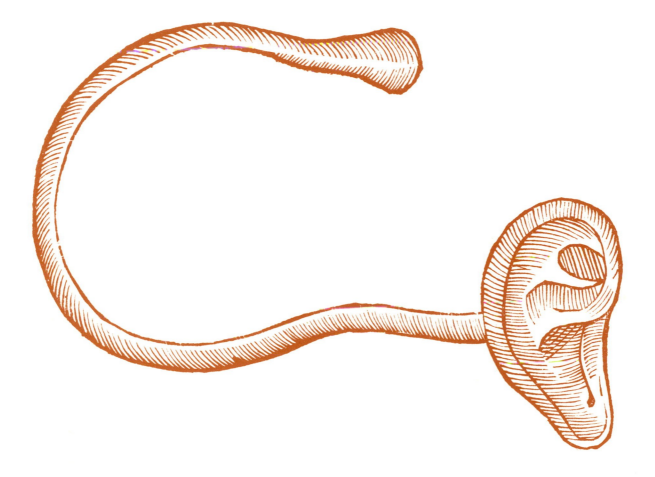

The Works of that Famous Chirurgeon: Ambrose Parey, 1678.

IV.

THE EYE

PRINCIPLES OF TREATMENT

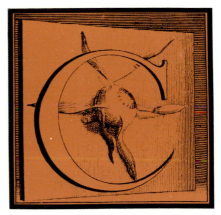

areful treatment is necessary for burns of the eye. Burns of the eye, the eyelid, and eyebrow requiring reconstructive operations have occurred in 253 of the burned patients recorded in the Michigan Burn Center, or 11½ percent. Although the eye burns are not common or life threatening, they require prompt treatment to avoid loss or impairment of vision. Protection and treatment of the globe, lids, and eyebrows provide the best chance of minimizing the damage caused by the burn.

The surgeon in charge of the emergency room or burn facility is usually the first to examine the patient and may have considerable experience in treating eye burns. However, an ophthalmologist should be consulted when injury to the conjunctiva or cornea has occurred. The following chapters include the opinions of the physician and prosthetist on the elements of early care and definitive reconstruction of the eye and related injury.

Irving Feller

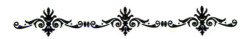

30

EARLY MANAGEMENT OF THE EYE, EYELID, AND EYEBROW

Irving Feller
Kathryn E. Richards

The blink is extremely fast, and this reflex usually prevents burns of the cornea and conjunctiva. It is not uncommon to see patients who have been burned in explosions with deep partial and full-thickness burns of the eyelids but little or no injury to the cornea. These patients also show unburned areas around the eye in the creases that result from blinking and rapid contracting of the periorbital muscles (Figure 1). However, patients who have been exposed to prolonged heat, explosions with minute projectiles, or chemical injuries may have injury to the cornea and globe.

Chemical burns require prolonged flushing with a physiologic solution and then treatment of the cornea and conjunctiva, depending upon the depth of tissue damage.

Patients with eye burns resulting from an explosion should have a thorough examination of the cornea and globe to determine the presence of a foreign body as well as corneal damage. Fluorescein staining of the cornea is required when injury is suspected. Evaluation and treatment by an ophthalmologist is advised.

Patients who had no eye damage at the time of the accident may suffer eye injury during the acute phase of treatment. The most common cause of complication is exposure of the cornea. Exposure keratitis may result from (1) loss of consciousness with lids remaining open, (2) prolonged exposure during anesthesia, and (3) ectropion from severe contractures which form during the acute period of treatment. Protection of the cornea is provided by keeping the lids closed when the patient's normal reflexes are diminished.

The most important aspect of care of the eye is to avoid exposure of the cornea. Early in treatment lid edema keeps the eyelids closed. Later tarsorrhaphy with or without release of contracted eyelids may be necessary to protect the cornea (Figures 2 and 3).

Hematologic spread of infection to the eye in the severely burned patient is rare but does occur. Both gram-negative bacteria and yeast have caused eye lesions when patients were severely ill with systemic infections. Early diagnosis and treatment is important.

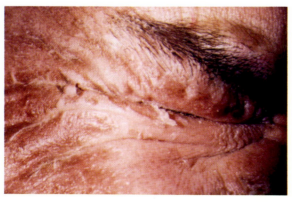 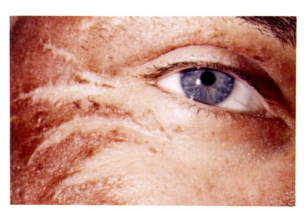

A   *B*

Fig. 1. The blink reflex is very fast and protects the eye from burns in most cases. **A.** Shows a patient with face burns with his eye closed. **B.** Skin creases were not burned.

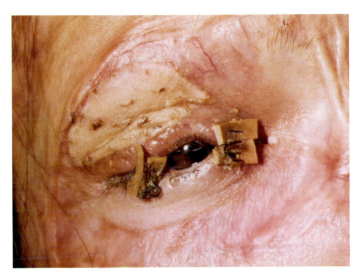

Fig. 2. A. Both medial and lateral tarsorraphies are needed when the eyelids are severely burned.

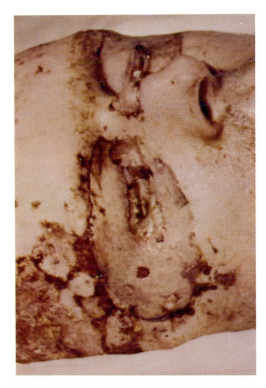

Fig. 3. Early skin grafting to the eyelids is extremely important. Tarsorraphy should be used in most cases to keep the lids from contracting when the grafts heal.

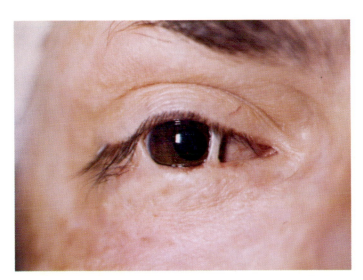

Fig. 2. B. The tarsorraphy remains in place until the danger of contracture is past.

31

CONSIDERATIONS IN CARE OF THE EYE

Joseph A. Moylan

Although ocular complications resulting from burns are not life-threatening, they may produce serious morbidity and even complete loss of vision. This important aspect of burn care may be inadvertently overlooked by the physician caring for a critically ill patient with a large thermal, chemical, or electrical injury. Of 1,400 admissions to the United States Army Institute of Surgical Research during a five-year period, 104 or 7.5 percent had ophthalmological problems in association with their burns. Eye damage may occur at the time of injury or may result later, secondary to exposure and infection. The physician caring for burn patients must be aware of the various ocular complications and should perform frequent and careful eye examinations during the patient's hospitalization.

HISTORY

The history is often helpful in alerting the physician to the possibility of an ocular problem. Blast injuries or explosions may produce lacerations or penetrating wounds of the cornea and globe. Direct ocular burns, although rare, are more common with chemical than with thermal injuries. Visual blurring or ocular pain should be noted. Specific neutralization of white phosphorus or hydrofluoric acid burns following copious water lavage may prevent further damage by the chemical agent.

OPHTHALMIC EXAMINATION

After obtaining the ocular history, the initial eye examination must be meticulous and complete. Performance of the examination as early as possible following injury, before the onset of lid edema, yields better results. When lid edema has developed, the examination is safely facilitated, using modified paper clips as lid retractors (Figure 1). The examination should include complete inspection, determination of ocular movements, assessment of gross visual acuity (which can be determined with a pocket-sized reading chart), ophthalmoscopic examination, and fluorescein staining for corneal abrasions. In both chemical and thermal burns, it is essential to examine the conjunctival sac and to remove any foreign bodies that might

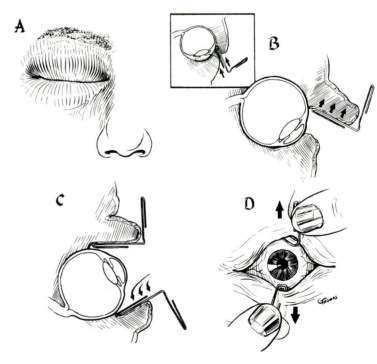

Fig. 1. A. Markedly swollen eyelids 48 hours postburn. **B.** With gaze directed caudad, the modified paper clip is inserted safely above the cornea. **C.** The superior "retractor" is elevated and the gaze is directed cephalad. The lower paper clip is inserted and retracted inferiorly. **D.** Visualization of the cornea and conjunctiva in spite of severe edema.

be present. Serial use of a slit lamp has been helpful in documenting depth of corneal ulcers and evaluating therapy. **The consultation of an ophthalmologist should be obtained if an eye complication is identified, and treatment coordinated with such a specialist.**

IMMEDIATE COMPLICATIONS

Conjunctival and corneal burns, as noted above, are rare and frequently caused by chemical burns. Initial evaluation may reveal the cornea to be opaque secondary to coagulation necrosis (Figure 2). The conjunctivae are often edematous and injected. Tearing is usually noted. Copious irrigation with water is the best early and readily available therapy for chemical corneal and conjunctival burns. It is most important to dilute and wash away the offending agent as soon as possible. This prevents continued contact and further damage. Neutralizing agents may be valuable in specific burns such as those due to hydroflouric acid or white phosphorus. Saline and antibiotic irrigation should be continuous for at least 48 hours post-injury. This can be accomplished by small catheters sewn beneath the eyelids. After 48 hours, ophthalmic antibiotics such as polysporin or neosporin should be administered five to six times each day until healing occurs. Thermal corneal and conjunctival burns are treated in a similar fashion with the exception of continuous saline irrigations.

Deep corneal lacerations and global penetrations in our series were all secondary to blast injuries and flying debris. Uniformly poor results with loss of vision occurred in the majority of cases despite early and adequate therapy. Many ultimately required global enucleation. Early therapy consists of simple suture closure or construction of a conjunctival flap following debridement. Topical ophthalmic antibiotics following bacterial sensitivity tests may be valuable. The poor results were primarily due to the damage from the initial injury. Infection from adjacent burns apparently plays a minor role.

The use of topical steroids in combination with antibiotics for complications secondary to burns is controversial because of the frequent ocular contamination by gram-negative organisms from the burn

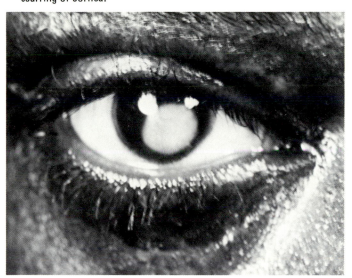

Fig. 2. Direct thermal injury to cornea demonstrating opaque scarring of cornea.

wound. The decreased inflammatory response ascribed to topical steroids appears not to be additionally beneficial when bacterial contamination can be controlled by antibiotics alone and may actually increase local susceptibility to infection. **Therefore, the use of topical steroids is best avoided.**

LATE COMPLICATIONS

Late complications account for more than 50 percent of the eye problems seen at the Institute of Surgical Research, Brooke Army Medical Center. These are primarily related to lid contractures secondary to either thermal or chemical injuries producing exposure of the globe (Figure 3). An ectropion develops because of scarring and shortening of the thin subcutaneous tissue above the tarsal plate. This process produces shortening of the lid, eversion of the lid conjunctiva, and exposure of the globe (Figure 4). Exposure conjunctivitis should be treated symptomatically with saline irrigation, methyl cellulose, and antibiotic eye drops until the primary cause, lid contracture, can be surgically treated. A culture of the conjunctival sac should be taken prior to the institution of antibiotic therapy. Polysporin or neosporin eye drops have been effective against the usual gram-negative organisms associated with burns. Failure to

Fig. 3. Severe ectropion involving the lower lid and producing conjunctivitis.

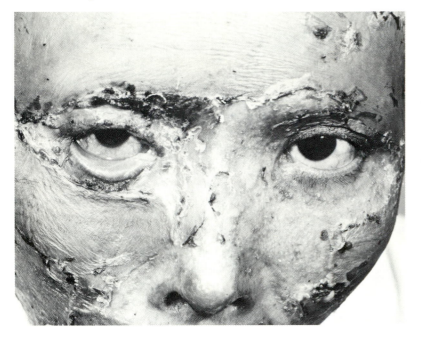

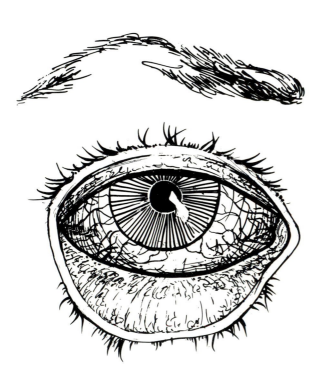

Fig. 4. Ectropion producing exposure conjunctivitis and corneal ulcer.

control an ocular infection within three days of initiation of therapy demands that reculture and antibiotic sensitivities be performed, followed by the institution of specific antibiotic therapy.

Ectropion allows drying of the cornea and permits repeated trauma to the area. The frequent administration of methyl cellulose drops prior to definitive surgical therapy decreases these complications. The increased occurrence of corneal abrasions and ulcerations following the development of a lid ectropion necessitates frequent fluorescein staining of the eye to detect these complications as early as possible. Antibiotics, cycloplegics, and eye patching are recommended for superficial injuries, while construction of a conjunctival flap or a subconjunctival flap may be required for a deep ulcer to prevent corneal perforation. Serial slit lamp examinations should be carried out to assess the effectiveness of therapy. Nonhealing of a superficial ulcer may also require coverage with a conjunctival flap.

Vigorous early therapy will reduce the severity of the contracture process. The use of topical antibacterial agents on partial- and full-thickness lid burns to control infection is important. Meticulous care must be taken when applying these agents to the lid and periorbital areas, as many can produce a contact chemical conjunctivitis.

Applying either homograft or heterograft skin may also be beneficial in reducing ectropion formation. Such homografts or heterografts should be carefully fashioned to fit the defect after eschar separation in both partial- and full-thickness burns (Figure 5). This coverage provides wound bacterial control, prevents desiccation, and allows healthy granulation tissue growth. These grafts should be changed when suppuration develops beneath the graft. Autografting should be accomplished as soon as there is a satisfactory graft bed.

Prophylactic lid closure or tarsorrhaphy early in the post-burn period in cases with full-thickness lid burns will provide protection of the cornea and, while not eliminating ectropion formation, may reduce its severity. This procedure may be performed on the ward using local anesthesia. An early tarsorrhaphy maintains length of the levator muscle, provides lid

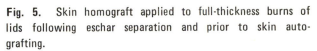

Fig. 5. Skin homograft applied to full-thickness burns of lids following eschar separation and prior to skin auto-grafting.

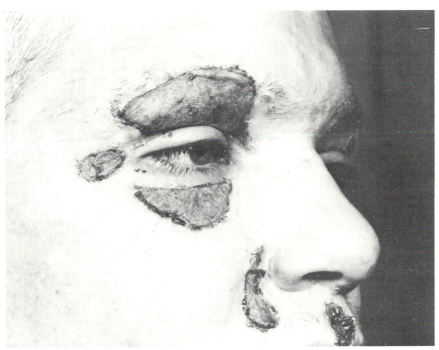

stabilization for homograft and autograft placement, and prevents eversion at the lid margin. The tarsor-rhaphy should be maintained until maturation of the healed lid burn wound has occurred, usually three to six months following autograft. Performance of a tarsorrhaphy with a central "peep-hole" allows the patient to be self-sufficient even when it is necessary to approximate the lids of both eyes (Figure 6A and B, next page).

Ectropion was diagnosed as early as the twenty-first post-burn day and as late as 90 days after injury in our five-year series. Surgical release of ectropion was required in over 85 percent of the cases and was usually carried out in the second post-burn month. Surgery can be timed to coincide with other operative procedures as long as ocular ulcerations do not pose a threat. The two surgical indications for ectropion release are corneal exposure and eversion of the punc-tum.

The operative technique for the treatment of eyelid ectropion is discussed in the chapter of the same title by John M. Converse.

SUMMARY

Ocular complications and serious morbidity may result from thermal injuries if they are improperly treated. The history is often helpful in alerting the physician to the possibility of an ocular problem. Frequent and meticulous eye examinations are important in the early detection of ocular damage. Immediate complications include direct corneal and conjunctival burns which are rare and usually due to chemical agents. Copious water or saline lavage is the best immediate treatment. In our series, corneal lacerations and global penetrations were treated with simple suture closure, conjunctival flap construction, or primary enucleation. Poor results were obtained because of the nature of the injury. Late complications are related to ectropion, producing exposure of the cornea and conjunctiva. These should be treated with symptomatic topical therapy until definitive surgery can be carried out. Tarsorraphy and/or surgical correction of the defect should be done on an emergent basis.

Fig. 6. Tarsorrhaphy with a central "peep-hole." In this illustration the ectropion has been released and skin grafts inserted. **A.** To perform a permanent tongue-in-groove tarsorrhaphy, a strip of conjunctiva is excised along the grey line of both lids, leaving a 4 to 5mm central area intact for the "peep-hole." A linear excision is made along the excised lid margin down onto the anterior surface of the tarsal plate of the upper lid to form the tongue. This tongue, which includes a segment of tarsal plate, is then sutured into the groove in the lower lid with sutures as shown tied over bolsters.

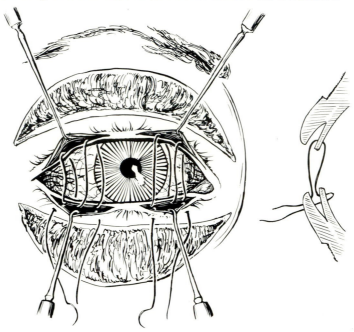

Fig. 6. B. The tarsorrhaphy suture should be left in place for at least 14 days.

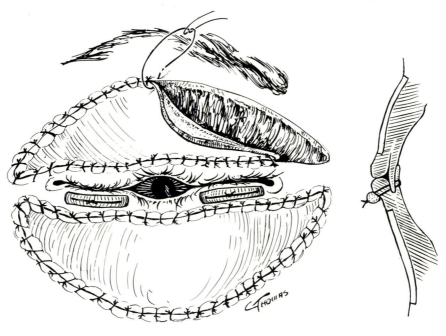

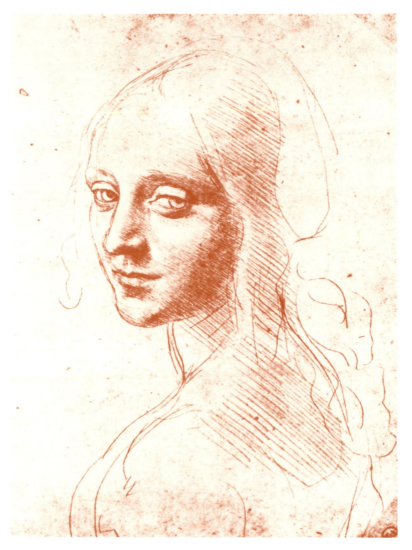

Leonardo da Vinci, 1452 — 1519.

A thing of beauty is a joy forever.
Anon

32

CORNEAL TRANSPLANTATION

Roger F. Meyer

In the past, penetrating keratoplasty has been considered almost hopeless in the treatment of severe corneal burns. The tissue damage which occurs with the healing phases after severe chemical burns, especially alkali burns, results in multiple problems. These include symblepharon formation, conjunctival and lid damage, abnormal tear function, damage to the corneal epithelium and Bowman's membrane with progressive pannus and failure of corneal epithelialization, and extensive corneal vascularization which predisposes to immune rejection. Recent advances in the field of keratoplasty, including the utilization of the surgical microscope, 10-0 monofilament nylon suture, meticulous postoperative care, and the fitting of therapeutic soft contact lenses have favorably influenced results.

Penetrating keratoplasty achieves its best results when the surgery is performed after the acute injury has been treated and the eye has remained without inflammation for several months (Figures 1A and B). However, keratoplasty may become necessary during the acute stage, if the central cornea sloughs and perforates. The surgical procedure is similar in both cases.

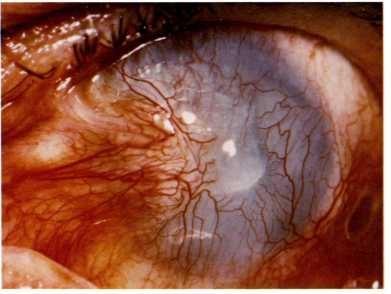
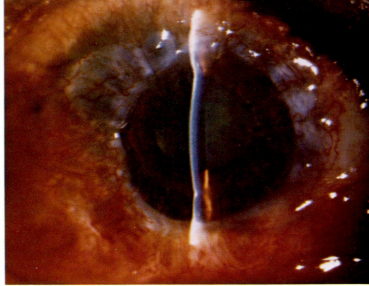

A   *B*

Fig. 1. A. Severely scarred cornea one year after alkali burn injury. Note dense conjunctival overgrowth covering entire surface of cornea. **B.** Postoperative result after successful penetrating keratoplasty. Conjunctival overgrowth has been resected and intraocular structures are visible through clear corneal graft.

THE SURGICAL PROCEDURE

At the time of the surgical procedure, the cornea is usually totally overgrown by conjunctiva. In this procedure, the surgeon makes an incision into the conjunctiva at the center of the cornea (Figure 2A), and dissects the conjunctival overgrowth to the limbus (Figure 2B). The conjunctiva is freed from the thickened subconjunctival tissue to both fornices and canthi. A surgical assistant lifts the dissected conjunctiva, and the subconjunctival tissue is excised to the sclera. With this approach, the subconjunctival tissue can easily be dissected from the sclera, creating a smooth surface of sclera surrounding the cornea. The dissection of the subconjunctiva should begin away from the limbus because the tissues are fused together at the limbus. The subconjunctival tissue is excised en bloc.

In those eyes without symblepharon, horizontal incisions through the residual conjunctiva are made at the nine and three o'clock positions and extended to both canthi. The conjunctiva is recessed approximately 4mm to 5mm from the limbus and sutured with 7-0 black silk interrupted sutures. Symblepharons are repaired by moving flaps of conjunctival tissue from the fornix where the conjunctiva is intact. These are sutured to the sclera and the lid surface is left raw.

A double Flieringa-LeGrand ring is sutured to the sclera for scleral support and fixation of the globe. A deep corneal incision is made with 7.5 or 8.0mm trephine (Figure 2C). Because extensive anterior synechia are often present in the inferior one-half of the anterior chamber, the chamber is entered with a razor blade knife at the eleven o'clock position (Figure 2D). The scarred cornea is excised with blunt-tipped corneal scissors (Figure 2E). A retrocorneal membrane is often present and must be excised using blunt and sharp dissection to separate its extensive attachments to the iris. When iridectomies are necessary, it is useful to clamp and crush the iris with the jaws of a fine needle holder so that excision of the iris does not result in bleeding.

If a cataractrous lens is found, it is removed through the corneal incision with a cryoprobe (Figure 2F). If vitreous is present in the anterior chamber or corneal wound, an anterior vitrectomy is performed. The anterior vitreous may be excised utilizing cellulose sponges and scissors or a vitreous suction cutter (Figure 2G).

Fresh refrigerated corneal tissue less than 24 hours old, generally from a young donor, or similar tissue stored for a short time in corneal bathing medium is used for donor material. This tissue is selected for the presence of good adherent epithelium, since normal donor epithelium appears crucial to success in patients with corneal burns. Every effort is made to preserve donor corneal epithelium during the procedure. The corneal graft is sutured to the host with interrupted 10-0 monofilament nylon sutures (Figure 2H). Interrupted sutures allow their selective removal in areas of greatest vascularization as required postoperatively. The anterior chamber is filled with balanced salt solution, and the wound is checked to be certain it is water-tight. Soluble corticosteroids are injected subconjunctivally at the end of the procedure.

POSTOPERATIVE TREATMENT

Postoperatively, intraocular pressure is checked daily with an electronic applanation tonometer, and treatment with carbonic anhydrase inhibitors is instituted in those eyes with elevated intraocular pressure. If, after a few weeks, intraocular pressure cannot be lowered by medical means alone, cyclocryotherapy is performed. Cyclocryotherapy is the procedure of choice after penetrating keratoplasty because it incurs less risk to graft transparency than intraocular surgical procedures.

Corticosteroids are used routinely during the early postoperative period to suppress iritis, vascularization, and graft reaction. Periodic attempts to reduce the frequency of administration will determine when therapy or prophylaxis is no longer necessary. Tear deficiency must always be suspected and treated, when present, with artificial tear supplements.

Fig. 2. Surgical procedure for corneal transplant.

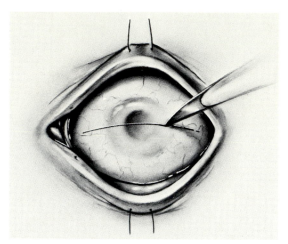

A. Initial incision into conjunctival overgrowth.

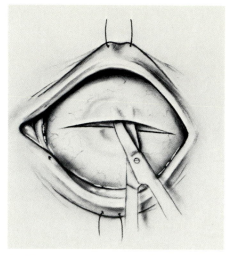

B. Dissection of conjunctiva from thickened underlying subconjunctival tissue.

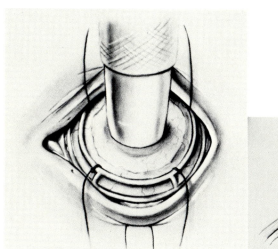

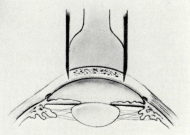

C. Deep corneal incision utilizing trephine.

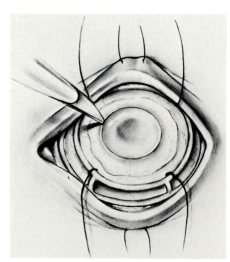

D. Entrance into anterior chamber along trephine incision utilizing razor blade knife.

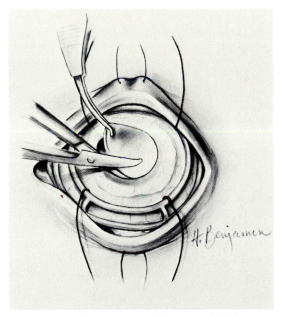

E. Excision of scarred corneal button with blunt corneal scissors.

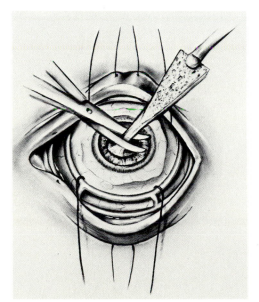

G. Excision of vitreous through dilated pupil with cellulose sponges and scissors.

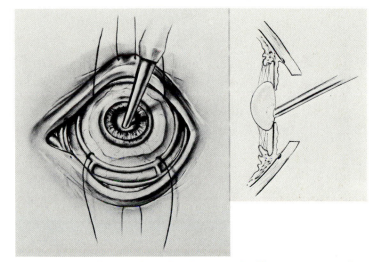

F. Application of cryoprobe to lens in preparation for cataract extraction.

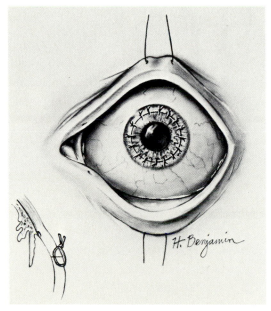

H. Donor cornea sutured into position with 10-0 monofilament nylon.

Epithelialization of the sclera and the corneal transplant is carefully observed each day with the use of fluorescein and a cobalt-filtered light source. When epithelialization of the graft is slowed, or if erosions develop in a previously epithelialized graft, treatment with a therapeutic soft contact lens must be instituted (Figure 3). The hydrophilic lens keeps the donor epithelium intact and protects it from the drying and lid damage commonly encountered.

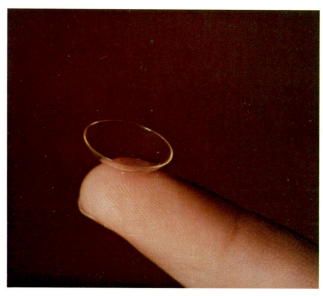

Fig. 3. Therapeutic soft contact lens, frequently used to promote epithelial healing of corneal transplants postoperatively in the rehabilitation of severely burned corneas.

Often, numerous lens changes are required before healing is observed. The patients must wear the lenses continuously for many months under close observation. The problem of recurrent epithelial erosion persists for years after grafting and must be closely followed. If epithelial erosions persist for even 48 hours, healing may result in surface opacities of the cornea with varying degrees of scar formation.

Healing of the corneal graft wound is relatively rapid due to extensive vascularization of the host cornea. Sutures are usually removed within two to four months postoperatively.

Lamellar keratoplasty should be reserved for minimal injuries after healing has progressed, or as a tectonic preparatory procedure prior to definitive surgery. Preparatory grafts are used to restore corneal thickness. They do not eliminate vascularization and should not be used for such a purpose. In both cases, preservation of the donor epithelium on the lamellar graft is essential for a good result.

Corneal transplants for chemical or thermal burns require much attention and supervision. They should not be performed in either uncooperative patients or patients who are unsuitable for soft contact lens wear. The postoperative course of penetrating keratoplasty for burns is beset with a variety of complications. Upon recognition they are amenable to therapy with different degrees of success. The value of prophylaxis against such complications must be stressed. Frequent, topically applied corticosteroids and antibiotics should be administered early in the postoperative period. The soft contact lens should be worn almost continuously under close observation at least until suture removal has been accomplished. With these precautions, an indefinite restoration of vision by corneal transplantation is possible, but continues to present a therapeutic challange.

SUMMARY

Penetrating keratoplasty for severely burned corneas of either thermal or chemical origin presents a therapeutic challenge. A broad therapeutic approach in the management of corneal grafts includes control of glaucoma, meticulous resection of subconjunctival granulation tissue, atraumatic keratoplasty and resection of membranes in the anterior chamber, control of tear deficiency and control of inflammation, as well as the use of soft contact lenses. Vascularization of the host cornea sets the stage for graft reactions which are frequent and need to be controlled with corticosteroids. Retention and postoperative protection of epithelium on the donor graft is essential. Recent advances in surgical technique, careful postoperative management, and the immediate application of soft contact lenses, when indicated, have improved the prognosis for penetrating keratoplasty after burn injuries.

Forms of Eyes artificially made of Gold or Silver, polished and enamelled, shewing both the inner and outer side.

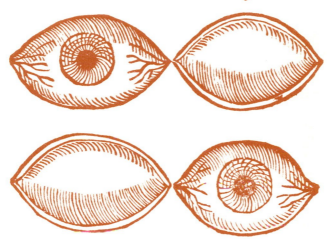

The Works of that Famous Chirurgeon: Ambrose Parey, 1678.

33

ENUCLEATION AND PROSTHETIC REPLACEMENT

John W. Henderson

When a blind, painful eye has resulted from a burn, and damage to the globe is too severe for surgical reconstruction, removal is indicated. Cosmetically, a prosthesis may be preferable to a globe with an unsightly, damaged anterior segment. The major aim in removal is to retain as much motility of the extraocular muscles as possible, as well as to replace the volume of the removed ocular tissue with some form of implant.

ENUCLEATION

The standard enucleation procedure is performed by incising the conjunctiva and underlying Tenon's fascia at the margin of the cornea, then dissecting between the sclera and Tenon's capsule with spreading scissor technique. The four rectus muscles are identified, tagged with sutures, and their insertions are detached. The optic nerve is then sectioned behind the eyeball and the globe removed, preferably with a 3 to 4mm length of attached nerve.

PROSTHETIC IMPLANT

After bleeding is controlled, the lining of Tenon's space is identified and an implant placed in the cavity. Our preference is for a Jardon implant constructed of a polyethylene sphere with overlying fine tantalum mesh. The implants are available in several sizes. The one most frequently used is 16mm in diameter. Tenon's capsule is then closed with a purse-string suture of 5-0 gut. Anterior to this, the rectus muscle tips are joined, superior to inferior, then medial to lateral, using the same suture material.

At this point, further undermining of the conjunctival borders is needed, and horizontal closure of this tissue is performed with a running fine-gut suture. A silicone rubber conformer, furnished with the implant, is then placed over the closure to prevent tissue edema. Since the conformer is similar in shape to the final prosthesis, adequate space is thus produced for later fitting.

About two weeks after surgery, prosthetic fitting can be initiated. The preferable material is plastic, and often a stock artificial eye can be used. However, the ocularist responsible may wish to prepare a mold for actual shape and then fabricate a prosthesis with more precise matching of iris color.

The implant described has the advantage of firm union to Tenon's capsule by ingrowth of fibroblasts into the tantalum mesh. This will maintain the action of the rectus muscles and minimize later migration of the implant into an improper position within the orbit.

The resultant motion of a prosthesis that has been properly fitted is quite satisfactory in the fine movements associated with lid action in the primary position. However, movements in the extreme lateral and medial directions are usually disappointing. The patient often avoids this by using head movements in gazing in extreme horizontal directions.

Numerous attempts have been made in the past to develop so-called integrated orbital implants to which the rectus muscles can be attached directly. A permanent opening in the anterior surface of the implant then allows the direct attachment of the prosthesis. However, since the conjunctiva was allowed to remain open anteriorly, in the vast majority of cases epithelium would grow backward to line the space around the implant, with inevitable extrusion. Most such implants have, therefore, been discarded. A compromise in which the muscles can be more directly attached to the implant has been developed by Allen of the University of Iowa. The conjunctiva is then closed anteriorly in the usual fashion. We have had no experience with this method.

EVISCERATION OF THE GLOBE

An alternative procedure useful in certain cases is evisceration of the globe with implantation of a ball implant within the sclera. Although some surgeons retain the cornea, remove the contents of the globe, and then place a ball implant in the space, we prefer removal of the cornea and, therefore, use a somewhat smaller ball. Wedges of sclera are removed above and below, a 12 to 14mm implant (Jardon type) placed, and the sclera closed with mattress sutures. The conjunctiva is then closed horizontally after undermining of the perilimbal tissue.

The advantage of evisceration is a fuller motion of the implant since the extraocular muscles are not disturbed. Objections to the procedure are the absence of recognizable tissue for pathology study and

the risk of leaving residual uveal tissue within the sclera, with the later possibility of sympathetic ophthalmitis. This can be avoided by meticulous inspection of the lining of the scleral cavity and removal of all pigmented tissue.

OTHER TECHNIQUES

In patients with extensive destruction of conjunctival and lid tissue from prior burns, cosmetic results may be less satisfactory. Contracted conjunctival cul-de-sacs may make mucus membrane grafts necessary in order to allow adequate space for a prosthesis. In addition, severing adhesions beneath the lids may be followed by placement of molded material in the anterior orbit and the lids temporarily closed with sutures. Conjunctiva will then proliferate to line the new space around the conformer.

When destruction of the conjunctiva has been so complete as to preclude cosmetic repair, the globe can be removed, an implant placed, and the lids fused. The resulting appearance of closed eyelids may be preferable cosmetically in certain patients.

It is the mission of history to make our fellow beings acceptable to us.
Ortega Y. Gasset

34

MAKING AN OCULAR PROSTHESIS

Frederick A. Waara

Ocular prostheses were originally made of blown glass in Germany, and shipped to the United States, but these shipments were stopped in 1938, prior to the U.S. involvement in the war. These glass eyes were made by German families who handed the skill down to their children and would not reveal their art to others.

The plastic materials now used in ocular prostheses were developed by Fritz Jardon and others in 1935, and the plastic ocular prothesis was developed in 1937. With continued improvement, mass production of plastic ocular protheses started in 1939, and in 1940, Fritz Jardon, with the American Optical, produced thousands of eyes for the U.S. and Russian armed services. (I had the privilege of being taught by Mr. Jardon, while I was employed with the University of Michigan Medical Center, Department of Ophthalmology, from 1953-1958.)

CONSTRUCTION

There are several methods of constructing plastic ocular prostheses. I will describe the procedure and materials that I have used over the years (Figure 1).

In cases where the eye has been enucleated or eviscerated or in cases of pthesical or microphthalmic eyes, the first step is to make an impression of the eye or socket. This procedure is similar to taking an impression for corneal-scleral contact lenses.

An impression should be made after all edema has subsided, which makes for a more accurate model for the prosthetic base. The impression is taken by placing a proper size fenestrated molding shell beneath the eye lids. These molding shells come in various sizes, and can be altered to fit the eye socket.

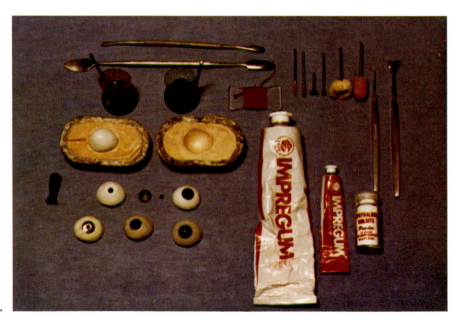

Fig. 1.

The impression material, 1.8mg Ophthalmic Moldite, is mixed with 6cc water for 30 seconds and placed into a 50cc syringe. With slow pressure, this is squeezed into the socket through a hole in the molding shell, until it overflows. The impression material takes approximately two minutes to set. When the moldite feels rubbery and not tacky, the molding shell and impression material are removed by hinging the shell out and away from the socket. The socket is cleaned of remaining moldite with a swab, and irrigated.

The impression material is removed from the molding shell, indicating the nasal side, and submerged into cold water to avoid dehydration of the impression material.

Other impression materials may be used in this procedure. Impregum dental molding material is used with impregum catalyst, measured in equal linear amounts on waxed paper, and mixed until it has a uniform color. The advantage of this product is its longer, five minute working time.

A stone paste is then prepared by mixing investing stone powder with water, to fill the base of a dental crown and bridge flask.

The set impression material is dried with a tissue and pressed into the wet investing stone in the flask base. When the base stone has hardened, the stone area is painted with Colorguard separator, and the upper half of the flask is placed on the bottom, and filled with investing stone. When the stone has hardened, the flask halves are separated, and the nasal side is indicated by marking the flask. The impression material is removed, and the stone portion of the flasks are again painted with separator.

The base of the ocular prosthesis is prepared by mixing 15cc white polymer and 5cc clear monomer, measured in graduated cylinders. The monomer is poured into a small glass jar, and the polymer is added to it. It is allowed to set until it has a dough-like consistency, and is neither hard nor tacky. It is placed into the flask and compressed under maximum pressure, if done by hand, or up to 4500psi if done with a pneumatic press. The excess acrylic is removed and a small amount is inserted back into the flask and pressed again to 4000psi to eliminate porosity.

The press and flask are submerged into preheated water at 160 degrees Fahrenheit for 80 minutes. It is transferred to preheated water at 212 degrees Fahrenheit for 30 minutes.

The base of the ocular prosthesis is removed from the flask base, buffed with wet flour pumice, and polished with Bendick polishing compound. It is cleaned with detergent soap, rinsed, and inserted into the patient's socket.

The pupil exit is determined by using a penlight to center the ocular prosthesis with the fellow eye. The placement is marked by an X with a wax pencil.

The diameter of the iris is measured to determine the size of the iris disk. The size of the iris varies from a microphthalmis to 14mm with an average size of approximately 11mm. The size of the pupil may vary from 1.5mm to 6mm with an average size of 3mm. Consideration must be given for magnification of the iris disk and pupil when the clear acrylic is applied over them to form the corneal and scleral areas. This causes as much as $1/10$ magnification.

The iris disk may be made from 2mm thick clear acrylic, or round stock acrylic, approximately $5/8$ inch in diameter. The iris disk should be beveled so that the posterior side is 1mm wider than the anterior side to allow for insizing. The iris disk is cut and beveled on a dental lathe, and a pupil hole is drilled in the center. The pupil is cut with an acrylic stone to size from a 1mm thick piece of black acrylic.

The base of the ocular prosthesis is counter-sunk by using an inverted metal burr to make a round depression slightly larger than the iris disk. The base is counter-sunk to within 2mm of the posterior portion of the base, but this may vary.

A black dot is painted in the middle of the counter-sunk area to cover the pupil area, and to indicate the thickness that the base may be ground from the back for fitting.

The posterior side of the iris disk is painted with acrylic syrup and acrylic paints to the same color as the fellow eye. When it is dry, the iris disk is set into the prosthesis base.

6cc white polymer and 2cc monomer are mixed to the same consistency as that used for the prosthesis base. The acrylic is pressed around the periphery of the iris disk. This fills any open areas and makes the iris and base into one solid piece. When the acrylic hardens, the excess is ground off with an acrylic stone, reducing the scleral area of the base by $1/3$ or more, and sizing the iris. The base is now ready for painting.

The iris stroma is painted in laminar fashion, alternating pigment and acrylic syrup to duplicate the colors, depth, and detail of the fellow eye. Several sable brushes, ranging from 0000 size to 11 size are used for painting the ocular prosthesis.

The veins are made from the separated fibers of red rayon thread. They are applied with monomer on each quadrant of the scleral area in a tortuous manner, and allowed to dry.

The base color of the scleral area is painted with a translucent combination of blue pigment and acrylic syrup, matching the fellow eye. Successive applications are added to reach the desired color. Yellow translucent color is painted over the blue to make the eye look lifelike. The pupil disk is now inserted (Figure 2).

Some dark-eyed people require an application of brown translucent over the blue and yellow to match their fellow eye.

15cc clear polymer and 5cc monomer are mixed in the same manner as previous mixtures. Both halves of the flask are painted with separator, and the prosthesis is placed in the corresponding flask, face up. The clear acrylic is placed over the painted prosthesis,

and pressed with the same steps and pressures as the base. The times and temperatures for the cooking and boiling are also the same.

The prosthesis is removed from the flask, and pumiced and polished. It is washed with detergent soap, rinsed, and inserted into the patient's socket. The gaze of the prosthesis is checked with a penlight. If not centered, alterations are made on the posterior portion of the prosthesis. The anterior clear portion may be altered to reduce the size of the cornea, which, in turn, reduces the magnification of the iris.

INSERTION OF THE PROSTHESIS

Initially, the patient is apprehensive, which causes some discomfort when the prosthesis is inserted for the first time. After a short period of time (one-half to one hour) the discomfort is minimal, if the eye is properly adjusted. If, after this acclimation period, there is still discomfort, minor adjustments may be made on the posterior portion of the prosthesis, or the edges may be rounded a bit more.

The patient is instructed on how to insert and remove the prosthesis. It should be removed and cleaned weekly to remove oil and mucoid deposits. A mild detergent soap washing or storage in 1:10,000 Zephren solution, or the germicidal duo-Flo (also used for hard contact lenses) make for an effective cleaning system. Periodic pumicing and polishing are also necessary.

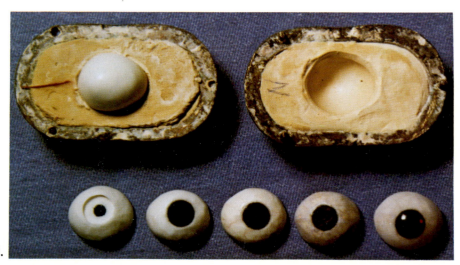

Fig. 2.

The form of an Iron Wier wherewith the deformity of an eye that is loft, may be fhadowed or covered.

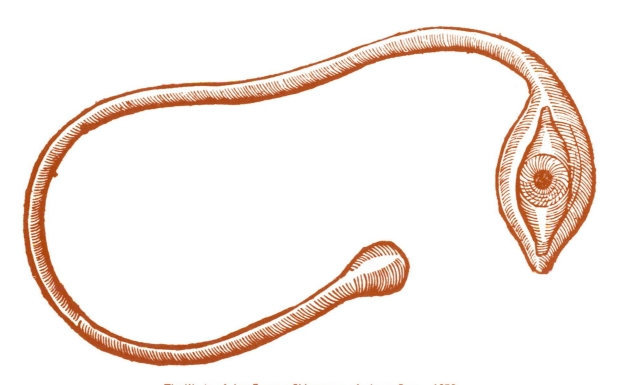

The Works of that Famous Chirurgeon: Ambrose Parey, 1678.

Five things are proper to the duty of a Chirurgeon; To take away that which is superfluous; to restore to their places such things as are displaced; to separate those things which are joined together; to join those that are separated; and to supply the defects of nature.

Ambroise Parey

V.

THE EYELID

PRINCIPLES OF TREATMENT

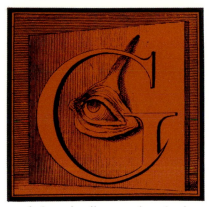

reat care must be taken to protect the cornea when a burn injury has damaged or destroyed an eyelid. The eyelids are extremely thin. Exposure to physical or chemical forces can result in partial or full-thickness skin loss. Fortunately, complete destruction of the eyelid is rare, but when it does occur, immediate care of the cornea should be carried out by the use of conjunctival and pedicle flaps from the nearest available uninjured tissue.

When full-thickness loss of skin of the eyelids has occurred, the eschar should be removed by multiple dressing changes. Split-thickness grafts should be applied as early as possible. Because the skin of the eyelids is thin, early eschar removal and grafting is possible. A tarsorrhaphy should be carried out in all cases where both upper and lower eyelids are burned and also when it appears that an ectropion may occur following the grafting of one lid.

Irving Feller

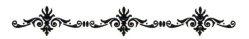

36

RECONSTRUCTION OF THE EYELID

Irving Feller

Ectropion of the eyelids may result from either full or partial-thickness burns. Early correction is necessary to avoid corneal damage. The following procedure has been used successfully to provide an early correction of the defect.

A. The line of incision is made 1/8 inch below the lid margin and carried down to normal tissue.

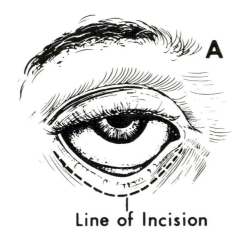

Line of Incision

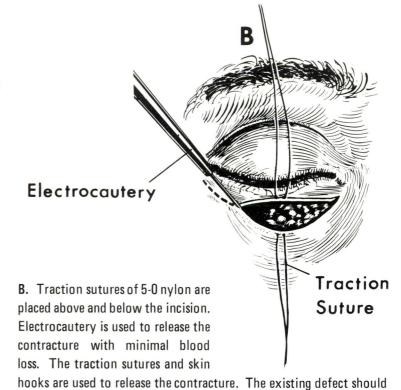

Electrocautery

Traction Suture

B. Traction sutures of 5-0 nylon are placed above and below the incision. Electrocautery is used to release the contracture with minimal blood loss. The traction sutures and skin hooks are used to release the contracture. The existing defect should be over-corrected by at least one-third to allow for contracture of the graft. Complete hemostasis is necessary before applying the graft.

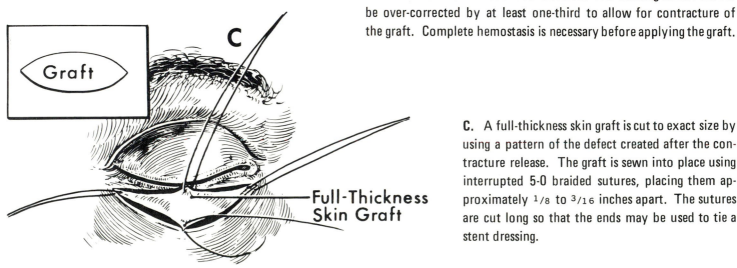

Graft

Full-Thickness Skin Graft

C. A full-thickness skin graft is cut to exact size by using a pattern of the defect created after the contracture release. The graft is sewn into place using interrupted 5-0 braided sutures, placing them approximately 1/8 to 3/16 inches apart. The sutures are cut long so that the ends may be used to tie a stent dressing.

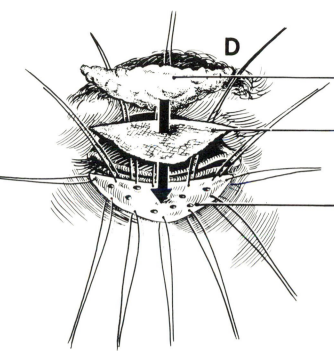

Cotton Dressing

Coarse Gauze
with Antibiotic
Ointment

Perforated Full-
Thickness Graft

D. When the suturing is completed, many small holes are made in the graft for drainage. A single layer of coarse gauze impregnated with an antibiotic ointment is applied, which in turn is covered with cotton soaked in a balanced salt solution.

E. The long ends of the suture are used to tie over the wet cotton. After the stent dressing is completed, the excessive solution is pressed from the cotton and the cotton is shaped to the curve of the globe.

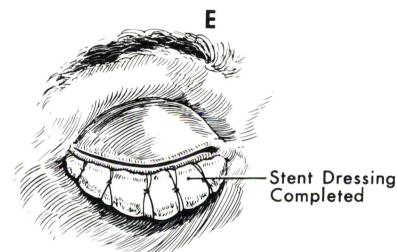

Stent Dressing
Completed

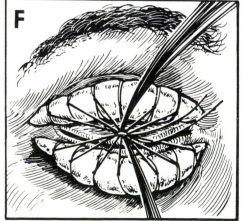

N.V. Marks

F. In some cases, both the upper and lower lids are involved. The same procedure is used to place the graft in both lids, i.e., steps A to E. An additional step can be added to keep the eye closed. The long ends of the suture can be used to tie the upper and lower lids together.

37

RECONSTRUCTION OF THE EYELID

John C. Mustardé

Apart from splashing by hot metals or liquids, the eyelids are seldom burned except when some part of the rest of the face is burned. Therefore, the management of the eyelids must be considered within the context of treatment for the rest of the face. The eyelids, however, are highly complex structures with a unique type of skin. Special additional measures are needed in their management if they are not to be permanently deformed, and if the underlying eye itself is not to suffer damage.

In many facial burns—and this particularly applies to scalds—the patient has sufficient time to blink or even screw up the eyes, protecting not only the cornea but even the pretarsal part of the eyelids to a considerable extent. Dry heat, however, will produce differing clinical pictures, depending on the duration of the exposure and on the degree of heat. Where there has been a flash from a nearby explosion, such as gunfire or an electrical explosion, the patient has no time for reflex blinking. Generally, since the upper lids are open, they tend to suffer less burning than the rest of the face and the cornea and conjunctiva. If the exposure to heat has been brief, but not instantaneous (for instance, an explosion from petrol vapor), the patient may have had sufficient time to close the eyes reflexly, but not to screw them up. This produces a picture of overall superficial burning of the lids and face, causing a fine fibrosis that gives rise eventually to a rather tight, mask-like appearance, with probably a slight degree of ectropion of the lower, and even the upper lids. Longer exposure to dry heat (e.g., flames in a burning building), produces a scald-like picture: the lid skin is partly protected by the intense screwing up of the eyes. At the furthest end of the scale are those patients who lie unconscious or semiconscious for a period of time exposed to a source of heat. In these patients, there will be burning of lid and face skin which may be deep enough to char the tissues and even result in total loss of the eyelids.

All eyelid burns tend to produce varying degrees of ectropion. Because of the risks to the underlying exposed cornea which ectropion of the eyelids produces—risks which may range from keratitis to ulceration and possibly loss of the eye itself—adequate treatment of the burned eyelid is of great importance. The overriding necessity in managing eyelid burns is to prevent a pathological state arising in the cornea. This does not mean that the cornea must always be capable of being covered, but that throughout the course of treatment there must be constant supervision of the state of the cornea, ideally by an ophthalmologist who can examine it minutely.

It is rare for the cornea itself to have been damaged. Usually there is only at most a temporary edema of the corneal epithelium, and perhaps a transient keratitis. The real danger lies in the risk of corneal ulceration. This arises partly from continued exposure and drying out of the cornea and partly from the presence of infection which inevitably supervenes in the eyelid burns themselves. The problem is much less likely to occur where the burns mainly affect the lower eyelids, since the cornea would be covered by the upper lid during sleep and when blinking takes place. Because of this, quite severe burns of the lower lid—including those where there is severe extropion—may be treated conservatively for a considerable time without any danger to the eye. However, if the upper lid has been severely burned, contraction of the superficial tissues may draw up the lid to such an extent that the cornea is not covered during sleep when the eye rolls upwards towards the upper fornix. Mere exposure of the cornea does not necessarily produce damage, but the combination of exposure and the potential of infection from the burns will mean that the cornea is more liable to damage. Thus, every effort should be made to control the infection and to correct the ectropion, at least in the upper lid, as soon as possible.

EARLY MANAGEMENT

The main problem for the surgeon in the management of eyelid burns is knowing exactly when operative correction should be carried out. It is extremely difficult with thin eyelid skin to tell with certainty the exact depth of burn at an early stage. It is better not to excise and graft burned areas as a primary procedure because quite often the burns are less deep than they initially appear. It may be two or more weeks before the eschar comes away and the severity of the burn really can be determined. During the very early period, the conjunctiva will probably be edematous, and this in itself may prevent the cornea from becoming unduly exposed. The instillation of antibiotic drops or ointment two or three times daily should be employed as a further precautionary measure. If these instillations cause the patient to complain of unpleasant blurring, a plastic eye shield may be used on the affected eye to obscure vision. **The eye should never be covered with a pad of cotton wool or other soft material. This will produce a condition of moist warmth, causing a rapid increase in any inflammatory condition which may be present.**
During this early phase a careful watch is kept on the condition of the cornea. If there is the slightest indication that keratitis is developing, the eye should be covered with a large watchglass which provides a moist chamber and reduces the drying effect on the cornea. The moist chamber can be constructed by laying a roll of tulle gras around the rim of the orbit and placing the watchglass on top, so that there is no stream of air passing across the eye. The watchglass will become steamed with moisture within a few minutes. It is necessary to remove it two or three times a day to carry out a toilet of the eye and to get rid of any discharge which may be produced by

the conjunctiva or by the burns of the lids. In lower eyelid burns it is extremely unlikely that these measures will be necessary. It is possible simply to wait for the eschar to separate from the burned lids, even though a gross degree of ectropion is caused.
Once the eschars are separated, if a granulating area is left it can be covered with a split-thickness skin graft (in the knowledge that producing healing of the lid in no way corrects or even minimizes the ectropion which is going to develop as the granulations and graft contract in the course of time). The same regime with regard to grafting of granulating areas can be carried out for the upper lid, but it is likely that a moist chamber may continue to be required if there is any risk of exposure keratitis to the cornea itself. It should be emphasized that early grafting of granulating areas seems to have little impact on the ultimate degree of ectropion that will result once the contractile phase in the lids has reached its climax, but at least the grafts will help to get the lids healed.

DEFINITIVE TREATMENT

One of the difficulties which now arises is deciding how long to wait with the lids in this state of ectropion before inserting skin grafts that will give full protection to the eye. If possible, grafting should be delayed at least five or six weeks (and preferably five or six months) after the lids have healed. **The overriding principle is that the cornea should be protected if it is at all irritated,** and it may be necessary to graft before this period of time has elapsed—an unlikely event as far as the lower lid is concerned, but a distinct possibility with burns of the upper lid.
The thickness of the skin graft to be used will depend primarily on whether it is the upper or the lower lid which has to be grafted and secondarily on the depth of the burn. As a general rule, ectropion of the lower lid may be corrected by the insertion of a sufficiently large full-thickness skin graft (Figure 1). This graft is preferably obtained, for reasons of color and texture, from the sulcus behind the ear. Such grafts will contract only slightly, and the rigidity of the lid caused by such a thick graft does not affect

Fig. 1. Correction of a moderate degree of ectropion following burn of the eyelid. **A.** The incision line 2 to 3mm from the margin is marked. Note that this line should extend beyond the actual canthi. **B.** The para-marginal excision is made, using the knife to undermine the skin slightly. **C.** By drawing the lid upwards and by continuing the undermining of the skin with the scalpel blade, the whole of the orbicularis muscle is freed from the overlying contracted skin. **D.** Estimated area which will require covering by a full-thickness free graft. **E.** Full-thickness free graft taken from behind the ear inserted into defect in eyelid. Note that a few incisions have been made in the long axis of the graft to allow drainage of blood or serum. **F.** A base of damp cotton has been tied over the graft to give even pressure and to assist in absorption of any secretion through the stab wounds. **G.** Final appearance three months after surgery. The graft has contracted the expected amount and there is no longer any ectropion.

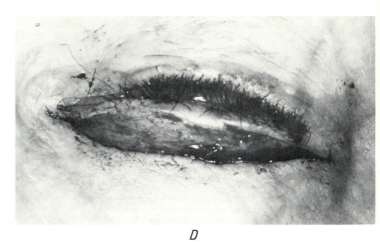

D

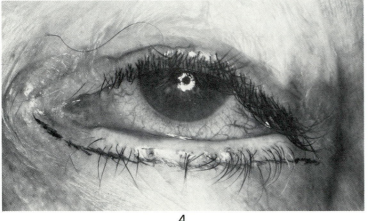

A

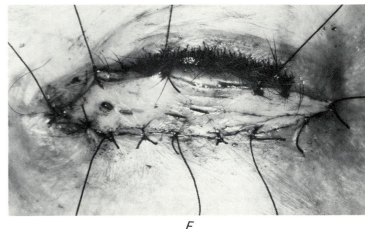

E

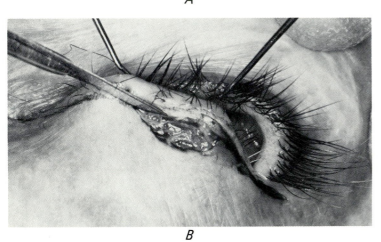

B

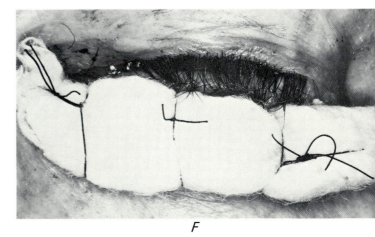

F

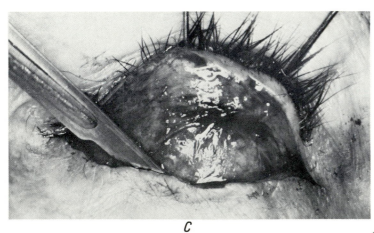

C

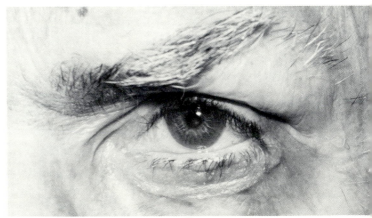

G

the function of the lower lid. Because suppleness and mobility of the skin graft is all important in the upper lid, only a split-thickness skin graft of moderate thickness should be used. Considerable contraction of a thin graft of this nature will, of course, occur, and an excessive quantity of skin (up to twice the final dimensions required) must be inserted. Although the graft will contract, it will retain a suppleness and ability to form the normal lid fold which would be quite impossible if a full-thickness skin graft were used (Figure 2).

If the burn involves not only the skin but also the muscle, a greater degree of fibrosis will have resulted. Several graftings will be necessary to achieve ultimate correction of the shortening and ectropion of the lids. Even in the lower lid it will be necessary to use split-thickness grafts rather than full-thickness skin grafts and to insert an excessive quantity of skin in the lid, knowing that it will contract to one-half or even one-third of its size (Figure 3). Eyelids in which the skin and muscle are destroyed become so severely contracted that the margin is drawn right out to the orbital rim. Such eyelids are sometimes erroneously described as having been completely burned away. This is not the case, of course, as the margin and the all-important tarsal plate and conjunctival lining are still intact and will form the basis for resurfacing of the lid. In total destruction of the eyelid an entirely different problem has to be met. This is dealt with in the chapter on full-thickness loss of the eyelids.

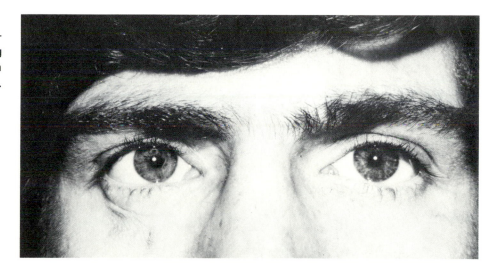

Fig. 2. Postoperative result (burns of right upper and lower eyelids) showing effect of grafting to correct ectropion. **A.** The lower lid has been grafted using full-thickness post-auricular skin.

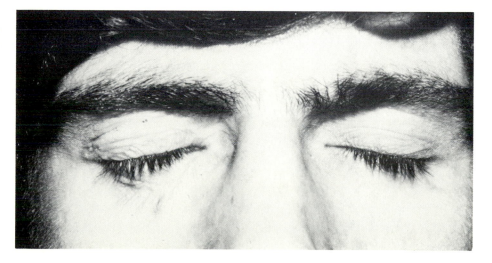

Fig. 2. B. The upper lid has been grafted using split-thickness skin from the arm. Note the broken folding of this thin graft.

Fig. 3. Severe burning of right lower lid, with partial destruction of orbicularis muscle as well as skin. **A.** Preoperative condition showing retraction of lid margin to the limits of the orbit.

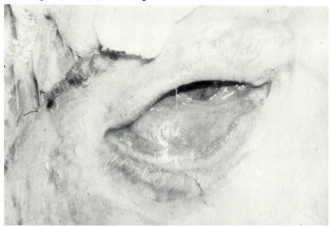

Fig. 3. B. The incision along the margin has been continued for 7 to 8mm beyond the canthi on either side. Gradual undermining of the skin (as shown in Fig. 1C) has allowed the lid margin to be drawn well over the upper lid so that an excessive amount of split-thickness skin graft can be inserted to cover the defect.

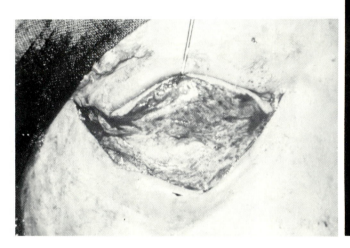

Fig. 3. C. Postoperative result (patient's right lower lid), showing that the skin graft has contracted to about one-half of its original size—largely because of the fibrosis in the destroyed orbicularis muscle layer. Note that the ectropion has been corrected.

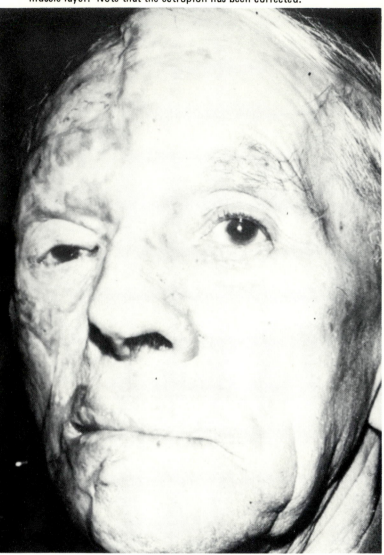

The technique of inserting these large split-thickness skin grafts in the lower or the upper lid is similar to the technique of inserting full-thickness grafts in the lower lid. It is worth reemphasizing, however, that **the incision close to the margin should run from a few millimeters beyond the canthus on either side to avoid a scar junction between the graft and the surrounding skin** which may pull down the margin at one or other canthus. As stated above, it may be necessary to repeat the grafting process once, or even twice. Full-thickness skin grafts used in these deeper burns, even in the lower lid, contract considerably because of the underlying fibrosis. They will become bulky and are best avoided.

Grafting of both lids at the same operation should be avoided. Although advocated by some, this procedure makes it impossible to carry the incision lines beyond the canthi in order to permit an adequate insertion of skin into both lids at the same time. It is also impossible to fully extend both lids, even if they are overlapped one above the other. If only a moderate ectropion is present, one might be prepared to deal with both lids simultaneously. But even in such circumstances it is still my preference to graft the lids separately. If grafting of both lids is required, several weeks should be left between the two procedures, and the upper lid should be grafted first in order to provide protection for the cornea.

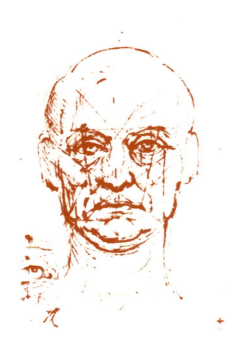

Leonardo da Vinci, 1452 — 1519.

38

ECTROPION

John Marquis Converse

The thinness of the eyelid skin and the intricate relationship between the skin and the pretarsal portion of the orbicularis oculi muscle explains the high frequency of ectropion, not only in burns with full-thickness skin loss but also in partial-thickness burns. The looseness of the eyelid tissues also predisposes them to retraction and ectropion when skin is destroyed in the vicinity of the orbit.

Full-thickness defects of the lid rarely occur in flash or flame burns; in chemical burns, however, it is not infrequent to see an area of full-thickness destruction of the lid.

The structures behind the lids are not usually injured in flash or flame burns. Corneal and conjunctival burns occur in chemical burns, however, and are particularly serious because spreading infection of the eye from a corneal ulcer may require enucleation of the ocular globe. The cornea was destroyed by acid in a number of our patients; infection led to endophthalmitis resulting in loss of the eye.

In long-standing ectropion, following flash or flame burns, corneal ulceration and scarring are seen as a result of exposure, drying, and subsequent infection. Most corneal lesions in burn cases are preventable if precautions are taken to protect the cornea from exposures. Soft plastic lenses are available for this purpose.

INTRINSIC AND EXTRINSIC ECTROPION

Because the eyelid skin is thin, it usually suffers greater tissue destruction than does the thicker skin of the face. As mentioned earlier, the eyelids consist of loosely attached tissues, which readily submit to the pull of contracting, healing, burned tissues over the periphery of the orbital rims. **A distinction**

should therefore be made between intrinsic extropion caused by the eyelids themselves and the extrinsic ectropion, caused by the loss of skin in the area around the eyes. This distinction is clinically important because it indicates the need for replacement not only of the eyelid skin but also of the adjacent skin.

Burn contractures may involve eyelid tissue alone, if the remainder of the face has suffered only a superficial burn; the thin and loosely bound eyelid tissues contract during healing, resulting in ectropion.

The eyelids are often spared in flash burns if the patient is wearing glasses, but when the skin of the remaining portion of the face is burned, scar contraction may cause extrinsic ectropion.

Even in deep burns of the eyelids where there is full-thickness destruction of the skin, a sufficient number of orbicularis oculi muscle fibers usually remain to ensure closure of the eye. Function of the levator palpebrae superioris muscle is rarely affected. When the eyelids have been involved in full-thickness burns of the skin, although the eyelashes and eyebrows are scorched, the eyelid margins are usually spared and the tarsal plates remain intact.

Deep burns involving the full thickness of the eyelid, or chemical burns in which the burning agent penetrates the conjunctival sac, result in symblepharon, an adhesion between the eyelid and eyeball; complete obliteration of the conjunctival sac is known as ankyloblepharon.

TARSORRHAPHY: CONTRAINDICATED

Tarsorrhaphy is not a substitute for skin grafting, which alone will restore the vertical dimensions of the eyelid, permitting palpebral occlusion. The eyelid margin is severely deformed when tarsorrhaphy is maintained during the contractile phase of healing (Figure 1). Some of our most difficult cases of eyelid reconstruction have been those in which the eyelid margin has been destroyed or distorted following tarsorrhaphy.

TIMING OF SKIN GRAFTING

The upper lid protects the cornea. The lower lid may be completely everted without resulting in corneal exposure. Unless the upper eyelid is turned inside out in total ectropion, the cornea may be protected by liquid plastic films, soft contact lens, moist chambers, and other devices. One should not be precipitous in skin grafting the eyelids, for the contractile phase continues for many weeks. After early skin grafting, secondary skin grafting is necessary with less satisfactory results. Raw areas causing extrinsic ectropion should be grafted and well healed prior to skin grafting the eyelids. A definitive skin graft can then be performed: the two upper eyelids in one operation and the lower eyelids subsequently.

In cases of moderate burn ectropion without dangerous corneal exposure, postponement for four or five weeks permits skin grafting under more favorable conditions and minimizes the danger of subsequent contraction. It must be emphasized, however, that in extensive skin loss of the eyelids, purposeful postponement of grafting may lead to dangerous exposure of the cornea and irrevocable deformity of the lids.

CHOICE OF GRAFTS

A full-thickness graft of eyelid skin provides the most satisfactory skin cover for the eyelids. Such a graft can be taken only from an unburned upper lid. Because the available area is limited, the method is usually applicable only in minor cases of burn ectropion.

A split-thickness graft from the inner aspect of the upper arm is relatively hairless and is the most suitable type of skin graft for replacing upper eyelid skin, for it remains thin and supple, permitting the

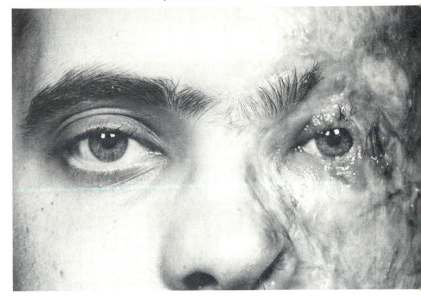

Fig. 1. Example of the type of distortion of the eyelid margins resulting from tarsorrhaphy in burns of the eyelids which complicated future reconstructive procedures.

graft to assume the horizontal folds characteristic of the lid. The color match as a rule improves in time, although some grafts remain white or yellowish-white in color. This inconvenience is of less importance in the upper lid than it is in the lower lid, because most of the upper lid is hidden in the normal forward gaze.

In most cases, the use of a thick full-thickness graft in the upper eyelid should be avoided because its thickness and lack of suppleness prevents the formation of the palpebral fold. In patients with hypertrophic scars of the lids and periorbital skin, full-thickness grafts may be indicated because they do not contract as do thinner grafts. Thin full-thickness grafts from the retroauricular or supraclavicular areas or the inner aspect of the arm are preferable; if these areas are not available, thick split-thickness grafts are an alternative.

A full-thickness graft from the postauricular or supraclavicular regions is the graft of choice for lower lid defects. Since the lower eyelid is less mobile than the upper, the lesser suppleness of the graft is an asset in maintaining the position of the lid. Although the thin, mobile skin of the lower lid is similar in structure to that of the lower lid, thin grafts are less satisfactory than thicker grafts in the lower lid, for the tendency toward ectropion recurrence is greater in the lower lid. The full-thickness graft, which contracts to a lesser degree, is preferable to the split-thickness graft. Full-thickness skin from the retroauricular region or the supraclavicular area is selected for grafts because of the favorable texture and the color match.

OUTLAY TECHNIQUE

The outlay technique, reported by Gillies in 1918, was popularized by McIndoe during World War II. Contraction of the skin adjacent to the eyelid can be anticipated in early grafting of extensive facial burns. The dental compound mold technique was advantageous in such grafting since it allowed for the introduction of an excess of skin graft into the defect and for the subsequent traction of the surrounding skin. The ectropic eyelid must be freed of scar tissue by an excision which must extend beyond the lateral rim of the orbit. Traction is exerted on a number of special everting vertical mattress sutures to distend the raw area of the lid. The wound edges are slightly undermined above, medially, and laterally for a distance of 0.5 to 1cm to further increase the size of the raw area. Softened dental compound is spread over the defect and introduced beneath the undercut edges of the wound. The compound is chilled and hardened by a stream of sterile ice water and is removed from the wound. The skin graft, raw surface outward, is then applied to the compound mold, placed into the defect, and the long ends of the end-on mattress sutures are tied over the mold. Pledgets of cotton and a pressure dressing are applied over the entire area.

The mold is removed on the fifth postoperative day. The excess overlapping skin graft is trimmed with scissors and the grafted areas are left exposed. Protection by a dressing or an eye shield during sleep may be indicated during the next five days.

The disadvantage of this technique is that a ridge frequently forms at the junction of the skin graft and the surrounding tissue. To obviate this complication the following technique is preferred.

THE OVERLAPPING TECHNIQUE

The overlapping technique, which I first reported in 1967, is illustrated in Figure 2. After an incision is made horizontally across the eyelid and extended laterally well into the temporal area, the eyelid is freed of scar tissue; by means of traction sutures, it is pulled downward, overlapping the lower eyelid (Figure 2A). A pattern of the defect is made and placed on the dermatome prior to removal of the graft. The graft is then placed over the defect (Figure 2C). Thus, a wide surface of skin graft is assured. The upper eyelids are grafted with split-thickness grafts cut at .014 inches to preserve their necessary mobility. A similar technique is used in later grafting the lower eyelid. When all four eyelids must be grafted, preference is given to grafting both upper eyelids in the same operating session, subsequently covering the eyes and eliminating vision for a few days. This does not cause inconvenience if the patient is forewarned. Both upper eyelids are covered with pressure dressings. When one eye is left open, synergistic ocular globe movement on the grafted side may disturb the graft.

LOWER EYELID SKIN GRAFTING TECHNIQUE

The lower lid is completely freed of all scar tissue until the margin of the lid resumes its normal outline and is reapplied against the eyeball. Incisions should be extended medially and laterally so that the graft can be applied in a sling-like fashion; it is carried medially to the nose and laterally above the lateral canthus (Figure 2D). This design is essential to maintain the support of the lower eyelid. It counteracts the effect of gravity and prevents a downward pull on the lid. One or more mattress sutures are placed through the margin of the lower eyelid, then through the margin of the upper eyelid. These sutures, anchored to the forehead skin by adhesive tape, exert an upward traction, maintaining the lower eyelid at the most favorable level for skin grafting (Figure 2D and E). A full-thickness retroauricular or supraclavicular graft, cut to pattern, is sutured to the edge of the defect (Figure 2E). A patient with burn ectropion of the eyelids before and after surgical correction by the overlapping technique is shown in Figure 3.

Fig. 2. Overlapping technique in skin grafting of burn ectropion of eyelids. **A.** Upper eyelids are freed of scar tissue and overlap lower eyelids, being maintained in this position by traction sutures. **B.** Pattern grafts of split-thickness skin placed over eyelid defects.

A   *B*

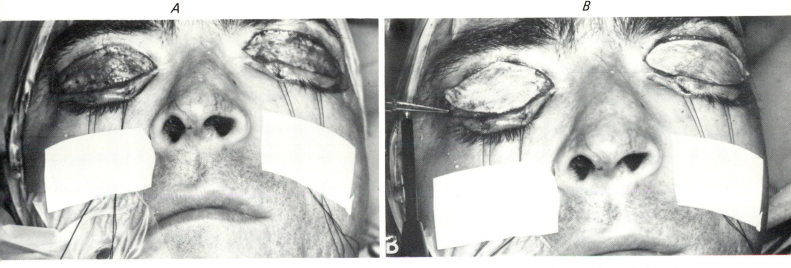

Fig. 2. C. Skin graft sutures in position. **D.** Lower eyelid defects ready for skin grafting. Lower eyelids are maintained elevated by traction sutures.

C   *D*

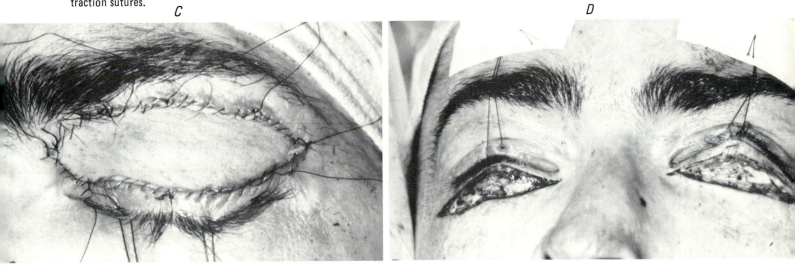

Fig. 2. E. Full-thickness retroauricular graft sutured in position.
(from J.M. Converse, Surg. Clin. N. Am. 47:323, 1967.)

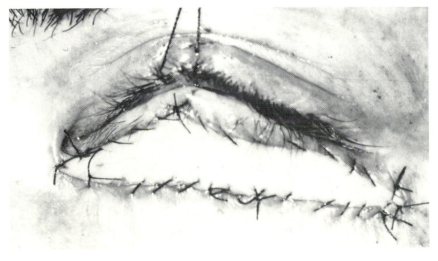

SIMULTANEOUS GRAFTING OF THE UPPER AND LOWER EYELIDS: CONTRAINDICATED

A particularly nefarious technique is that of freeing both upper and lower eyelids from their ectropic position, denuding the eyelid margins, performing a tarsorrhaphy and placing a split-thickness graft over the adjoining raw areas of the upper and lower eyelids (Figure 4A). Later the eyelids are separated by incising through the tarsorrhaphy junction line. **Two complications occur following this** technique: (1) an inadequate amount of skin requires secondary skin grafting of both lids and (2) the eyelid margins remain irremediably deformed. Figure 4B shows the patient after numerous secondary skin grafting procedures.

Epicanthal folds occur occasionally. After a period of waiting to allow for restoration of eyelid mobility and softening of the skin grafts and scars, the technique of double-opposing Z-plasties, which I reported in 1966 (Figure 5) has given us satisfactory results (Figure 6).

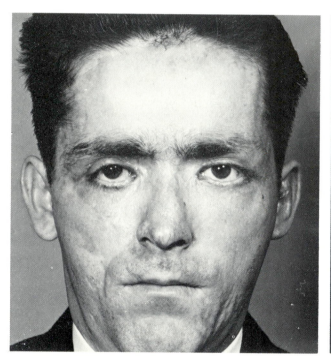
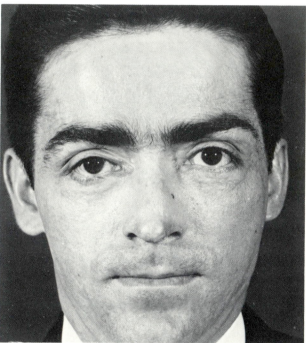

Fig. 3. Repair of burn ectropion by overlapping technique. **A. and B.** Burn ectropion showing inability to occlude eyelids.

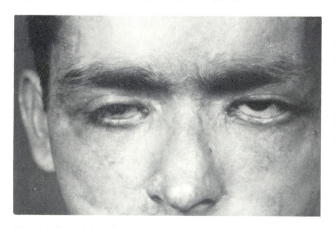
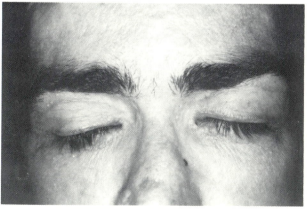

Fig. 3. C. and D. Result obtained following repair by technique illustrated in Figure 2 in a first stage; in a second stage, double-opposing Z-plasties were done to eliminate the epicanthal folds (see Figure 5) as shown in Figure 6.

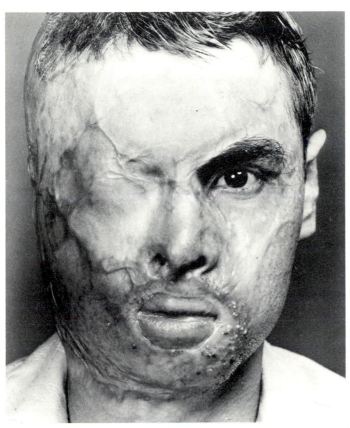

Fig. 4. Extensive burns of face involving scalp, eyebrow, eyelids, cheek, and lips. **A.** Preoperative appearance. Note that a complete tarsorrhaphy of lids was performed and a split-thickness graft placed over the continuous raw area of upper and lower eyelids. **This, in our opinion, is an undesirable procedure.** It destroys the eyelid margin and fails to provide a sufficient surface area of skin graft to eliminate ectropion.

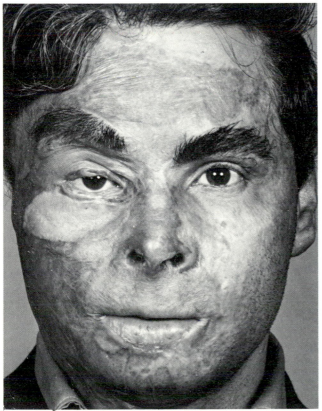

Fig. 4. B. Tarsorrhaphy was cut through and eyelids separated. Upper eyelid was grafted by means of overlapping technique (see Figure 2). Lower eyelid was also grafted in a later stage by means of overlapping technique. Note size of graft that was required to correct ectropion. After these procedures, the medial canthus was still in an advanced position and the lacrimal puncta were not in contact with lacrimal lake. A skin graft was placed in the medial canthal region and succeeded in replacing the canthus in a satisfactory position. Additional reconstructive procedures consisted in transposition of scalp flaps; a scalp flap was utilized to restore the eyebrow, and a full-thickness graft restored adequate length to the upper lip. The ectropion of lower lip was relieved by Z-plasties and small full-thickness grafts. Additional skin grafts were added to the right cheek. (from Kazanjian and Converse's *Surgical Treatment of Facial Injuries*, J. M. Converse, Ed., 3rd Edition, Williams & Wilkins Co., Baltimore, 1974.)

Fig. 5. Double-opposing Z-plasties. **A.** Design of the double-opposing Z-plasties.

Fig. 6. Double-opposing Z-plasties for correction of epicanthal fold following burns. **A.** Linear contracture is accentuated by finger traction and an ink line is traced over it.

A

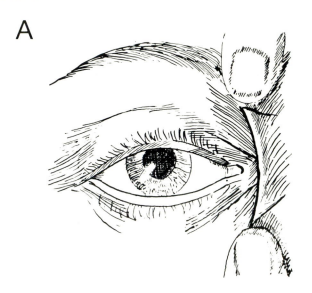

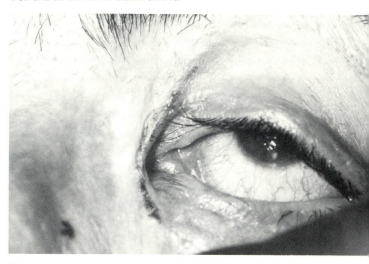

Fig. 6. B. Design of double-opposing Z-plasties.

Fig. 5. B. Position of the flaps at completion of the operation. This procedure is as effective as Z-plasties done with longer flaps and is achieved with shorter flaps, an advantage in anatomically confined areas such as the medial canthus. Another advantage of the shorter flaps is that it permits the use of the Z-plasty with healed burned tissues of diminished blood supply. The design of the flaps may be done in a reverse manner as shown in Figure 6. (from Converse, J.M. and Smith, B., Naso-orbital Fractures and Traumatic Deformities of the Medial Canthus. *Plast. & Reconstr. Surg.*, 38:147, 1966.)

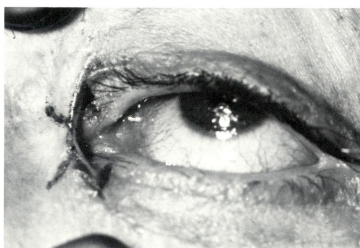

Fig. 6. C. Flaps have been transposed and are ready for suture. (from Kazanjian and Converse's *Surgical Treatment of Facial Injuries*, J. M. Converse, Ed., 3rd Edition, Williams & Wilkins Co., Baltimore, 1974.)

B

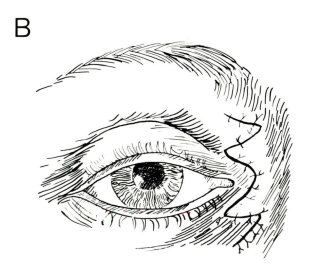

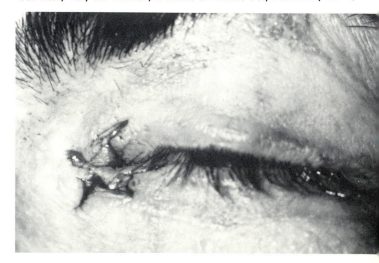

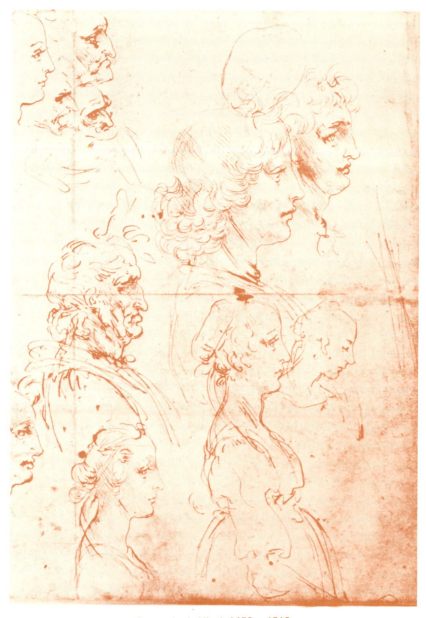

Leonardo da Vinci, 1452 — 1519.

39

FULL-THICKNESS LOSS OF THE EYELID

John C. Mustardé

Full-thickness destruction of the whole eyelid, including the conjunctival and tarsal layers as well as the more superficial layers of skin and muscle, seldom occurs without the underlying eye being extensively damaged and ultimately destroyed (Figure 1). When there is the slightest possibility of saving the eye, the only practical course of action is to undermine and bring forward the conjunctiva from the remains of the upper and lower fornices. Even though the lids have been extensively burned, if the eye can be saved there will be some conjunctival fornix left both above and below. This can be brought forward and sutured in the midline, forming a conjunctival layer covering the damaged and exposed cornea. A pull-out 6-0 monofilament nylon suture should be used, and a medial and lateral gap left between the union of the conjunctival layers to allow discharge to drain from the newly produced conjunctival pocket. The raw surface of the conjunctiva must be covered immedi-

ately with a skin layer. Although in theory a free skin graft would suffice, it is better if possible to use a flap to cover over the raw surface of the conjunctiva and the exposed Tenon's capsule. If there is any possibility of saving the eye this procedure must be carried out as an emergency measure as soon as the patient is fit enough for surgery. Until such time, the eye should be kept moist and free from infection by using a glass chamber.

As soon as it is possible to operate, a flap of skin should be brought from the most appropriate and usable site. Ideally, a midline forehead flap could be brought down to cover the exposed raw surface of the conjunctiva (Figure 2A to F). The pedicle of the flap should not be divided until the area of the orbit immediately around the eyelids has been grafted or covered by flaps (if this area has also been burned) because the blood supply to the flap from the conjunctival surface alone may be insufficient to support

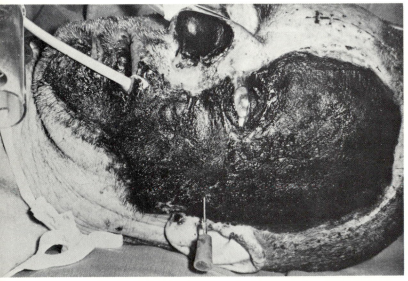
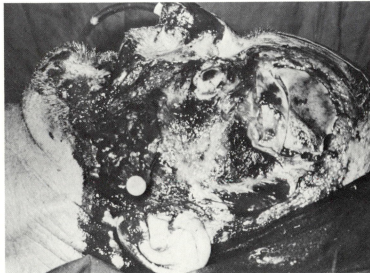

Fig. 1. Full-thickness destruction of eyelids in a patient lying unconscious. **A.** The tissues of the underlying eye have been coagulated and the eye is destroyed. **B.** Two weeks later, the necrotic lids have sloughed. (Photograph by permission of Mr. Ian Jackson, F.R.C.S., Consultant Plastic Surgeon, West of Scotland Plastic Surgery Unit.)

Fig. 2. Full-thickness destruction of both lids: technique of reconstruction.

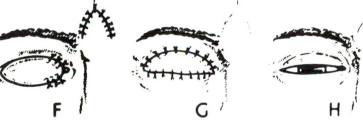

A. and **B.** The conjunctiva in the fornices is freed and sutured across the cornea in order to protect it.

C., D., and E. Skin cover is obtained by the use of a midline forehead flap comprising skin and subcutaneous tissue.

F. Division and return of the pedicle of the flap two weeks later. **G.** The upper part of the flap is replaced two months after stage **F** by a thinner split-skin graft. **H.** Three months after insertion of the split-skin graft, the lids can be opened and the lid margins established.

it at this time. If the forehead is not available, a flap may be brought from the inner aspect of the arm or from the neck, or from any of the standard sites which may be used to produce flap skin for use on the face.

The final management of the reconstructed eyelids should be left until all areas of the face are healed and free from infection. At that time the flap skin and part of the subcutaneous tissue over the area which will constitute the new upper lid can be excised (Figure 2G and H). This area is now covered with a full-thickness postauricular skin graft. Then three months later the junction between the upper and lower lids

can be carefully opened and the mucosa sutured to the skin edges. On the lower lid it may be necessary to insert a mucosal graft along the edge, using nasal mucosa, to avoid excessive contraction if the lower lid is very thick.

The levator action in such a totally reconstructed lid will be considerably diminished, and the **attachment of the conjunctiva from close to the limbus directly on the lids may prevent full movement of the eye.** If eye sight is good enough to warrant it, free grafts of buccal mucosa can be inserted in the upper and lower fornices in the manner for correction of a symblepharon.

Fig. 3. Technique for reconstructing full-thickness defects of the lower lid.

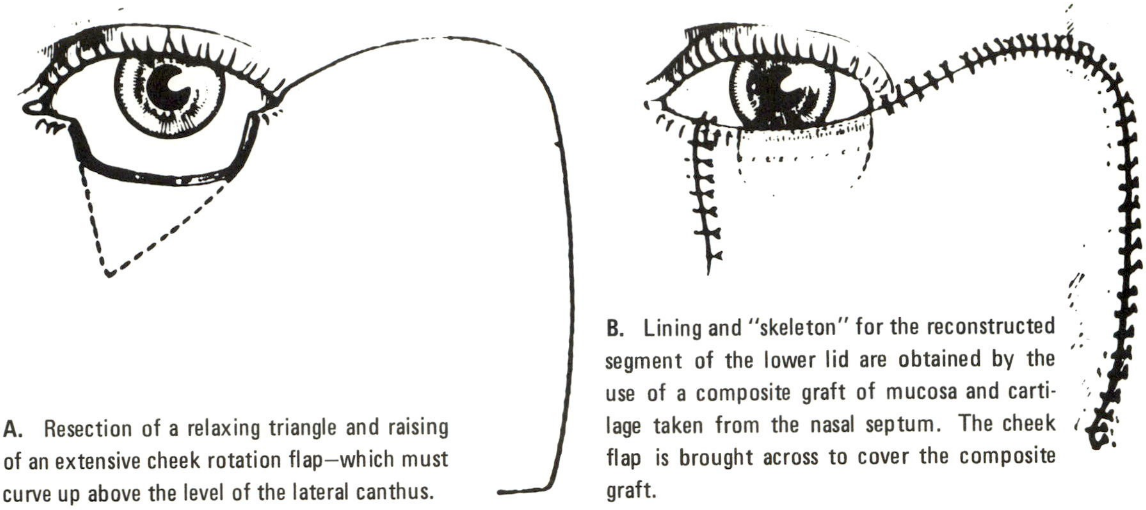

A. Resection of a relaxing triangle and raising of an extensive cheek rotation flap—which must curve up above the level of the lateral canthus.

B. Lining and "skeleton" for the reconstructed segment of the lower lid are obtained by the use of a composite graft of mucosa and cartilage taken from the nasal septum. The cheek flap is brought across to cover the composite graft.

LIMITED FULL-THICKNESS LOSS OF EYELIDS

Occasionally there may be burns of the eyelid, caused by the splashing of molten metal or other hot substances, that result in a small area of full-thickness necrosis but leave the underlying eye either undamaged or savable. In such instances it may be extremely difficult to tell at an early stage whether the full thickness of the lid has been destroyed or not. A conservative regime should be adopted, including a careful daily toilet to the eye using antibiotic drops or ointment and an attempt to keep the necrotic lid tissue dry. This minimizes infection and encourages the necrotic tissue to mummify and slough in due course. The immediate regime to be followed after that will depend on whether the upper or the lower lid is affected.

Lower Lid Defects. If the **lower** lid is affected, it is better to allow the edges of the defect to undergo secondary epithelization so that the defect in the lid becomes established, even if it causes some distortion of the rest of the lid tissues. No harm should come to the eye by waiting, and after it is deemed that the scars have settled, in four to six months, the defect in the lower lid can be corrected by one of the standard

eyelid reconstruction techniques.

I favor rotation of the soft, thin orbital skin lateral to the lateral canthus. This can be brought across to form a new sector of the lower lid by a cheek rotation flap (Figure 3A). The new sector, which will now lie on the lateral side, should be lined by a free, composite graft of nasal septal mucosa and cartilage (Figure 3B). If only a minimal amount of the margin alone has been destroyed, the missing part of the lid can be reconstructed using a bipedicle Tripier flap brought down from the loose skin of the upper lid above the pretarsal zone. This should be lined with nasal mucosa and cartilage. The pedicles of the Tripier flap can be returned in two weeks' time.

Upper Lid Defects. When the area of full-thickness necrosis is situated on the upper lid, a waiting regime should again be adopted, but the patient must be kept under constant supervision so that any evidence of exposure keratitis may be detected early. Should exposure keratitis become evident or threaten, the eye should be covered with a moist chamber (as I described previously) and an antibiotic ointment instilled into the conjunctival sac. Such a regime will require the cooperation of an ophthalmologist. It may also be necessary to use a

Fig. 4. Technique for reconstructing full-thickness defects of the upper lid.

A. Full-thickness flap of lower lid outlined.
B. Flap rotated upwards on pedicle broad enough to preserve vascular arcade. Cheek flap brought across to repair gap in lower lid.
C. and D. Lower lid flap sutured into upper lid defect. A small additional segment of lower lid has been constructed.
E. Division of vascular pedicle and revision of lid margins after two weeks.

mydriatic depending on the degree of inflammation in the eye itself. One is aiming all the time at allowing the defect in the lid to heal and the tissues to lose their edematous, inflamed, and friable character before definitive reconstructive surgery, but the overriding consideration must always be the safety of the underlying eye.

If, despite all precautions to prevent corneal damage, it is evident that the eye is in danger, the cornea must be covered by a conjunctival flap brought from the lower fornix and sutured into the upper fornix at the edge of the defect in the upper lid. If this is not suitable because of the extent of the lid burn or the inflammatory condition of the tissues, a full-thickness skin graft should be taken from behind the ear or the opposite upper lid. It is advisable to construct the flap brought up from the lower lid so that it comprises skin as well as conjunctiva, as in the Cutler Beard lid reconstruction technique. This will limit the degree to which the conjunctiva can be brought up, and retraction on the lower lid will tend to pull the flap away from the soft, edematous tissue of the upper lid.

Six weeks later the intervening pedicle of the conjunctival flap can be divided. It may be that such

a repair of the upper lid will be satisfactory enough to preclude further surgery. Should this not be the case a formal repair of the temporarily reconstructed sector can be carried out by rotating up a full-thickness flap of the lower lid on a pedicle which must include the marginal vessels (Figure 4A to D). The pedicle of such a lower lid flap can be divided after two weeks, and the margins of the upper and lower lids finally revised (Figure 4E).

It should be noted that in the foregoing descriptions of full-thickness reconstruction of the lids, no mention has been made of using a hair-bearing skin area to simulate eyelashes. **I strongly believe that it is unwise to place a hair-bearing area on the edge of a reconstructed eyelid where it is impossible to tell how the scar tissue, which is inevitably present, will distort the direction of the follicles.** The risk of having some of the hairs turn in to the cornea is too great to make such a procedure worthwhile. If the patient is concerned about the loss of lashes, it is far better to advise them to use one of the natural-looking false eyelashes. These can readily be applied and are esthetically preferable to what may be a disorderly jumble of hairs curling in various directions.

VI.
THE EYEBROW

PRINCIPLES OF TREATMENT

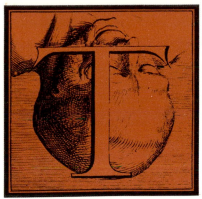

The method of choice for surgical reconstruction of the entire eyebrow is related to the thickness of hair and the width of the brow prior to its loss. For almost all women and many men, the thin, narrow brow that results from scalp-hair transplants by Mustarde's technique is of the proper width and thickness. In reconstructing the wider and heavier brows of some men, a scalp flap can more readily be tailored to the proper shape. This is especially true when a portion of one heavy brow or an entire heavy brow is to be reconstructed. When both brows are lost, the creation of heavy brows with a scalp flap usually will not be esthetically pleasing.

Orienting the direction of the hairs in a graft or flap is of special importance. Trimming and plucking some of the hairs, and using theatrical makeup wax to help control their direction, is of help in obtaining the best esthetic result.

It is probably best to have a pair of eyebrow hairpieces made up early in the rehabilitation period. These can be glued in place and will have a satisfactory esthetic appearance for many patients. Some women with thin eyebrows will have a satisfactory appearance by drawing on the shape of the eyebrow with an eyebrow pencil. A cosmetician will be of help.

Irving Feller

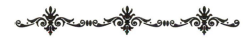

41

EYEBROW REPAIR: HAIR TRANSPLANT

John C. Mustardé

When eyebrows have been destroyed, the manner of reconstruction will depend on the degree of soft-tissue destruction rather than the extent of eyebrow hair loss. In comparatively superficial burns, where there is no significant loss of tissue in the region of the eyebrow, free grafting of strips of hair-bearing skin taken from the scalp, or from the opposite eyebrow, will provide a reasonably adequate new eyebrow. Some surgeons take comparatively wide hair-bearing strips, but it has been my experience that such wide strips tend either to fail, or that if the skin survives many of the hair follicles do not. To overcome this problem, I use narrow hair-bearing strips taken from the temporal area in a vertical line so that the hair will point towards the lateral extremity of the eyebrow. Two, or possibly three, such strips are inserted into incisions made in the skin of the eyebrow region (Figure 1A and B). These grafts are held in place by through-and-through mattress sutures, which can also be used to tie a dressing over the eyebrow and provide an adequate but gentle pressure. Some of the hair will fall out even with a complete

Fig. 1.

A. Eyebrow reconstruction by means of hair-bearing scalp grafts which are three follicles wide.

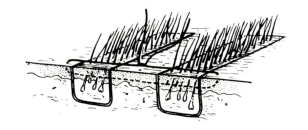

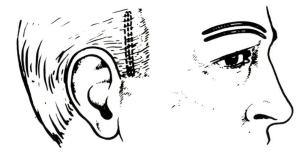

B. Two of these hair-bearing grafts can be inserted into two parallel incisions with a 2 or 3mm strip of skin between them.

take of such grafts, but new hair should soon begin to appear. Three months after grafting, it should be possible to excise the intervening scarred strips and replace them with narrow hair-bearing grafts.

Burns of the eyebrow causing more extensive loss of soft tissue will leave a flattened appearance of the eyebrows. **Correction requires not only the addition of eyebrow hair but subcutaneous tissue as well.** This can be achieved by the use of an *island* pedicle flap which can be brought down from the temporal regional on a subcutaneous pedicle comprising the artery and vein to the area (Figure 2A). These vessels are dissected out under direct vision through a face-lift type of preauricular incision. The small island flap is brought out to the skin surface through a tunnel made beneath the skin of the temporal region, over the supraorbital ridge, and sutured in place (Figure 2B). There is a tendency to make these island flaps too wide. However, it is probably better to do

this than to risk damaging the blood supply to the flap. At a later date the excessive width of the eyebrow can be reduced.

It may happen that the temporal region is itself burned, or is otherwise unsuitable for use as a donor site. In such instances, a hair-bearing area of skin must be brought down from another region of the scalp, using a pedicled flap of standard design. After two weeks the pedicle of such a flap can be divided and replaced in its original position—often leaving only a small defect on the scalp.

Eyebrows constructed by any of the above techniques contain hair which, unlike normal hair, will continue to grow indefinitely, and they must be trimmed from time to time. Irregularities in the "lie" of these new eyebrow hair follicles are probably never permanently corrected. Application of Vaseline or similar substances may be used to temporarily fix the hairs in a reasonable position.

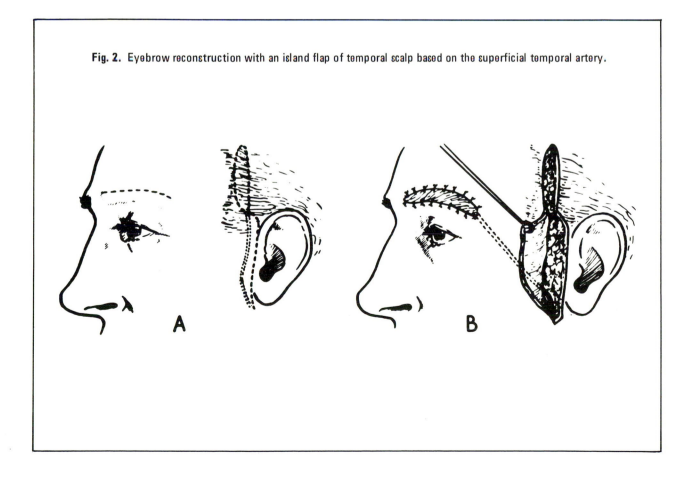

Fig. 2. Eyebrow reconstruction with an island flap of temporal scalp based on the superficial temporal artery.

42

EYEBROW REPAIR: SCALP FLAP

Desmond A. Kernahan

When the eyebrow is destroyed by a full-thickness forehead burn, and the area is resurfaced with split-thickness skin grafts, the resulting absence of the eyebrow constitutes a marked cosmetic disfigurement. The adhesion of the scarred and grafted skin to the bone of the supraorbital ridge will probably preclude reconstruction of the eyebrow using a full-thickness hair-bearing free graft, because there will not be a sufficiently vascular bed on which to place it (Figure 1).

Reconstruction, therefore, involves the introduction of hair-bearing skin carried on a pedicle. This pedicle must be of sufficient length to bring hair-bearing skin from the scalp down to the eyebrow region and to ensure that the distal extremity of the flap, which will constitute the new eyebrow, will have hair growing in a direction most nearly imitating the complex arrangement of the hair of the normal eyebrow.

If available, the hairy skin of the temporal region fills these needs most adequately, because the blood supply is profuse and a long, mobile pedicle can be raised with safety. The pedicle donor site, being narrow, can be closed by approximation, leaving a minimal secondary deformity either in the hairline or at the junction of the temporal hair-bearing skin and forehead. Alternatives to this pedicle transfer are the use of an arterial island flap as described by Monks and Esser, or a transfer of a portion of the opposite normal eyebrow on a glabellar flap. The disadvantage of an arterial island flap is that the superficial temporal artery and its major branches must be followed with exactitude to the skin area to be transplanted. Where this area is as small as the eyebrow, this can be extremely difficult. When this is successful, it involves only a single procedure. There is a much greater chance of success if the pedicle can be 2cm in diameter. Similarly, the transfer of a portion of a normal opposite eyebrow involves raising a very narrow flap based medially in the glabellar area and rotating it 180 degrees to the opposite supraorbital area, both practical considerations liable to prejudice a satisfactory result. Two other factors detract from the usefulness of this flap. It is not possible, due to the limitations in placing the base of the pedicle, to provide sufficient length to reconstruct the outer portion of the eyebrow adequately. At best, this method is limited to reconstruction of the medial portion of the eyebrow. Also, the normal eyebrow may be disfigured.

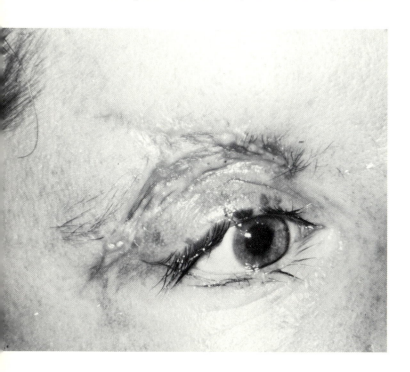

Fig. 1. Localized full-thickness destruction of the skin of the upper eyelid with loss of the eyebrow.

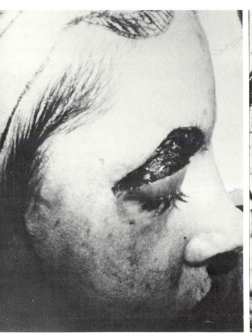

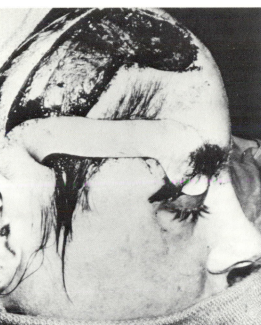

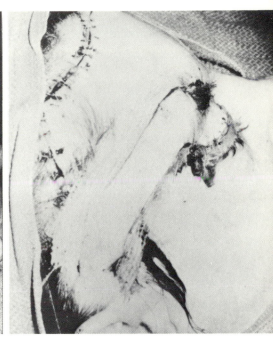

Fig. 2. A. Defect recreated by excision of scar and flap planned within hair-bearing scalp. (Some non-hair-bearing skin incorporated for upper portion of eyelid.

Fig. 2. B. Flap elevated, transposed, and sutured into eyebrow and eyelid defect.

Fig. 2. C. Closure of donor defect by direct approximation and undersurface of flap lined with split-thickness skin graft.

SCALP FLAP RECONSTRUCTION

An aluminum foil pattern is made of the opposite, normal eyebrow, reversed, and placed in the mirror image position on the contralateral supraorbital region. This area is delineated and excised. The distance from the medial extremity of this area to a point overlying the superficial temporal vessels, in the pre-auricular area, just above the tragus, is then measured with umbilical tape, accommodating the thickness of the pedicle of the flap by allowing some slack.

While the auricular end is held in place, the tape is swung up into the hair-bearing temporal skin. At a suitable point, the future eyebrow is marked out using the aluminum pattern. A pedicle 1.5 to 2cm wide is then marked out along the line of the tape, incorporating the superficial temporal artery and its branches as completely as possible. The artery is located by palpating for its pulsation which can be enhanced by having the patient run in place. The margins of the pedicle and the flap on the end of it are then incised down to the areolar layer and the flap elevated, transferred, and sutured into position at the recipient site in the supraorbital region. The donor site of the pedicle can then be closed by undermining and approximation. The underside of the pedicle is dressed with a thin split-thickness skin graft to avoid infection and also to avoid the strangulation of blood supply which might occur from trying to tube a narrow pedicle.

The pedicle can be divided in stages, without anesthesia, at eight and ten days and the inset completed a day or two later under local anesthesia. The unused portion of the pedicle is discarded (Figure 2).

Because hair growth will continue after transfer of temporal hair-bearing skin, it will be necessary to trim and shape the reconstructed eyebrow at regular intervals. It may also be desirable to use a waxy material to keep the hairs in place.

VII.

THE NOSE

PRINCIPLES OF TREATMENT

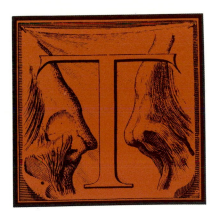

he nose, like the ear, is susceptible to severe damage from burns. The problems that result are (1) tissue loss, (2) occlusion of the nares, (3) hypertrophic scar tissue formation, and (4) scar discoloration.

The restoration of tissue loss is carried out by autografting with split or full-thickness grafts, pedicle transfer of skin and subcutaneous tissue, or composite grafts. Scar contracture occlusion of the nares can be corrected by excision followed by pedicles and autografts. Splinting is required until healing is completed. Both hypertrophic scar formation and scar discoloration can be managed by a combination of shaving and autografting of the excised area.

Irving Feller

44

EARLY MANAGEMENT OF THE NOSE

Irving Feller
Kathryn E. Richards

The early care of the burned nose includes frequent daily dressing changes to debride the eschar and so decrease the loss of partially damaged tissue by infection. Careful placement and taping of nasogastric tubes is necessary to avoid pressure damage to the nares. Because the blood supply to the nose is exceptionally good, spontaneous rupture of partially destroyed blood vessels may occur during the debriding process. Control of this hemorrhage is best accomplished by ligating the vessel with absorbable suture. Keeping crusts from forming in the nares will make for better patient comfort. The nose should be autografted as early as possible to decrease deformity.

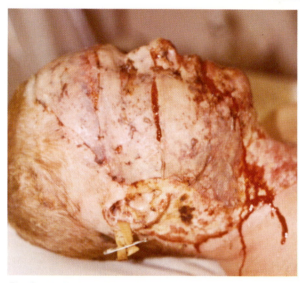

Fig. 2. A. Early grafting after debridement decreases the deformity.

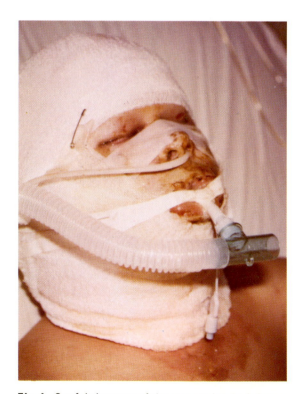

Fig. 1. Careful placement of the nasogastric tube is important to avoid pressure necrosis to the burned nose.

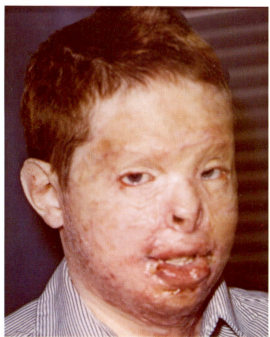

Fig. 2. B. The nose is now covered with autografts and reconstructive procedures can begin when the tissue softens.

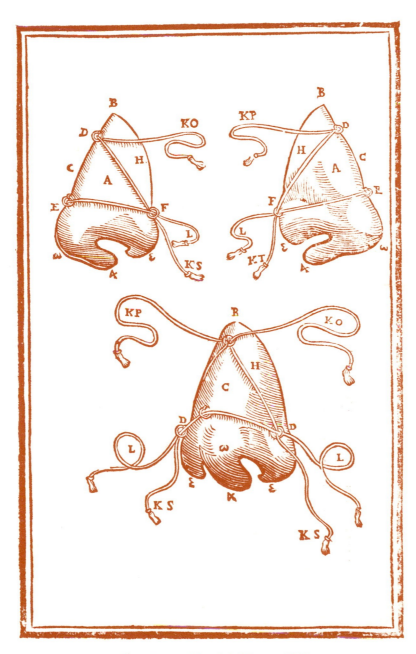

De curtorum chirurgia insitionem, 1597.

45

REPAIR OF PARTIAL LOSS OF THE NOSE

Jack Penn

Before assessing the technical problems of repair, it is necessary to consider the socioeconomic aspects involved—expense, time, the importance of perfect function, textures and color match, and the psychological makeup of the patient. In an elderly breadwinner, where time and money may be more important then an attractive appearance, a quicker and less presentable result may be preferable to a long-term striving toward perfection. The method of repair should be chosen with regard for the technical difficulties involved, as well as complications or restrictions that might, on occasion, result.

It is also necessary to assess what tissues are lost and how they may be replaced. Six methods are commonly used to repair partial destruction of the nose: (1) split-thickness skin graft, (2) full-thickness skin graft, (3) composite graft including fat, cartilage, or both, (4) local skin flap from the cheek, (5) local skin flap from the forehead, and (6) distant skin flap.

SPLIT-THICKNESS GRAFT

The split-thickness skin graft offers many advantages. It is easy to apply, there are many possible donor sites, and it will take even in the presence of a certain amount of mild infection, making it very useful as a temporary covering for a raw area. In some cases it may be used as the permanent graft. However, when taken from the body, the color does not perfectly match that of the face, there is inevitable contraction which may have an effect in everting the alar verge, and the graft contrasts considerably with the sebaceous skin in the vicinity. Nevertheless, the contour and delicacy of the nose as a whole may be preferable to that found following use of a pedicle skin flap.

The split-thickness graft is also particularly useful in instances where the entire face has been burned. Because all skin must be replaced by free grafts, there is no need to match the normal facial skin (Figure 1).

Operative Technique. The burned skin of the nose is removed and the alar wings are turned down to allow the application of as much split-thickness skin as possible, in order to allow for contracture. Dental composition (stent) is heated in water and molded to cover the raw area. It is then cooled until it has set, giving an accurate impression of the recipient site. A split-thickness skin graft is removed from a non-hair bearing area of the arm or the leg. If it is important to match facial skin, the graft may be taken from the neck, although the skin is extremely thin and will contract considerably. Overtie sutures are placed around the periphery of the raw area and the skin graft is wrapped over the mold which is then placed with the cut portion of the graft against the bed. The mold is now kept in position by overties. The excess skin graft may be trimmed away. After five days, the overties may be cut and the mold removed.

FULL-THICKNESS GRAFT

The full-thickness graft is a most useful skin replacement where only the skin of the dorsum is involved, and where texture and color match are important. The best donor area is at the back of the ear. This graft has the advantages of being very similar in texture and color to the normal skin of the upper two-thirds of the nose and it is not necessary to make allowance for contracture after application. However, it is vulnerable to infection and hematoma, but is safe if these complications are avoided.

Fig. 1. **A.** This pilot had the entire skin of his face and anterior neck burned. The patient's appearance prior to skin grafting. **B.** The patient's appearance after split-thickness skin grafts have been applied to the forehead, eyelids, cheeks, nose, lips, and anterior neck. The eyebrows have been reconstructed with pre-hair-bearing scalp grafts.

A

B

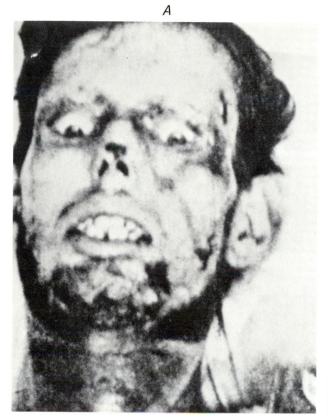
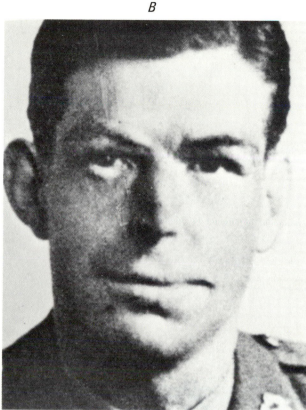

Operative Technique. After excision of the scar, the shape of the area to be covered by a full-thickness graft is defined. The requisite amount of skin to cover the raw area is removed from either one or both ears. In doing so, delicate handling of the graft tissue is essential. It is neither necessary nor desirable to remove any underlying fat which may adhere to the skin. To do so would traumatize the deeper layer of the skin unnecessarily. The graft is then meticulously applied to the raw area using fine sutures along the entire periphery of the graft. It is advisable to place basting sutures in the center of the graft to avoid hematoma and to ensure that there is close contact with the bed. It is not necessary, and is, in fact, harmful for over-firm pressure to be applied on the graft. If overties for pressure are used, the material of the mold should not be hard. Actually, it is usually unnecessary to have a mold on the nose at all, although the graft may be covered under gentle pressure by means of micropore tape strips. No pressure is preferable to pressure which is extreme.

Tension on the graft in all directions opens up the spaces for revascularization but twisting of the graft is undesirable and may vitiate the result (Figure 2).

COMPOSITE GRAFT

Composite grafts may be utilized for the reconstruction of the alae, the tip of the nose and, sometimes, for the columella. This form of replacement has bulk, has an excellent color and texture, and can be shaped accurately to fit the complicated contours of the lower third of the nose. However, it requires a most meticulous technique and an exact fit. Prevention of hematoma and infection are mandatory. Although these grafts are most useful in burns of the tip of the nose or the alae due to the application of cautery or acid, they are inadvisable in cases of radiation burns, owing to endarteritis of the surrounding tissue, and should not be utilized unless a sufficient area is removed to allow free vascular circulation.

Composite grafts are taken from the earlobe, the helix of the ear, or from the nasolabial fold, depending on the shape and texture of the recipient site. If the patient has a large earlobe, a portion of it could be utilized very effectively to supply cover, lining, and body for an alar wing or columella. Because of its flexibility, it is often superior to the helix containing cartilage, although in small wedge replacements the application of a composite graft from the helix is very useful. The use of nasolabial fold skin is somewhere between a full-thickness graft and a composite graft, as it has more dermis than fat and is particularly useful for the tip of the nose, where the sebaceous appearance of the nasolabial fold near the nose closely approximates the tip of the nose.

Operative Technique. Magnification when operating on composite graft replacements is very useful. This enables the surgeon to make his cutaway clean and straight. It also enables him to remove the tissue from the donor area cleanly and accurately, and to suture it into place meticulously with the finest sutures on atraumatic needles. It is advisable not to bury any sutures below the surface of the skin, and cauterization should be carried out to a minimum. The handling of the tissue must be meticulous, and no crushing or squeezing of the graft should be tolerated. The composite graft requires no pressure dressing (Figure 3).

LOCAL SKIN FLAP FROM THE FOREHEAD

The use of local skin flaps for burns of the nose should be confined essentially to the reconstruction of the alae in instances where local destruction has caused a snarling deformity. They are particularly useful in radiation burns because the imported blood supply from the adjacent area of the cheek is usually adequate to maintain viability. The color and texture of the cheek are similar to that of the lower third of the nose, and it constitutes a one-stage procedure. Because most people requiring this type of flap are older, there is usually an adequate supply of loose skin in the nasolabial fold region. This tissue can be brought from a vertical to a horizontal position based on the alar groove, allowing for closure of the donor area without undue deformity (Figure 4). The alar

groove is usually obliterated, but this can be corrected at a second stage if this is desired by the patient.

LOCAL SKIN FLAP FROM THE CHEEK

Use of a local skin flap from the forehead is an extremely good method for the reconstruction of the partially or totally destroyed nose. If not scarred, the skin of the forehead has all the elements needed for normal appearance of the nose, including its texture and color, and the excellent blood supply which it carries it. Nevertheless, it is not a good method for the replacement of skin loss only, because the tissue is too bulky and lacks refinement in shape when the framework is intact. It is, however, of extreme importance when through-and-through loss occurs affecting particularly the lower third of the nose where both alae, the tip, and the columella have been destroyed.

Patients requiring this form of treatment are those with local destruction by heat or acid, those who have had tumor removal in this region, or epileptics who have fallen into a fire or on a hot plate. This flap is also useful in instances where excessive radiation treatment has been given, as enough tissue is usually available to reconstruct the nose even after wide excision of the radionecrotic area.

Operative Technique. In order to have symmetry in the reconstructed nose, it is advisable to reconstruct both sides rather than one, even if it means a sacrifice of normal tissue. The forehead flap will require a width of not less than 7.5cm. The amount of height necessary varies according to the height of the forehead, but amounts to 7.5cm if the total area is required for the covering of the nose and the creation of a lining. A height of approximately 5cm is necessary if only the lower third, together with lining, is to be reconstructed. The pattern of the flap is shown in Figure 5A.

The skin flap to form the new nose is elevated off the forehead superficial to the frontalis muscles. As soon as the hairline is reached, the incision is deepened to the periosteum where the flap is easily

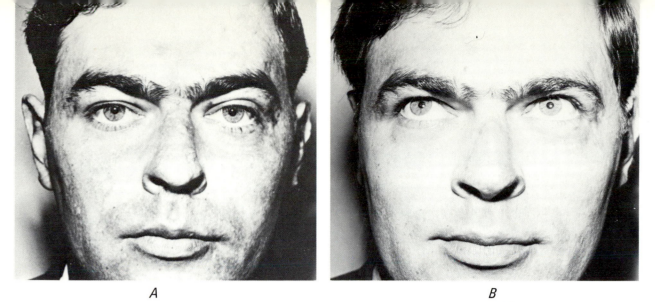

Fig. 2. This patient sustained superficial burns of the face so the nose spontaneously became re-epithelialized. A better cosmetic result was achieved by covering most of the nose with a full-thickness skin graft. **A.** Preoperative appearance. **B.** Postoperative appearance following full-thickness skin graft to the nose.

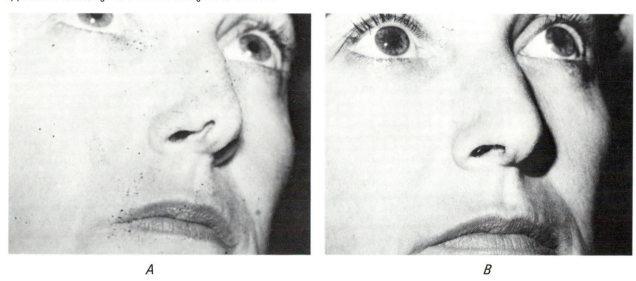

Fig. 3. This traumatic defect of the right nostril rim was reconstructed with a composite auricular graft of skin cartilage and skin. **A.** Prior to reconstruction. **B.** Following reconstruction of the alar margin with a composite graft.

Fig. 4. Reconstruction of the right ala of the nose utilizing a nasolabial skin flap with the end folded upon itself to provide external skin coverage and nasal lining. **A.** Preoperative appearance. **B.** Postoperative appearance.

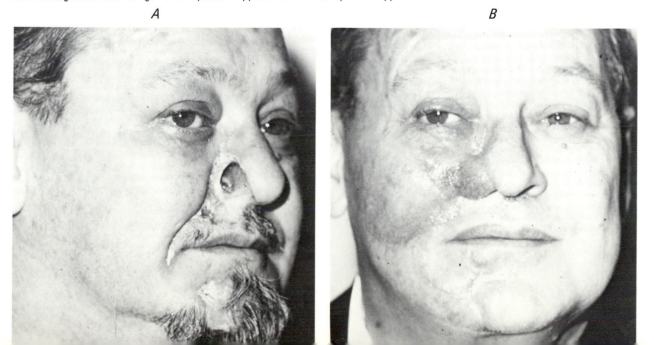

elevated through the areolar tissue between the periosteum and the galea aponeurotica. After excising the burned area of the nose, the pedicle is brought down, thus constructing the columella, the lining, and the two alar wings. The raw area on the forehead is covered with a split-thickness skin graft.

The second stage, three weeks later, consists of separating the nose from the carrying pedicle by making a deep 'V' incision through the pedicle down to the tip of the nose and returning the pedicle to the forehead. The nose itself is repaired by suturing the deep 'V' in such a way that the contour is correct (Figure 5B and 5C).

After some months the skin graft on the forehead matures to normal thickness, but may be slightly different in color. This may be corrected by abrading the epidermis off the graft and replacing it with a thin split-thickness skin graft taken from the neck.

In Figure 6, a patient with radionecrosis of the nose has had the nose reconstructed in this manner. The contour and color match are good and there is minimal deformity on the forehead where the skin graft remains.

In the very young it is important to make the new nose as large as possible so that the patient will 'grow into the new nose' (Figure 7).

DISTANT FLAPS FOR NASAL RECONSTRUCTION

The best type of flap to be utilized for large partial losses of the nose is the forehead flap, but there may be instances where the forehead is not usable, either because of scarring or a very low hairline. There are several methods that may be used in taking a flap from an alternate site. The one utilized by the author is the zigzag arm pedicle or thoracoacromial pedicle (Figure 8).

The arm pedicle is particularly useful because the skin is soft and pliable in both men and women—in men because there is no hair on the arm on the inner side, and in women because it can more easily be hidden by a dress. Zigzagging the pedicle allows for elongation and ease of application, for although the skin will stretch, the scar of the pedicle will not, and by elongating it in a zigzag fashion it allows for contracture of the scar without deformity to the pedicle.

The pedicle is based on the tip of the shoulder, which is extremely mobile, and the distant end is brought up to the nose where it is attached. When viability at the nasal end is obvious (and this can be tested by placing a small rubber tourniquet around the base of the pedicle), the pedicle is separated. The upper part is fitted in to form the nose, while the lower section is returned to the donor site.

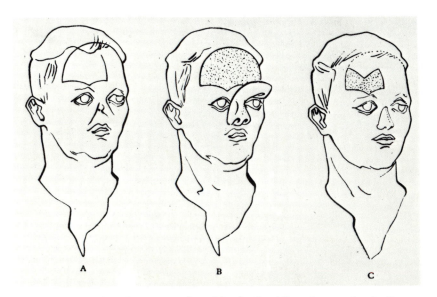

Fig. 5. Total nasal reconstruction with a forehead flap. See text for details.

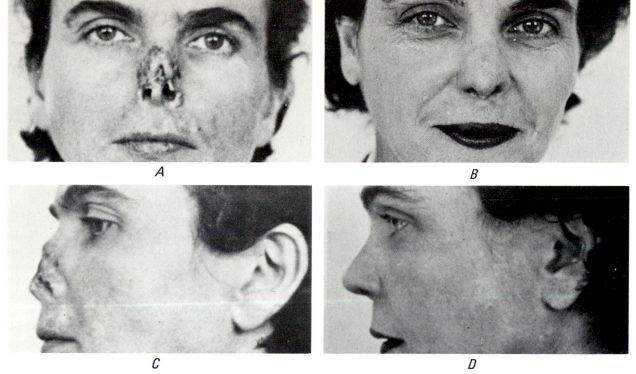

Fig. 6. The distal half of the nose in this patient was destroyed due to excessive irradiation. The nose has been reconstructed with a forehead flap. A skin graft was used to cover the flap donor site on the forehead. **A.** Preoperative appearance. **B.** Postoperative appearance. **C.** Preoperative appearance. **D.** Postoperative appearance.

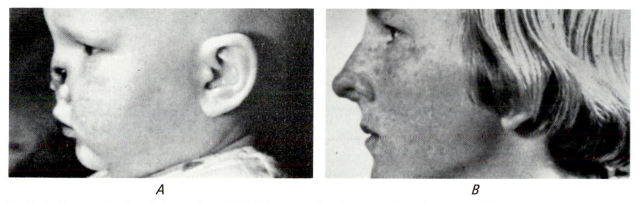

Fig. 7. In the reconstruction of the nose in a child it is important that the new nose be as large as possible so that the patient will grow into the new nose. **A.** Preoperative appearance in infancy. **B.** Appearance of the nose when this patient became a teenager.

Fig. 8. Reconstruction of the nose utilizing a thoracoacromial skin flap. See text for details.

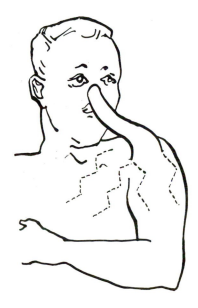

46

NOSE-TIP RECONSTRUCTION USING BIPEDICAL GRAFT

Irving Feller

It is not uncommon to find that the tip of the nose is destroyed in severe facial burns while the remaining nose skin is only injured full or partial-thickness. In these cases definitive repair can be accomplished by advancing a pedicle of skin from the proximal part of the nose to the tip.

During the early treatment, the non-viable tissue at the tip is excised and when the full-thickness loss of skin and underlying tissue is confirmed, the eschar is debrided and a split-thickness graft applied. The reconstructive procedure is delayed until the graft and the healed partial-thickness burned skin areas have softened and developed a good blood supply. The timing for this process varies from a month to more than one year for some patients. This procedure works well for small and moderate sized defects. Large areas of nose loss require pedicle grafts.

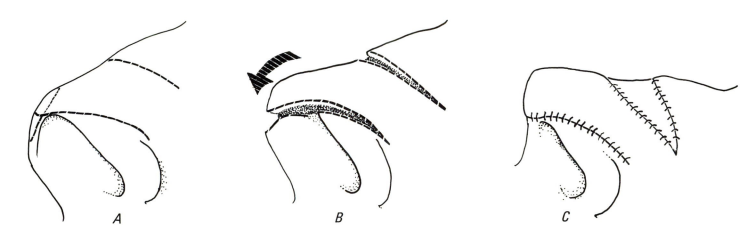

Fig. 1. A. At the time of operation, the pedicle is outlined on the nose. **B.** The pedicle is then elevated and moved over the tip. **C.** The distal suture line is then closed and the full-thickness graft is sewn into place using fine sutures, cut long for a stent dressing.

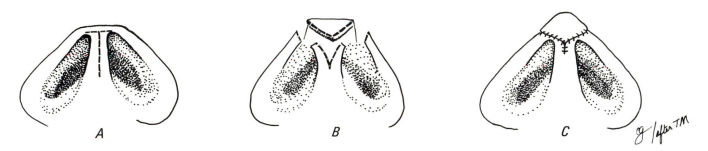

Fig. 2. The columella is widened by; **A.** incising the skin vertically; **B.** perforating the edges; and **C.** suturing the advanced pedicle into place.

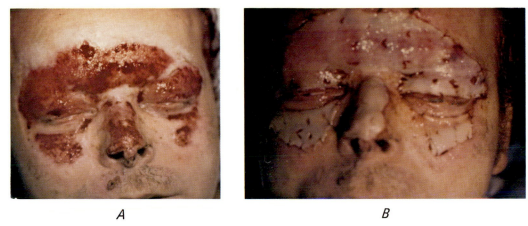

A   B

Fig. 3. The injury is shown in **A** and the initial split-thickness skin graft is illustrated in **B.**

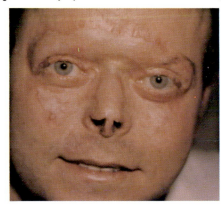

Fig. 4. The loss of tissue from the tip of the nose is seen several months after the primary healing.

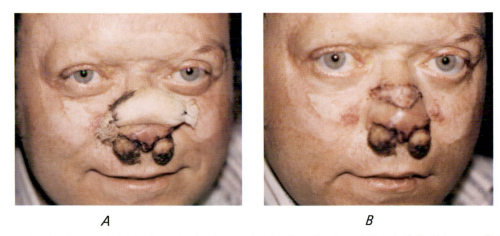

A   B

Fig. 5. A. The pedicle flap is moved distally from the tip. A stent dressing is used to immobilize the full-thickness graft that covers the defect resulting from the pedicle advance. **B.** Cannulae are left in place after the dressings are removed to maintain patent nares.

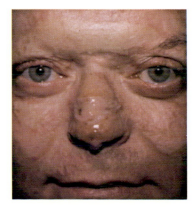

Fig. 6. The repair is illustrated showing the healing pedicle and full-thickness graft. The tip has been reconstructed.

47

NOSE REPAIR: USE OF THIN PEDICLE FROM THE NECK

Irving Feller

When extensive full-thickness loss of the nose has resulted in a large defect, a thin tube pedicle can be used for reconstruction. The use of forehead and arm pedicles works very well. Another area for making the pedicle is the neck. If the neck skin is not burned full-thickness and is not scarred, it can be used as the donor site. The patient should understand and agree to its use because surgical scars will remain in the exposed area and many months are necessary to complete the procedure. The operation can be carried out using general anesthesia for the first stage and local anesthesia for the subsequent procedures.

A thin tube pedicle, one centimeter in diameter, is formed as is illustrated in Figure 1A, B, and C. A combination of partial primary closure and autograft is used to close the bed of the donor site. In Figure 2 the transfer of the pedicle is shown. Four steps were needed to bring this pedicle into position (Figure 3). A fifth operation was used to attach the pedicle to the nose (Figure 4) and a sixth was necessary for final form. All of these procedures, except for the first, were carried out with local anesthesia. Figure 5 demonstrates the pre- and post-operative appearance in a patient who required the reconstruction.

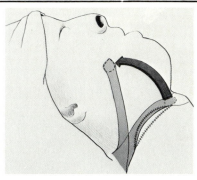

Fig. 2. After three weeks, one end of the pedicle is detached and moved to the cheek.

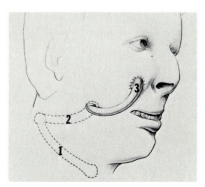

Fig. 3. In succeeding steps, each three weeks or more apart, the pedicle is advanced toward the nose.

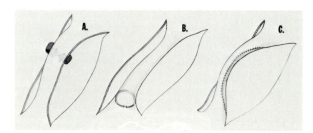

Fig. 1. A. The pencil thin pedicle is formed by elevating the full-thickness skin with a minimum amount of subcutaneous tissue. **B.** The tube is then created by sewing the outer edges together. **C.** The base of the defect is grafted with a split-thickness graft.

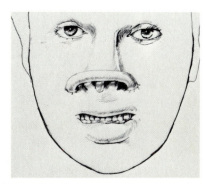

Fig. 4. The pedicle finally comes to rest on a bridge across the end of the nose. Another procedure is necessary to attach the pedicle along its full length and to provide the proper contours.

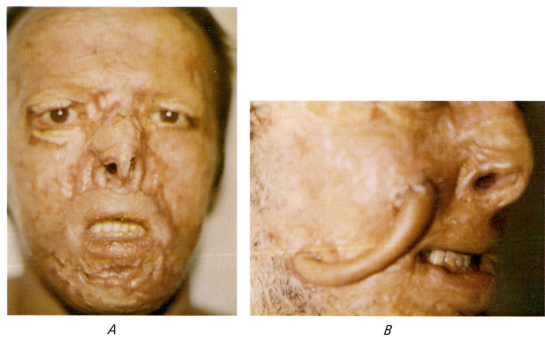

A	*B*

Fig. 5. A. This young man suffered full-thickness burns of his face in a truck accident. A considerable nose deformity resulted. **B.** A thin pedicle was made on the neck and transferred first to the cheek.

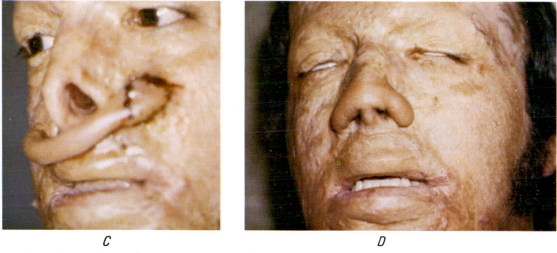

C	*D*

Fig. 5. C. The pedicle was then transferred across the front of the nose. **D.** And then was attached to the nose along its full length.

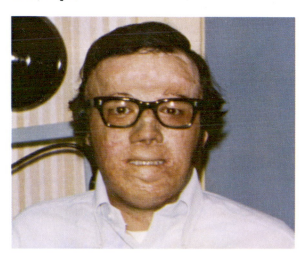

Fig. 5. E. The patient's appearance is shown several years after the final stage.

48

NOSE REPAIR: USE OF PEDICLE FROM FINGER TIP

Irving Feller

Some patients who require pedicle grafts to correct nose defects will have other areas that have to be amputated. The following is a demonstration of this principle in the patient who required a repair of his nose following a severe burn and also required amputation of the fifth finger of the hand on the same side.

At operation the bones were removed from the fifth finger, and the finger was used as the pedicle to the nose. After four weeks, the pedicle was separated from the hand, completing the amputation. A third operative procedure was necessary to complete the reconstruction.

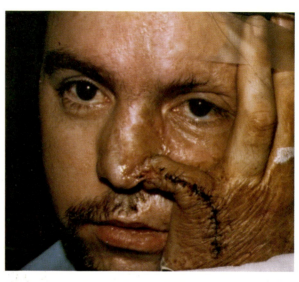

Fig. 2. Amputation of the left fifth finger was indicated because of severe contracture deformity which interfered with his job. After removal of the bones of the fifth finger, the soft tissues were sutured to the nose.

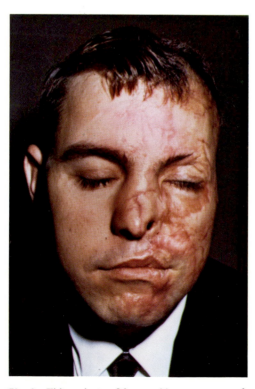

Fig. 1. This patient, a 24-year-old young man, suffered loss of the left nare when he was burned in an automobile accident. His left upper extremity including his hand was also burned full-thickness.

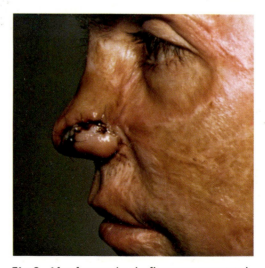

Fig. 3. After four weeks, the finger was amputated, thereby completing the pedicle transfer. A third operation was required to incorporate the pedicle into the nose.

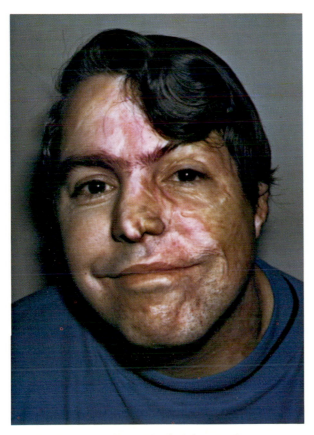

Fig. 4. The patient six months after the procedure.

49

STENOSIS OF THE NARES

Irving Feller

Stenosis or occlusion of one or both nares rarely occurs. Because this contracture occurs most frequently when the whole face is burned, there is usually little or no normal tissue in the area to use for pedicle grafting, making reconstruction difficult.

A combination of a small pedicle graft when possible with a split-thickness graft provides the best correction when followed by the prolonged and judicious use of splints. When pedicle grafting is not possible, thick split grafts and splints will suffice, but the period of splinting will be longer and the need to correct recurrences is not uncommon.

The procedure involves the excision of the scar to open the defect. When possible a pedicle is rotat-

ed into the defect to widen the nares. Split-thickness grafts are then applied and plastic tubing is sewn into place as the splint.

The splint should be left in place for several months or until there is evidence that the scarring process is softening. Tube changes may be necessary if the suture holding them causes infection. The following case study illustrates these concepts.

In some cases a Z-plasty may be used even though the area has been burned. It is necessary to wait until the scar has softened before this procedure can be carried out.

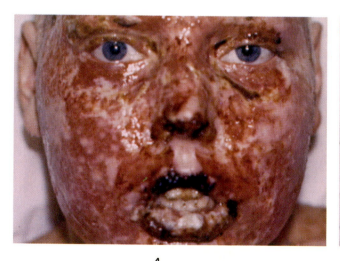
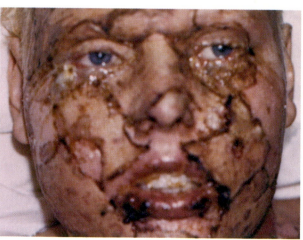

A   B

Fig. 1. A 17-year-old young lady suffered severe burns during a seizure. **A.** Her face was burned full-thickness. **B.** Early debridement made it possible to apply split-thickness skin grafts by the third week following the accident.

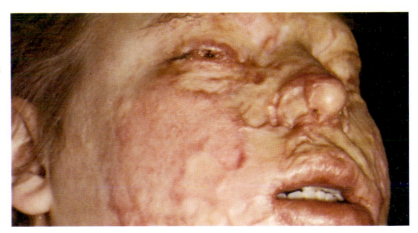

Fig. 2. In spite of early autografting, the nares stenosed, occluding both sides.

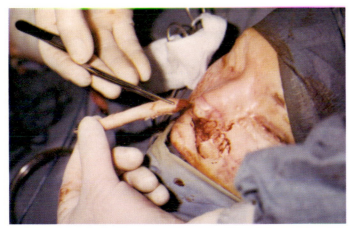

A

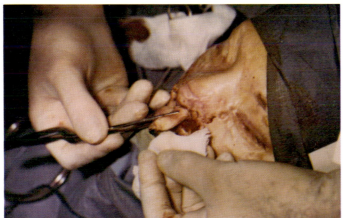

B

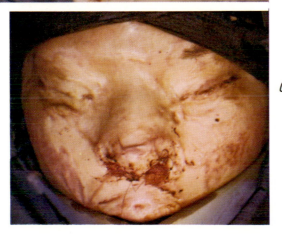

C

Fig. 3. Reconstruction required excision of the scar and grafting with a full-thickness piece of skin which was sewn over a cotton stent so that the cut surface was approximated to the raw surface of the defect. **A. and B.** The stent and graft are being placed. **C.** The outer edges of the skin grafts are sewn to the margins of the nares.

Fig. 4. Because the patient demonstrated massive hypertrophic scar formation that resulted in stenosis, a long-term stent is necessary to avoid recurrence. This photo illustrates the use of a clear plastic tube stent which is held in place by a stainless steel suture.

50

NOSE: COSMETIC PROSTHESIS

Denis C. Lee

Partial damage to the nose is a frequent problem of patients suffering facial burns. This damage usually results in loss of the alar cartilages and surrounding tissues.

Often, it is easier to replace a complete nose with a prosthesis than a partial nose. Replacement of the lateral nostril areas usually requires two small prostheses, which are easily lost or damaged.

It is important that nasal prostheses be paper thin at the margins so that they blend into the nose and may be easily concealed with makeup if desirable. Of course, the thinner the prosthesis the less durable it is. Often the patient must be supplied with several annually.

Patients sincerely interested in cosmetic restoration could be taught to prepare and apply their own prostheses, saving them a great deal of time and money. Preparation of the nasal prosthesis is basically the same as the ear. An impression is taken of the face with a hydrocolloid. Cotton is placed in the nose carefully so as not to distort the nose. Straws are placed in the mouth in case the mouth is covered with impression material.

Plaster is then poured into the hydrocolloid mold to make a plaster cast of the nasal defect and surrounding area.

The missing areas are then replaced with clay. Pictures are usually available of the patient to ensure exact duplication of the nose. A mold is then made covering the clay with more plaster stone.

The clay is removed and replaced with tinted silicone rubber, catalyzed, and the two sections of the mold are clamped until the silicone has cured. The prosthesis is then removed and trimmed.

If the color is off, the prosthesis may be tinted while on the patient to ensure a good color match.

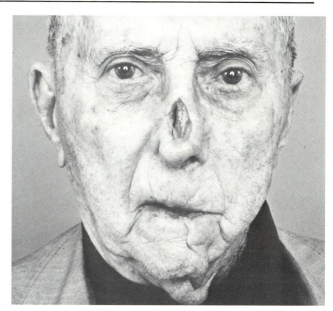

Fig. 1. A. Partial loss of the nose.

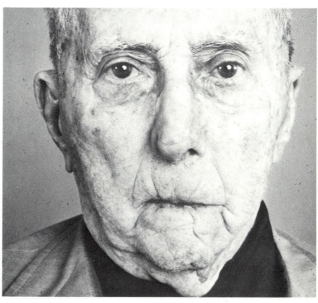

Fig. 1. B. Partial nose prosthesis in place.

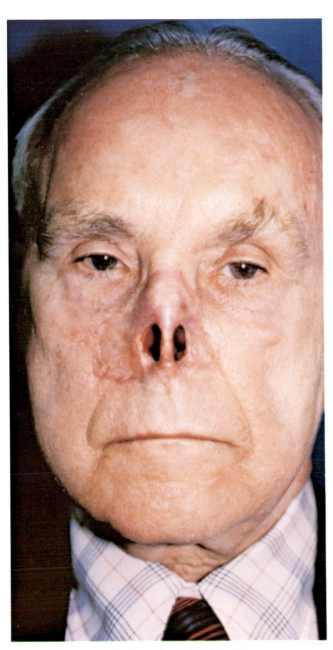

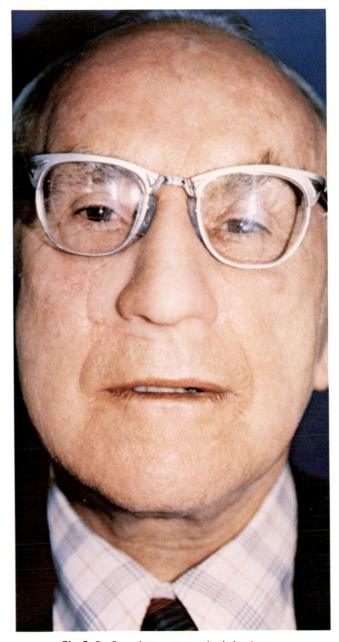

Fig. 2. A. Loss of entire nose.

Fig. 2. B. Complete nose prosthesis in place.

VIII.
THE FACE

PRINCIPLES OF TREATMENT

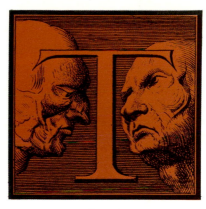

T he burn scar deformity of the face is the most difficult to repair for many reasons. Perhaps the most significant is the importance of the face in our society. Evidence of this is the fact that billions of dollars are spent annually for cosmetics and hair dressing by both men and women to "improve" their appearance. Therefore, a small burn scar deformity on the face will have considerably more impact on the patient's emotional well being than a larger one on other parts of the body.

A second problem comes from the fact that the face has very specialized tissues for defining shape and form, special functions and facial expression. The eyelids are covered by the thinnest skin on the body. The cornea and conjunctiva are unique tissues for sight. The shape of the nose and ears is formed by a special combination of connective tissues and cartilage. The surface tissues of the lips are also unique and the muscles are very specialized.

Scarring or destruction in part or in whole of any of the above tissues results in defects that are difficult at best to repair. It is not possible to restore exactly what has been damaged or lost, and it is important to help the patient understand what can and cannot be accomplished by reconstructive surgery. It is also important to guide the patients to therapy of the emotional problems when they occur, so that they can continue with their lives, fully appreciating that they are the same person that they were before the accident even though their face has been altered. It is gratifying to see that these patients who have had a good rehabilitation program express the fact that they are better off emotionally after the accident than they were before because they more fully understand and appreciate themselves.

The following chapters deal with the principles and practices of facial reconstruction by surgeons skilled in the field. These surgical procedures should be learned and practiced under careful supervision.

Irving Feller

52

EARLY MANAGEMENT OF
THE FACE AND LIPS

Irving Feller
Kathryn E. Richards

Conservative initial care of the severely burned face is important. When a full-thickness injury to the face is present, daily examination of the eyelids for evidence of retraction and the nose for signs of pressure necrosis if an oxygen or a nasogastric tube is in place, and early grafting should be carried out.

The initial care of the severely burned face is directed to minimizing tissue damage and destruction from infection and so conserving as much of the surface as possible for functional and cosmetic healing. Frequent cleaning of the burned surface with soap and water—gentle washing three to four times daily—the use of an antibiotic ointment after each cleaning; and frequent dressing changes provide a means for debridement of the eschar and, thereby, avoiding infection to the underlying damaged tissues. If topical agents are used they should not be toxic to the eyes. Even as the gradual debridement with frequent dressing changes is important, sharp excision

of eschar on burned parts of the face is not indicated. A conservative approach is advised to save all tissue that is not destroyed. This tissue will make itself known as the eschar separates.

The facial hair, except the eyebrows and eyelids, are shaved every three to five days. The eyelids should be kept clear of exudate and tarsorrhaphy used as soon as contracture is suspected. The nares must be kept clear of debris. Tube stents can be used to keep the nares open and allow for normal breathing. Changing the stents daily provides a means for cleaning the parts. Antibiotic ointments are applied to the lips more frequently than the dressing changes since they are exposed and require the protecting cover until healing is complete. These procedures will protect the tissue and hasten debridement to allow for early autografting. Figures 1 through 4 illustrate application of these principles.

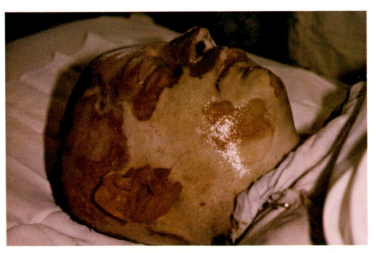

Fig. 1. The badly burned face should be kept clean. This includes attention to the eyes, nose, ears and shaving all hair except the eyebrows and eyelids.

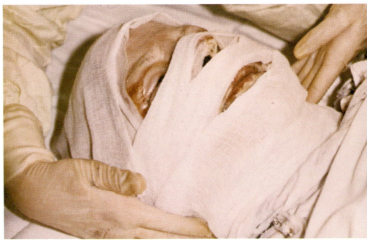

Fig. 2. A well applied dressing allows the patient to see, speak, and eat. The dressings are changed at least twice a day to keep the wound clean and to hasten debridement.

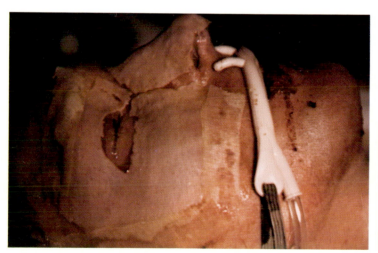

Fig. 3. Early autografting is very important to limit damage by infection and to decrease the cosmetic and functional deformity.

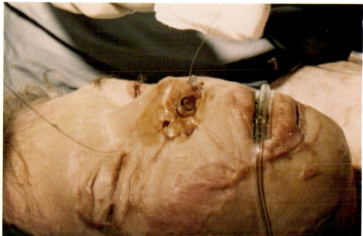

Fig. 4. Early tarsorraphy is often necessary when the lids start to contract. Split-thickness grafts are necessary to correct the contracture.

53

DEPIGMENTATION AND HYPERPIGMENTATION OF THE FACE

John B. Lynch

At the time of initial examination, wounds of the cheek and forehead may be erythematous, blistered, and infused with dirt and debris. These characteristic clinical findings are common in patients exposed to flash and flame burns and, in general, should be treated very conservatively. Minimum irrigation with psyiologic solutions to remove dirt and debris should be performed with extreme gentleness to avoid additional trauma to the area. Burns about the cheeks, forehead and face that may on initial evaluation appear to be full-thickness often heal because of the good vascularity in this area. For this reason, additional trauma should be avoided at the time of initial cleansing and debridement and, if the wounds are clean, blisters should be left intact for the first two or three days to avoid producing a raw, weeping surface which can become desiccated and dehydrated, converting a partial-thickness wound to one that requires grafting. In some patients where direct contact with stoves, flames, or fires have occurred, obvious full-thickness burns will be clinically apparent at the time of examination. These frequently involve eyebrows, eyelids, and the nose and ears, which portends an ominous prognosis regarding deformity after healing of the original burn.

Initial mechanical treatment should be limited to very gentle cleansing and meticulous avoidance of additional trauma. Most of the topical antibacterial agents commonly used in burn treatment contain a caution to avoid application in or near the eye. Sulfamylon or silver sulfadiazine can be applied to burns of the cheek and forehead, but more frequently the use of Neosporin ointment is preferred because of the proximity to the eye, even if Sulfamylon or silver sulfadiazine are being utilized on other parts of the body. **The objective of treatment is to maintain a moist surface with a lubricating ointment to prevent the development of dry, hard crusts on the burn wound surface.** If allowed to develop, these crusts can crack during facial movement and produce localized fissures with bleeding in deep partial-thickness burns. In full-thickness burns, after definite separation of eschar has occurred, split-thickness skin grafts should be applied early to minimize the contracture occurring in open wounds. Sheets of medium or thick split-thickness skin grafts are recommended. **Mesh grafting and other expansion techniques should not be used on the face because of the cobblestone appearance resulting from the use of expanded grafts of this type.**

Surgical debridement of wounds of the face should be extremely limited and conservative and preferably performed daily after the patient has been bathed in the Hubbard tank for softening of the eschar. Conventional surgical debridement of full-thickness eschar on wounds of the cheek or forehead should be delayed for at least two weeks in order to ensure that the area to be debrided is definitely a full-thickness injury. After debridement has occurred, either spontaneously or by a sharp dissection, it is desirable to apply sheets of skin grafts at the earliest opportunity.

DEPIGMENTATION AND HYPERPIGMENTATION

After healing of burns, patchy areas of depigmentation in partial-thickness burns are disconcertingly common. When these occur in a burn that has healed spontaneously and with a smooth surface, the most satisfactory solution for female patients is the use of cosmetics. Many men will not wear them and further will not request any treatment for patchy areas of depigmentation. If more definitive treatment of depigmented areas is requested by patient and appears to be indicated, the best solution is excision of the depigmented areas and primary closure if the defect is small enough to lend itself to this approach. The use of tattooing has been advocated, but it is extremely difficult to get a permanently satisfactory color match and, in general, the effort required is disproportionate to the end result. Dermatologists are continually working with new agents for pigmenting skin in patients who have similar problems secondary to vitiligo, but they cannot be unequivocally recommended at the present time.

More disconcerting than depigmented areas are hyperpigmented areas that occasionally develop following healing of extremely deep partial-thickness burns or full-thickness burns where skin grafting has been required. Often spotty and irregular, these areas give a patchwork appearance to the cheek or forehead and, in addition, may be associated with some thickening, irregularity, and hypertrophy of other scars in this area. The treatment of hyperpigmented areas by cosmetics is less satisfactory than that of depigmented areas and, in addition, is usually unsatisfactory if the hyperpigmentation is associated with thick, irregular hypertrophic scarring that produces an uneven surface. In these patients, the use of extremely superficial dermabrasion is effective in removing the hyperpigmented areas but the long term outlook is uncertain. The hyperpigmentation frequently tends to recur following dermabrasion alone and may be more irregular and less acceptable than the original defect. Dermabrasive smoothing of the hypertrophy in postburn scars of the cheek or forehead has been attempted from time to time and, in the majority of patients, is not completely satisfactory in eliminating irregular areas of hypertrophic scarring over the cheeks and

forehead unless followed by application of skin grafts. A word of caution is necessary prior to dermabrasion for irregularity in scars over the cheek and forehead. The scars are frequently thinner than one would anticipate from clinical evaluation, and dermabrasion frequently results in scattered areas of full-thickness loss. These areas will usually heal spontaneously, but often secondary irregular hypertrophic scarring results.

SUMMARY

Facial burns involving the cheek and forehead occur very frequently. Initial treatment should be limited to minimal debridement required for elimination of dirt and foreign particles on the wound surface. If blisters are present, it is profitable to leave them intact for the first two or three days. If cloudy fluid collects in the blisters, they should be opened. Although Sulfamylon or silver sulfadiazine can be applied to the broad surfaces of the cheeks or forehead, the use of Neosporin to keep the wound soft and to avoid the development of hard, dessicated crusts is preferable. Debridement should be conservative, because wounds that initially appear to be quite deep may heal spontaneously over the cheeks and forehead. For at least two weeks, debridement should be limited to conservative daily debridement following soaking. After two weeks, if thick, adherent, obviously full-thickness eschar is present, it should be surgically debrided in order to obtain a surface for skin grafting at the earliest possible time to minimize the tendency for wound contracture. Treatment of secondary deformities consisting of irregular scarring, contractures, hyper- or hypo-pigmentation of the cheek and forehead is individualized for each specific patient.

The canons of art are merely the expression in specialized forms of the requirements for depth of experience.
Whitehead

54

PIGMENTATION CHANGES OF THE FACE

Lorenzo Mir y Mir

After the skin has been burned, there is often a change in its pigmentation. This occurs both when the burned surface becomes spontaneously epithelialized and when it has been grafted. It appears to make little difference whether the skin graft is applied soon after the burn or much later.

Our experience indicates that the final coloration of the skin is often poor due to **hyperpigmentation** in some patients, while in others the poor esthetic result is due to a **hypopigmentation** or achromia. In still other patients, the pigmentation may be close to normal.

DERMABRASION OF HYPERPIGMENTED SKIN GRAFTS

I have been investigating pigmentation changes of the skin in the burned patient since the late 1950s. At present, our most reliable results are achieved in removing pigmentation from hyperpigmented skin, especially hyperpigmented skin grafts. Through dermabrasion of the hyperpigmented skin graft, at least 12 and preferably 18 months or more after grafting, it has been possible to remove excessive pigmentation. **This time interval is most important.** When the dermabrasion is performed, there will be a temporary depigmentation, which is then followed by hyperpigmentation to a lesser degree than before.

The dermabrasion should be superficial—just deep enough to whiten the skin graft (i.e., only the epidermis is removed). Patients are advised not to expose the dermabraded skin to the sun for at least three months and if possible to lengthen this period to six months because premature exposure to the sun's ultraviolet rays could lead to a recurrence of the hyperpigmentation.

Results from dermabrasion of hyperpigmented skin grafts have been excellent in almost every case (Figures 1 and 2), although in a small percentage of cases the result has not been as good as we would have liked.

There is no similar treatment for hypopigmentation of the skin in the burned patient. The use of cosmetics for camouflaging hypopigmented skin is discussed in another chapter.

PHYSIOLOGIC EXPLANATION OF EFFECTIVENESS OF DERMABRASION

Lerner has demonstrated that the hormone melatonin, which is produced in the pineal gland, and thus acting through the bloodstream and at the peripheral nerve endings, stops the process of melanogenesis in the melanocytes of the skin. Thus vitiligo, according to Lerner, is a consequence of an excessive production of melantonin in the cutaneous nerve endings.

Theoretically, by waiting 12 to 18 months until the hyperpigmented skin graft is reinnervated, the melatonin in these cutaneous nerve endings which are now present prevents a recurrence of the skin hyperpigmentation. It is also theorized that by superficial dermabrasion the nerve endings which produce this hormone are less likely to be damaged.

COLOR MATCH FROM PREVIOUS DONOR SITES

Lopez-Mas and others have described the improved color match of split-thickness skin grafts which are taken from the donor site of a previous split-thickness skin graft. Based on the observation

Fig. 1. This twenty-year-old girl had sustained full-thickness burns of most of the facial skin at one year of age. Multiple split-thickness skin grafts were utilized to replace the scarred contracted facial skin. **A.** Patient's appearance two years after the last skin graft. The skin graft of the left mid-cheek is hyperpigmented. **B.** Appearance of the patient six months after the left half of the face was superficially dermabraded, and just prior to dermabrasion of the right half of the face. The decrease in pigmentation is especially evident in the left cheek and at the junction of dermabraded and non-dermabraded skin graft in the midline of the chin. Although the skin will appear hypopigmented soon after dermabrasion, this is not of concern as it will acquire a normal or near normal pigmentation after a few months.

A   B

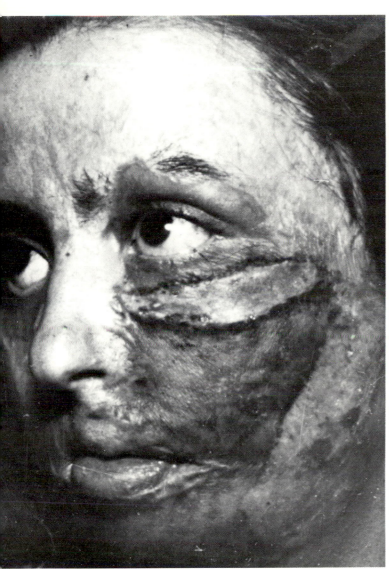
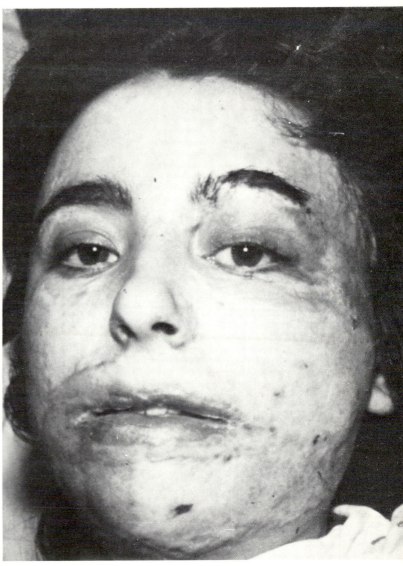

that donor sites which have gone through a noncomplicated healing process have some uniformly permanent and hypopigmented areas, these areas have been used for split-thickness grafts to the face. Either an old donor site is used, or a donor site is prepared by taking a thin split-thickness skin graft from it, then waiting six months before taking a second graft for the face. Evaluations by the authors revealed that no severe hyperpigmentation has occurred, although some patients who had prolonged exposure of the grafts to the sun developed discrete irregular pigmentation. However, these were never more pigmented than the original donor site.

Fig. 2. A. Post-irradiation scar of the chin after x-ray treatment of a hemangioma in infancy. **B.** Full-thickness skin graft in place after a wide extirpation of damaged skin.

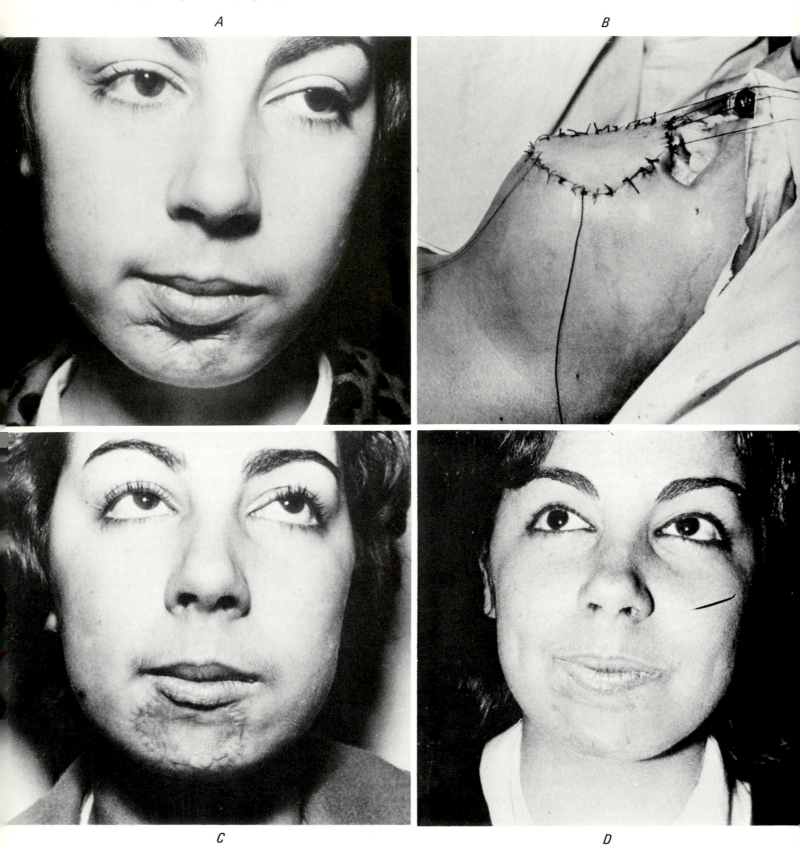

Fig. 2. C. Hyperpigmented skin graft two years after operation, now ready to be dermabraded. **D.** The near normal pigmentation of the skin graft, one year after dermabrasion.

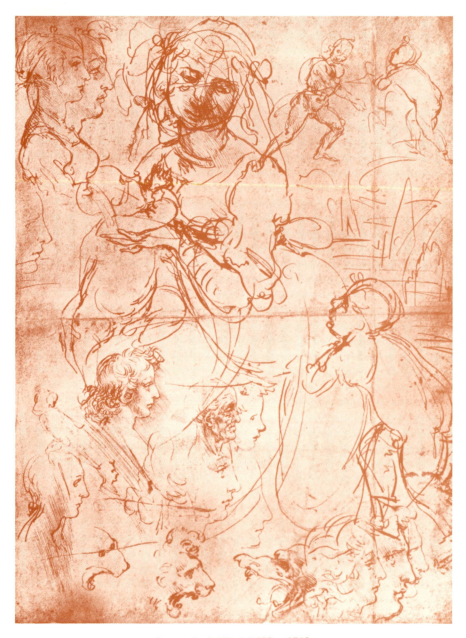

Leonardo da Vinci, 1452 – 1519.

55

RECONSTRUCTION OF FACIAL BURNS

Zvi Neuman
Menachem Ron Wexler

Most facial burns are a mixture of partial-thickness and full-thickness loss. Between the second and third week following burn injury, the wounds are usually either healed or ready for grafting. The primary goals are to close the burn wound, eliminating a source of infection, and to diminish scar tissue formation, secondary contractures, and severe deformity. In the facial skin, contracture appears very early during the healing process because of the presence of loose areolar tissue.

The preference for skin grafting instead of flaps is based on the advantages of readily available skin, early closure of the burn wound, and the resulting reduction of morbidity and hospital stay. The best donor sites with good color match are the retroauricular areas, and inner surfaces of the arms. **Skin grafts, unlike flaps, are without bulk and do not mask facial expression.** They take readily, if applied according to all principles of plastic surgery. The thicker the graft, the better the cosmetic result, and therefore the fewer secondary surgical procedures. Restoration of facial contour and expression, with minimum scar formation, is primary. A second aim is to hide scars, whenever possible, in natural skin lines and shadows.

It takes many months and years for a hypertrophic scar to settle down, soften, and lose its activity. It is of great importance, therefore, to be able to create a patient-doctor relationship which will help to eliminate useless procedures. Courage, patience, and hope are important elements that should be instilled in the patient by all those who surround him during the treatment. Surgeons, nurses, psychologists, and social workers should cooperate to overcome the effects of the burn catastrophe.

Planning the reconstructive procedure is necessary before beginning surgery. This will enable the surgeon to graft in esthetic units, obtain adequate color match, hide scars, and finally obtain both good contour and expression.

Late secondary procedures, such as dermabrasion, overgrafting, and scar excision, are stages in the final rehabilitation of the patient. **The longer these procedures are postponed, the better the results.** Deep abrasion with the Kurtin wire brush permits the removal of scar epithelium and superficial scars. When overgrafting is performed, the skin grafts, taken from the above-mentioned donor sites, are carefully sutured into place. The healing will occur without too much scarring, thus ensuring good cosmetic results. With the wire brush we are usually able to remove the epithelial layer, including a thin layer of scar tissue. Formation of sebaceous cysts under the skin graft is quite rare. But, even if they are found, they do not affect the ultimate cosmetic result. The thin layer of scar tissue which is left behind prevents secondary scar contracture. It should be pointed out that this method is not always applicable in male patients because of the hair follicles that remain embedded deep in the scar.

Skin grafting in patients with dark skin results in deep, dark pigmentation in the skin grafts. They will require rotation, advancement, or even distant flaps to cover the defects.

Upper eyelids are usually covered by split-thickness skin grafts, using double the amount of skin required for the recipient area and with the eyelids fixed by temporary canthorrhaphy. Upper eyelids require thin skin because of their mobility. For lower lids, full-thickness skin grafts are used. Here the aim is stronger support on a lid with less mobility. Superficial scars or scars that develop between graft and recipient areas on the face are dermabraded and over-grafted, using very thin skin. Again, the surgeon should **not** excise all scar tissue in order to prevent later contracture.

CASE STUDIES

In the following cases, the early and late procedures will be illustrated and discussed:

Case 1. The patient was burned by a kerosene stove following a fall due to epilepsy, suffering a deep burn of forehead and a narrow strip on the left upper eyelid. These were grafted using skin from the lateral aspect of the neck. Nevertheless ectropion of the eyelid developed and the lid was regrafted after three months, using a split-thickness skin graft taken again from the lateral aspect of the neck (Figures 1, 2, 3, and 4).

Fig. 1.

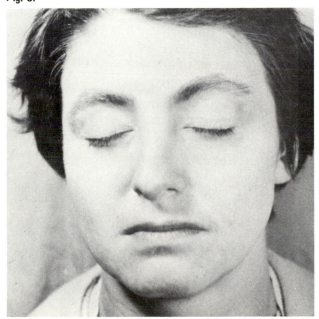

Fig. 2.

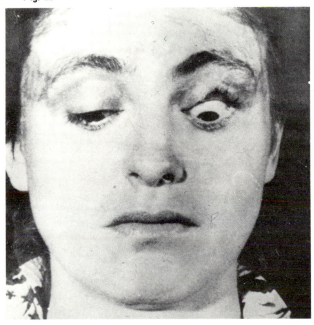

Fig. 3.

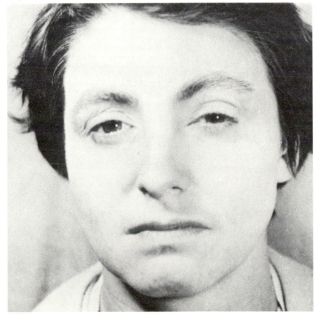

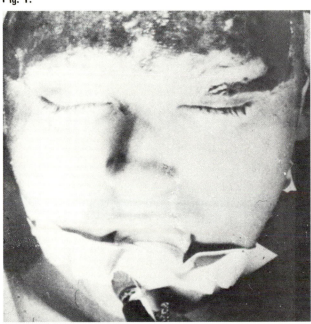

Fig. 4.

Case 2. The following patient is a girl burned at the age of 12 in an open kerosene stove fire. She was treated in another hospital and the wounds of the face were left to heal spontaneously. This took about eight weeks. At the age of 13 (Figure 5), hypertrophic scars were still hard. Scars of the nose were excised and the dorsum was grafted using full-thickness retroauricular skin (Figure 6). The same patient aged 17, following dermabrasion of scars of cheeks and overgrafting (Figure 7).

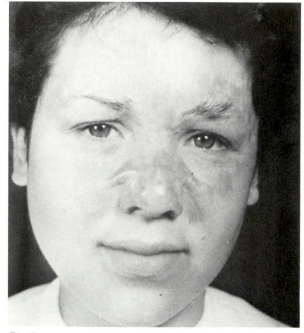

Fig. 5.

Fig. 6.

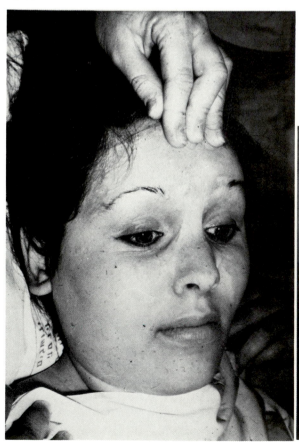

Fig. 7.

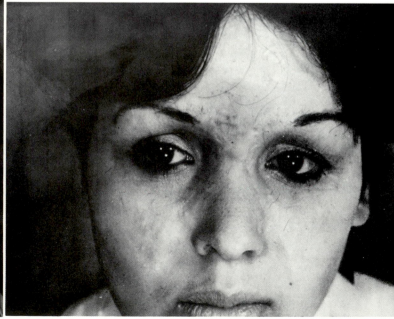

Case 3. The patient is 47 years old. He suffered from a facial burn at the age of three. When admitted to our department he suffered from an extensive scar all over the right side of the face with an ulcer in the middle of his right cheek, which did not heal for four months (Figure 8). The following steps were undertaken: (1) Excision of the scars of the right cheek, and an advancement-rotation flap from the neck was used to cover the defect. Histology of the ulcer showed a basal cell carcinoma adequately excised. (2) Excision of the scar of the nose and defect covered by a full-thickness retroauricular skin graft. (3) A supraclavicular skin graft was inserted into the lower lip to create a flexion crease (Figure 9).

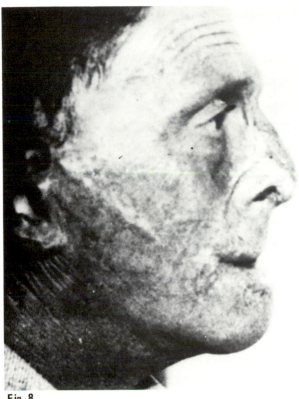

Fig. 8.

Fig. 9.

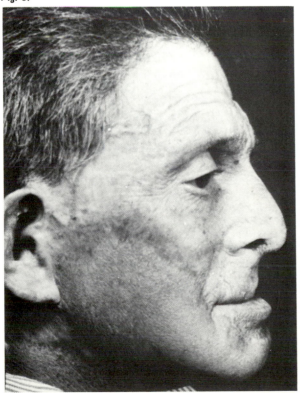

Case 4. The next patient is a little boy aged nine from Cyprus, burned two years before admission (Figures 10 and 11). The procedures undertaken were the following: (1) Skin grafts to eyelids and forehead, taken from the arm. (2) Skin graft to nose (retroauricular). The final results show the patient before he left for home two months after surgery (Figure 12).

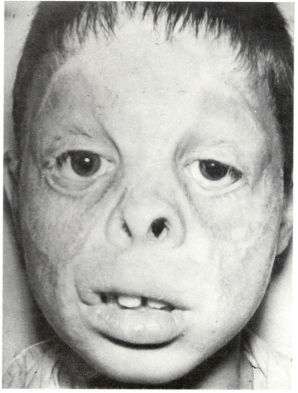

Fig. 10.

Fig. 11.

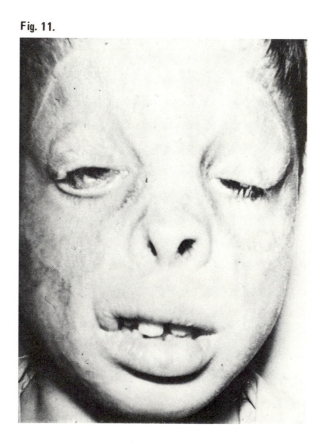

Fig. 12.

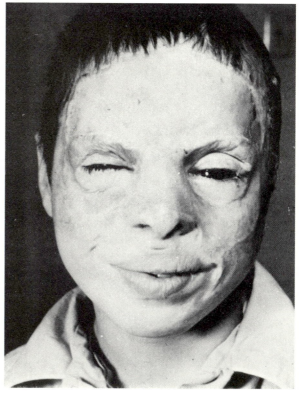

Case 5. The next patient, aged 27, was treated in another hospital for an old burn of the right side of the face. The skin graft applied was taken from the thigh and became dark brown (Figure 13). Attempts to abrade the forehead and cheek were unsuccessful (Figure 14). The procedures undertaken were as follows: (1) Excision of the skin graft and rotation-advancement of a neck and retroauricular flap was used to cover the defect. (2) Dermabrasion and over-grafting improved part of the forehead scar (Figure 15).

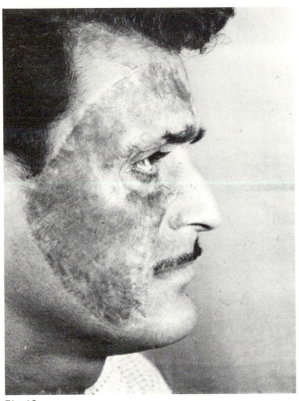

Fig. 13.

Fig. 14.

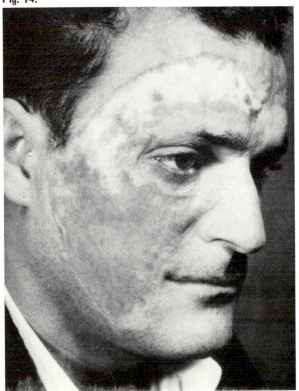

Fig. 15.

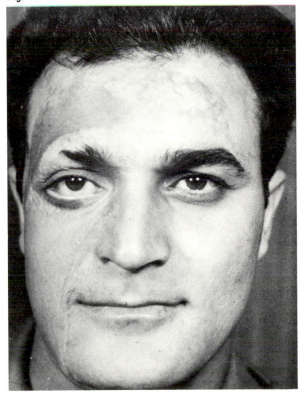

56

DERMAL OVERGRAFTING OF
THE FACE

Noel Thompson

Use of dermal overgrafting to treat disfiguring facial scars was first described by Wilfred Hynes in 1957 as "shaving" and skin grafting. An identical technique used to treat unstable lower-limb scars had, however, been independently reported by George Webster at a meeting of the American Society of Plastic and Reconstructive Surgeons in 1954.

It is generally accepted that free skin grafts become vascularized within 48 hours of transplantation by direct anastomosis of graft and host vessels at the recipient site. Hynes pointed out that mature scars possess a much richer capillary circulation than is generally supposed and are, in fact, capable of vascularizing skin grafts with much more reliability than subcutaneous fat. Removal of the thin, superficial epidermis from the scar discloses a multitude of easily visible fine punctate capillary bleeding points. These are available for anastomosis to the vascular elements in the graft, so that the latter's dermal capillary plexus is restored speedily and with certainty. With careful technique, failure of graft take is almost unknown.

In scars, the surface epidermis is thin, devoid of papillae, and without the epidermal appendages found in normal skin (i.e., hair follicles, sebaceous glands, and sweat ducts) projecting into the underlying dermis. Thus the possible, but always minor, complication of epidermoid cyst formation from buried epithelial elements is almost completely eliminated. Such cyst formation can occur only from the epithelial elements in the applied skin graft, a hazard present in all types of skin grafting procedures. Because of its simplicity and reliability, dermal overgrafting constitutes the treatment of choice in the cosmetic improvement of extensive scars in burn patients (Figure 1).

INDICATIONS FOR DERMAL OVERGRAFTING

The mature burn scar of good quality cannot be improved by dermal overgrafting. Where persisting hypertrophy with surface irregularity or altered pigmentary values are present, the use of overgrafting will result in caucasians in a flat, pale, minimally depressed, slightly glossy grafted surface of uniform texture and color. In dark races, the color values are usually good, but may be uniformly darkened, usually to a limited degree.

The best results are obtained by deferring treatment for about one year after primary healing has been obtained. Active, florid scars accept the graft with equal certainty, but tend to again become thickened and raised.

Although chiefly used to improve the surface appearance, the method has particular applicability to the treatment of scars touching important structures, such as exposed frontal meninges in burned epileptics or major vessels of the upper neck. In such cases, a thick split skin graft is used to give maximum protection.

Minor contractures affecting the angle of the mouth, nasal alae, or palpebral fissure, may be relieved when extensive adjacent superficial scars are treated by dermal overgrafting. The entire thickness of the residual scar tissue is divided using a number of parallel cuts at right angles to the direction of contracture before applying the surface skin graft.

TECHNIQUE OF DERMAL OVERGRAFTING

The scarred area is outlined using pen and ink. By keeping in mind the aesthetic units of the face, particularly pleasing results are obtained by extending the boundaries of the area to be treated to the hairline posteriorly, the jawline below, and the nasolabial groove anteriorly. The entire surface to be denuded of epidermis is then painted with marking ink and allowed to dry so that any unremoved surface epithelium is more readily seen. This is important because it is essential that epidermal cells be completely removed.

Surface epidermis can be removed by sandpapering, dermabrasion, dermatone, or by freehand graft knife. I prefer the freehand graft knife because it makes splitting the epidermis impossible. Dermabrasion carries with it the potential risk of ground in epidermal cells acting as centers for epithelial proliferation in the recipient site bed. The free capillary host bleeding that results is readily controlled by pressure with a gauze swab soaked in saline-epinephrine (1:200,000) solution, reserving pinpoint electrocoagulation for persistent points of hemorrhage. It is imperative that hemostasis should be absolute before the surface graft is applied.

Where cosmetic values—rather than functional resistance to pressure—alone are concerned, as in facial scars, the skin graft is cut thinly and applied without tension to the "shaved" recipient site, sutured at the periphery and at other scattered points (using a fine interrupted nonabsorbable suture), and the peripheral excess graft carefully trimmed. Pressure is applied, usually with tieover sutures and a dressing of petrolatum gauze reinforced by cotton wool firmly

wrung out in saline. When the cotton wool dehydrates after a few hours, it achieves the consistency of papier-maché, effectively immobilizing the grafted region. Surface adhesive strapping reinforces the fixation. The take of the graft is so certain that elaborate immobilization is not needed.

The graft is dressed on the seventh day, all sutures are removed, and the area is left exposed.

COMPLICATIONS

Complete take of the graft is the rule, in the absence of hematoma formation or infection. The former results from inadequate hemostasis; the latter is a failure of aseptic technique.

Co-optation of the margins of the graft to the periphery of the treated recipient site may not always be perfect. When a stepped edge is present at the junction with host tissue, it is trimmed flush by a scalpel blade or by dermabrasion under local anaesthesia as a secondary procedure.

In the early weeks following grafting, minute, white, miliary cysts may appear on the graft surface. These are invariably epidermoid inclusion cysts arising from elements of epidermal appendages (usually hair follicles) in the graft or in the underlying host dermis, where it is present. The cysts respond to simple unroofing by gentle scraping of the surface (without anaesthesia) and show no tendency to recur after a few months.

Fig. 1. **A.** Preoperative appearance of healed facial burn in a girl nine years of age. **B.** Postoperative appearance at age 11 years, after dermal overgrafting. Trimming of the uneven margin of the graft was done subsequently under local anesthesia. (Photos courtesy of Wilfred Hynes, F.R.C.S.)

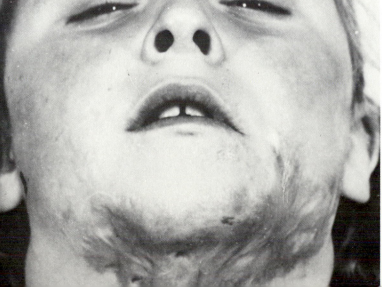
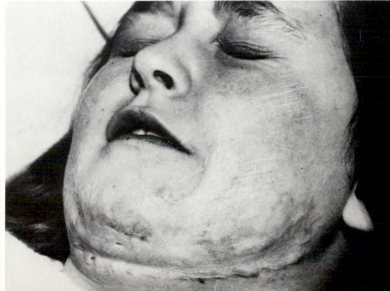

57

MULTIPLE EXCISION OF THE FACE

John E. Hoopes

HISTORICAL REVIEW

A review of the evolutionary history of multiple excision (**excisions successives**, gradual partial excision, serial excision) provides, in itself, a most interesting commentary on the progressive and sequential nature of developments in plastic surgery and emphasizes the essential relationship between technical and conceptual progress. The technique was born at the turn of the century, developed falteringly until World War II, achieved its zenith of popularity during the 1940s and 50s and currently finds limited applicability, particularly in the management of cervicofacial burn sequelae.

In essence, the multiple excision technique consists of performing the maximal excision that will allow primary closure; the procedure is repeated after a healed wound has been achieved and sufficient time (e.g., six months to one or two years) has elapsed to permit further stretching of the skin. The excision generally is elliptical in design and is outlined entirely within the scar, except at the final stage. John Staige Davis exhibited few reservations in describing the advantages of the technique:

> I have used gradual partial excision with closure successfully in removing extensive scars, large pigmented moles, x-ray and radium burns, localized scleroderma, keloid, etc., and have found that by this procedure these cutaneous disfigurements may be eliminated without mutilation, and that better results may be better obtained than by any other method with which I am familiar.

Ferris Smith must be considered the champion of multiple excision. He is credited with pursuance of the principle to its ultimate utilization:

Methods other than multiple excision mask a loss, restore function to a large degree, but leave much to be desired from a cosmetic standpoint. These are procedures of necessity rather than procedures of choice. The end results of pedicled flaps, rotated forehead flaps, and free skin grafts are such that they should never be considered procedures of choice for facial repair.

Smith emphasized the importance of distinguishing, for planning purposes, between functional and cosmetic procedures and between procedures of necessity and procedures of choice; he obviously felt quite strongly that " a desirable cosmetic result is rarely obtained with transplanted skin flaps and grafts." His publications illustrate that excellent results are obtainable by means of multiple excision, utilization of Z-plasty for the purpose of transferring abnormal skin to an area from which it can be removed by serial partial excision, and skin grafting with subsequent gradual removal of the graft. These publications do not, however, comment on the period of time required for completion of reconstruction and/or the number of operative procedures involved. Richard Stark advocated the concept, but his advocacy also contains the major deterrent to employment of the technique:

> Large burn scars of the face are best treated in the same manner as large benign nevi: multiple partial excision with either a rotation or advancement skin flap from the neck or postauricular region if it is unscarred and otherwise suitable.

Wallace Steffensen and Eugene Worthen realistically defined the limitations of multiple excision. Current thinking tends to recognize their observation that "the law of diminishing return works overtime with serial partial excision" and their admonition that one "be not a slave to a principle, or it may make a slave of you." Lack of widespread acceptance of the technique is indicated by the fact that relatively few publications, other than those of Ferris Smith, suggest this method of approach.

DISADVANTAGES

The technique of multiple excision possesses both inherent disadvantages and disadvantages specific to the correction of burn scar deformity. Multiple hospitalizations and operative stages are required, with substantial periods of time of necessity intervening between these stages. Correction of a major facial deformity utilizing only multiple excision may require years. A relative soft tissue redundancy in the proposed area of serial excision is essential, and this redundancy seldom coexists with post-traumatic deformity. Particular attention must be directed to the prevention of distortion in critical areas; i.e., hairline, eyebrows, eyelids, nostrils, and mouth. Successful employment of gradual partial excision requires that the maximum quantity of tissue possible be excised at each stage; wound closure in the presence of excessive tension rather commonly leads to unsatisfactory, hypertrophic scarring. Steffensen introduced the objection that multiple excision is contraindicated in areas overlying bony prominences in children on the basis that excessive soft tissue tension can result in growth retardation.

The outstanding characteristic of a healed burn wound, whether healing has been achieved primarily or by grafting, is a deficiency of skin. In addition, the healed severely traumatized tissues possess low biologic quality and do not tolerate excessive tension and/or sophisticated transfer techniques. Cervical skin is more subject to full-thickness burning than facial skin, and it is somewhat unusual to encounter a patient who demonstrates severe burn scar deformity of the face without involvement of the neck; transferring severely scarred neck skin to the cheek serves no useful purpose. Many procedures described as multiple excision in reality consist of excision of the burn scar and resurfacing by means of a cervical rotation or advancement flap.

ESTHETIC UNITS

The significance of esthetic units of the face cannot be overemphasized in terms of optimal camouflage of facial scars. The topographic anatomy of the face creates a number of esthetic units; and, whenever possible, an area corresponding precisely to one esthetic unit should be resurfaced in one stage in order to achieve the optimal cosmetic result. Scars lying within an esthetic unit immediately call attention to themselves; scars located at the periphery of an esthetic unit frequently pass unnoticed.

SUMMARY

The gradual decline of the multiple excision technique was initiated by a number of factors; by acceptance of the limitations of multiple excision, by the recognition of the concept that split-thickness skin graft color-match bears a direct relationship to the proximity of the donor site to the recipient site, by the development of the mechanical dermatome which permitted the taking of split-thickness skin grafts from the flush areas of the neck, and by emphasis on the importance of visualizing the face in terms of esthetic units. The multiple excision technique has now found its level and is limited to the removal of localized facial scars with surrounding normal skin (Figure 1), burn scar alopecia of the scalp, and hypertrophic scarring in the nasolabial fold regions.

Fig. 1. A. Hypertrophic scar of the left cheek caused by a burn at the age of six years. B. A two-stage multiple excision was performed at two and three years post-burn. In spite of the one-year interval, wound tension was substantial at the time of the second procedure.

A   B

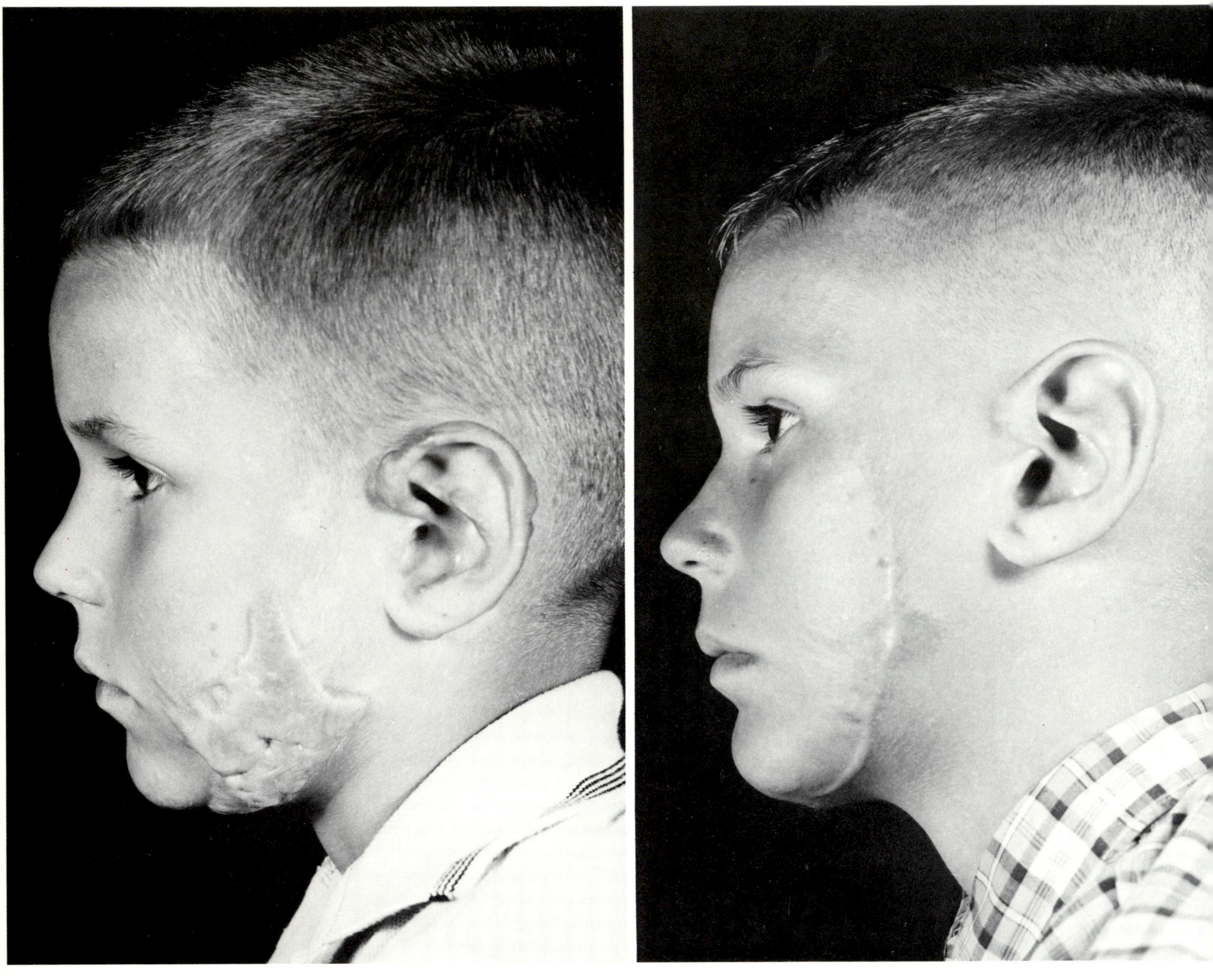

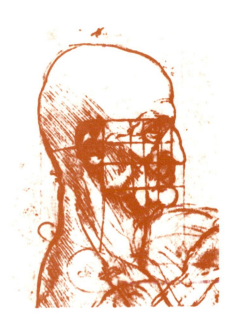

Leonardo da Vinci, 1452 — 1519.

Those who do not remember the errors of past are condemned to repeat them.

Santayana

58

EXCISION OF FACIAL SCARS

John B. Lynch

EARLY REACTION TO SCARRING

After deep burns have healed, either spontaneously or with the application of skin grafts, there is a characteristic hypertrophic scar phase. This is manifested clinically by thick, elevated, indurated hypertrophic scar tissue, which may be fiery red in color. During this phase, some discomfort in the form of itching, stinging, and similar symptoms is often present.

These symptoms can be minimized by regular application of bland, lubricating ointments, although an occasional patient's itching may be so intense that antipruritic medication is required. In selected patients, the symptoms can often be minimized by injection of steroid preparations (triamcinalone acetonide) directly into the scar if burn scars are relatively localized. It should be emphasized that this period of scarring is to be anticipated following most burns and does not necessarily represent keloid formation. This intense hypertrophic reaction is seen frequently following very deep partial-thickness burns that heal under the influence of the currently utilized topical burn agents. This reaction is also frequently encountered where incomplete take of primary skin grafts is obtained on full-thickness burns and supplemental grafting is required. With the passage of several months, maturation of the scar tissue becomes evident by regression of the redness, softness and improved texture of the scars and subsidence of the symptoms of itching and burning. The application of pressure in the form of elastic bandages or compression splints is helpful in hastening the resolution of the scar hypertrophy.

BURN SCAR EXCISION

The residual scarring can produce either functional or cosmetic deformities or both, which may require reconstruction. If the resulting scars are relatively localized or produce linear bands, simple scar excision with or without Z-plasty may be all that is required. More often, however, the burn scars tend to be broad and are frequently rough and irregular and involve so much tissue that only excision and resurfacing of the defect is feasible.

Donor Site. Excision of burn scars with skin grafting is a definitive, major reconstructive procedure. As such, the patient should be hospitalized, and general anesthesia will ordinarily be required. Selection of donor areas for the skin graft is of importance in that the reconstructed skin should be unscarred and free of defects or blemishes. The desirability of saving good donor sites for possible reconstruction should be kept in mind at the time of original grafting during the acute phase. Using the neck or supraclavicular area as donor areas in an attempt to improve the color match has been advocated from time to time. However, if the face requires resurfacing for burn scars, the neck is frequently involved with scars as well. Also, the size of graft required for resurfacing a forehead or cheek often makes adjacent donor areas unsuitable.

Excision. All burn scars should be adequately excised to ensure that any contracture that has occurred will be adequately corrected. The shrinkage that occurs after the burn wound heals will usually result in relaxation of the skin after a scar has been removed. For this reason, the scar should be excised first and then the skin graft removed to fit the resulting defect. The excision of the scar should be planned to incorporate triangles at the corners and along straight edges to minimize the possibility of secondary contracture of straight line scars that may necessitate additional Z-plasty or other touch-ups at a later date.

Grafting. Delaying the application of skin grafts for 24 to 48 hours after excision of scar has been advocated from time to time as a method of insuring hemostasis and enhancing graft take. This method is useful in release of functional contractures of the extremity, but for definitive reconstructive procedures involving excision of burn scars from the face, I feel that immediate application of very thick skin grafts with a complete take of the graft will give the best possible results. The resurfacing skin graft should be one sheet to avoid additional seams when this is possible. Obviously, **mesh grafting or other similar techniques are contraindicated in reconstructive procedures of this type.** The repair should be made with a very thick split-thickness graft (.018 to .024 inches in adults). The texture of the skin will be superior to that achieved when thin grafts are used and the tendency for secondary contracture with production of secondary deformities is less. The morbidity of the deep donor areas can be minimized by covering them with a second thinner graft (.008 to .012 inches) to obtain early healing.

Minimizing Hypertrophic Scarring. Often after resurfacing, there is a disconcerting tendency for temporary hypertrophic scars to develop at the suture lines. This tendency can be minimized by insuring that all contracture has been corrected by complete scar excision, by using a graft of adequate size that fits snugly but without tension, and by incorporating triangular Z's to minimize straight line contractures during the postoperative period. Lines of scar excision should be planned to utilize normal expression lines whenever possible. Additionally, the use of firm supporting pressure for a period of many weeks is helpful in patients showing a tendency toward excessive scar hypertrophy.

Indications and Technique. Excision of burn scars and skin grafting is frequently indicated about

the face, either to correct mild contracture, such as ectropion of the eyelids or mouth, or to resurface broad, irregular, raised areas of scar on the cheeks, forehead, or nose. Occasionally, burn scars in the beard area in men cause difficulty in shaving and may contribute to a recurring folliculitis which may require resurfacing of large areas of hair-bearing tissues.

If excision and skin grafting of the cheek is being performed to correct eyelid ectropion, excision of the scar should be followed with application of full-thickness grafts to the lower eyelid and very thick split-thickness or full-thickness grafts of the upper eyelid. For release of contractures about the lips, mouth, and chin, thick split-thickness grafts are preferred. Occasionally, temporary lip tarsorrhaphy is helpful in correcting severe contracture of the lip. On the other hand, if resurfacing is to eliminate broad, irregular, thick scarring, the area should be resurfaced as a unit unless the scarring is extremely localized. For example, the entire forehead, entire nose, entire cheek, entire upper or entire lower lip should be covered as a single anatomic unit for optimum results. Incisions should be placed in expression lines when possible, and in general, lines should be straight instead of semicircular, since semicircular lines can produce late secondary deformities (Figures 1 and 2).

Meticulous hemostasis must be obtained and skin grafts sutured into the defect meticulously with careful edge approximation. Although full-thickness grafts should usually be used on the lower eyelids, thick split-thickness grafts are satisfactory for resurfacing the forehead and cheeks.

SUMMARY

Excising broad areas of burn scars and resurfacing with skin grafts is required for functional or cosmetic reasons in many post-burn patients. If obvious contractures of flexion surfaces are excluded, this procedure is required most frequently about the hands and face. This is a major definitive reconstructive procedure requiring complete excision of all the scar, meticulous hemostasis, application of thick split-thickness skin grafts, and meticulous postoperative care to insure the best possible result.

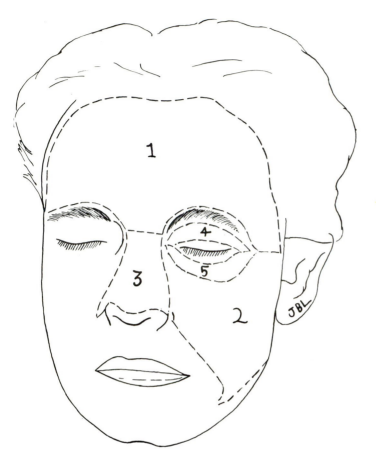

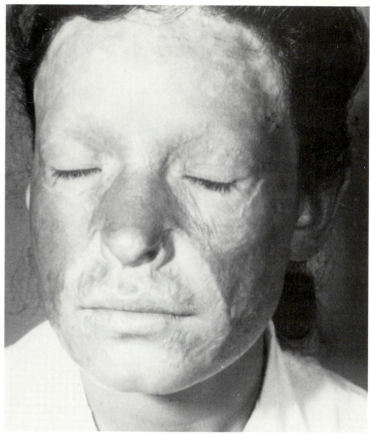

Fig. 1. Outlined are the anatomic areas of the forehead, cheek, and the adjacent areas of nose and eyelids marked by the dotted lines. Note that resurfacing of the forehead should extend to near the lateral canthal area and proceed in an almost transverse fashion back to the hairline and should extend in the midline down to the root of the nose where the scar will be more acceptable than having it transversely across the forehead above the eyebrows. In resurfacing area 2 on the cheek, the inferior border should lie slightly below the inferior border of the mandible, as scarring along the mandible often tends to remain hypertrophic for an inordinately long time.

Fig. 2. Appearance of a patient with extensive burn scars of the face where a resurfacing of the forehead, nose, cheek, and eyelids has been performed. At a later date, eyebrow reconstruction was performed.

204

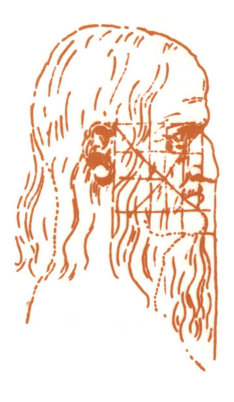

Leonardo da Vinci, 1452 — 1519.

While there is life there's hope; the dead, I ween, are hopeless.
         Theocritus (3rd Century B.C.)

He is the best physician who is the best inspirer of hope.
        Samuel Taylor Coleridge

59

DERMA-CORRECTIVE COSMETICS

Michael G. Westmore

Derma-corrective is a term Marvin Westmore and I use to describe our techniques for camouflaging scars and discoloration of the face and body. These techniques have been developed both through extensive research and study with actual patients.

Before attempting a cosmetic solution, those who require assistance must first be analyzed to determine their skin condition, skin coloring, and skin texture. The physician must be satisfied that sufficient healing has taken place before the patient begins any camouflage or beautification (Figure 1).

It should be mentioned that few men will wear cosmetics despite severe deformity, although they will accept the use of hairpieces and glasses. Sometimes a thin application of the cosmetic will be acceptable to a man who is reluctant to wear more elaborate makeup.

Generous cleansing and lubrication of skin with cremes, moisturizers and lubricants is essential to the treatment of burned skin because of the loss of natural oil and water. Cosmetics or skin care products which are drying must be avoided. We prefer cosmetic products that have had the known allergens removed and are thus hypoallergenic.

UNDERTONE MAKEUP

The first step, after conditioning the skin, is the application of an undertone makeup. Undertone is the generic name of creme and stick cosmetics used to camouflage a discoloration of the previously burned skin before applying the normal cosmetic foundation. In men who may object to wearing of cosmetics, a light application of undertone and powder will aid in balancing a natural skin tone.

Fig. 1. A. The skin grafts are very smooth and white. The areas around the eyes and mouth are not burned; therefore the skin is a fair, natural pink tone. The problem was to select a foundation makeup that would blend with the patient's natural complexion and warm-up the white grafted skin. Note the loss of eyebrow hair and hair of widow's peak.

A

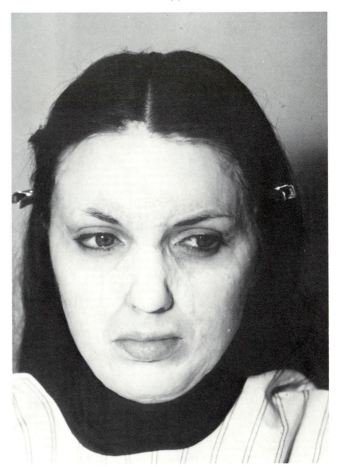

Fig. 1. B. The entire face was cleaned with a cleansing lotion applied from a cotton patt. **C.** Moisture creme was applied to the face on a piece of white sponge. The moisture creme provides a better surface for adherence of the makeup.

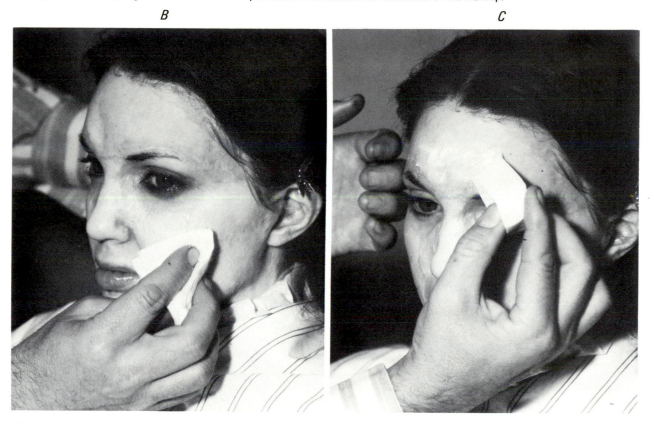

Fig. 1. D. Due to the light coloration of the skin grafts it was not necessary to apply an undertone makeup. The "beige" creme makeup foundation patted on gave sufficient coverage. **E.** Completed makeup: emphasis placed on eye makeup. Rouge blusher was applied for natural warmth and facial contour. Areas of lost hair are filled in with pencil.

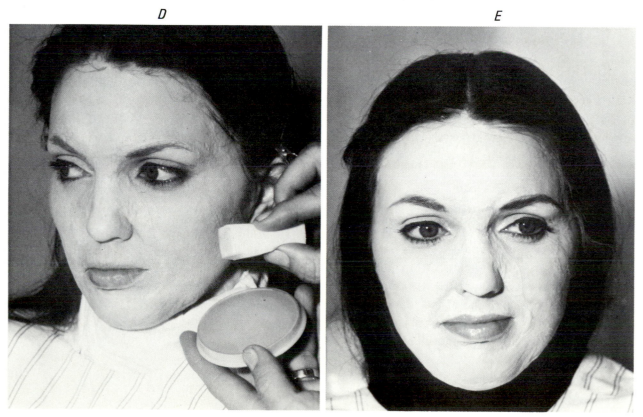

There are several shades of undertone which may be applied to disguise or diminish discoloration; the most widely used **for blocking purple and redness are warm and cool tones of yellow ochre.** The deeper the redness the less the warmth in the undertone. Warmth refers to a slight hint of pink or orange in the yellow ochre and cool refers to a greenish cast. Skin **discolorations of brown and yellow are concealed with a peach or amber undertone.** Due to the extreme variations of skin discoloration, it will be necessary to experiment with different colors to find the one which will perfectly blend with the natural skin tone. As healing progresses and the scarred areas become less erythematous, the undertone colors can also be changed and lightened.

THE STIPPLING TECHNIQUE

Essential to the successful use of cosmetics is the method with which they are applied. The stippling method, which uses a smooth or coarse sponge and a rapid, patting motion to apply the makeup, allows the makeup to evenly cover and blend over the affected area.

Partial-Thickness Burns. The skin of a partial-thickness burn will eventually return to its normal state, but while it is healing there will be a surface redness. This can be easily eliminated by stippling over the redness and blending out the edges with an undertone color of ochre. A light powder and normal cosmetic foundation are then applied.

Full-Thickness Burns. Skin-grafted burns are the most difficult to analyze and to cosmetically correct. Skin grafts do not have a pore structure and the smooth skin will not easily hold makeup. When cosmetics do not adhere, a thin coat of **pure castor oil** must be stippled over the area before applying the undertone makeup. Healed partial-thickness burns with their very tightly closed pore structure also require a thin castor oil coat before undertone.

In situations where the skin graft has a reddish, purple, or pale blue cast, a yellow undertone is selected. If the cast of the skin graft is yellowish or brown, an undertone ranging from peach to amber is

chosen. Because of the grease contained in the undertone and in the castor oil, the makeup should be sufficiently powdered and then all the excess powder removed by blotting with a damp sponge or cotton ball.

FOUNDATION SELECTION AND APPLICATION

A foundation which most complements the natural skin tone, but does not contain pink or rose, should be selected.

In **minor burns,** when a foundation makeup is not desired, the undertone makeup should offer sufficient concealment. Where the undertone is covering sufficiently, light liquid foundations can be applied and blended up to the undertone but not necessarily applied over it. For men, who are usually reluctant to wear makeup, a light, thin application will not appear as a cosmetic.

Following skin grafting, the foundation must have enough coverage to camouflage the undertone. We have found that creme, stick, or Pan-Cake foundation will have to be applied to provide this opacity.

When a foundation is applied over an undertone, it must be patted or stippled on with a piece of white latex sponge. The **fingers should not be used** to apply the foundation over the undertone, **because their warmth has a tendency to lift or move the makeup.**

NATURAL MAKEUP FOR CAMOUFLAGE

Following the application of a woman's selected foundation, moist eye shadow can be applied to the eyelids and moist rouge may be applied to the cheeks. Both of these products may be used to further disguise facial scarring and to bring forth natural beauty. When a subtle application of color is desired, the dry, brush-on types of rouge and eye shadow may be used to enhance the features after powdering. Colored eye shadows and rouges are very effective because they aid in diminishing the defect and drawing an inquisitive eye away from the problem area. Blue and green eye shadow are best for disguising eyelid problems. In selecting cheek rouges, peach or amber are best for fair complexions and coral or orange for dark complexions.

Generally, advice concerning natural cosmetic application and selection should be sought from one of the local demonstrators of the recommended cosmetics listed at the end of this chapter.

CONTOUR MAKEUP

To help correct the loss of facial expression due to a burn, the face should be balanced with an undertone makeup before foundation makeup is applied. Highlights and shadows are blended onto the foundation before any powder is applied.

A shadow is a foundation makeup, at least two shades darker than the normal foundation which is used to diminish an area. A highlight is a foundation or lightener, at least two shades lighter than the normal foundation, used to bring forth an area. In either case the correction used must be light or dark enough to provide a contrast with the normal foundation and to effectively cosmetically contour a flat or expressionless area. This type of makeup takes a great deal of practice to keep the image from appearing theatrical. **The key to this technique is subtleness** through the art of blending.

After the highlights and shadows have been applied and blended, the powder is patted on and any excess removed with a damp sponge. If additional contour is necessary, it may be applied with the use of dry shadows. Shades of brown and gray will help deepen the areas, while white, toast, or mushroom shades will bring forth highlights. Following contouring in a woman, a dry rouge can be applied to the cheeks and jawline to further develop a natural effect.

Extreme Cases. In extreme cases of facial disfigurement it may be necessary to fill voids with derma wax or to have a form-fitting facial prosthesis constructed. This would be applied first, then followed with any of the cosmetic solutions which have been described.

COSMETICS TO SIMULATE THE BEARDED AREA OF THE FACE

A major problem for men is the non-hair-bearing skin graft in the bearded area. In most instances the graft will appear to be clean shaven, necessitating that the patient shave around it several times a day, but even then the beard-growing area will not match the skin graft. When a normal, shaved beard line needs to be simulated, the theatrical technique of applying a stipple beard will blend the scarred area with the natural beard area. This is a technique that requires practice. It consists of patting a makeup color onto the non-hair-bearing skin with a coarse or pored sponge. A makeup color that will match the natural beard line must be selected and may range from a very light brown to a heavy blue or gray. These colors will have to be purchased from a theatrical makeup supplier. After stippling the makeup on the face, it must be powdered and the excess powder removed with a damp sponge or cotton. The powder will set the makeup and keep it from smearing. More information on this technique can be found in theatrical makeup texts.

ARTIFICIAL HAIR GOODS AND EYEGLASSES

False Beards and Moustaches. There are several areas in which artificial hair goods can replace permanent or temporary losses. Where possible and comfortable, good hairlace beards and moustaches can be used to disguise grafted skin. False beards and moustaches can be matched and constructed to an individual's hair color and styled to complement his personality. With practice, false hair goods can be applied, dressed, and cleaned by the wearer. Directions for the wearing and caring for these pieces may also be obtained from the manufacturer or found in theatrical makeup texts.

Wigs. Wigs may be used by males and females alike to disguise and cover the head. With an amount of creativity, they can be styled to cover and detract from the burned scalp. We highly recommend the new prestyled synthetics since they are both easy to care for and inexpensive.

Eyeglasses. Eyeglasses, with their attractive frames and colored lenses, can be used skillfully to disguise a problem around the eye area. Many eyeglass companies specialize in artistic frames, which should be chosen to complement the facial shape as well as for their attractiveness. The color of the frame should blend with the patient's own coloring. For additional effect, the upper frame may be the eyebrow. The most practical colored lenses are gray, dark green, and brown; these colors not only disguise but also offer the eyes maximum protection from the sunlight.

Eyebrows. Eyebrows can skillfully be reproduced with an eyebrow pencil, if it is impossible to perform a hair graft. The colored eyebrow pencil should match the patient's own hair coloring and should be applied in individual hairline strokes. To accomplish this, the pencil must be sharpened with a razor blade. The same companies that construct hairlace beards and moustaches can also construct stylish false eyebrows. Males should have false brows made, since penciling is not an acceptable solution for a man.

Eyelashes. False eyelashes, for both the top and bottom lids, have become so common that they are now foolproof accessories. To appear natural, a false lash should be selected for its uneven flair and thinness; thicker lashes are used for feminine glamour. A clear base or individually applied lashes heighten the natural appearance.

CONCLUDING REMARKS

Whatever the problem, small or large, the key to corrective cosmetics for the burned patient is learning those techniques which are most complementary to individual needs. The patient must have a desire to learn and practice, and I can say with assurance that when a person can confidently apply and wear corrective cosmetics he or she will have a brighter outlook not only on meeting old friends, but making new ones as well.

REFERENCE SOURCES

M.G. Westmore Cosmetic Studio
15910 Ventura Boulevard
Encino, California 91316

The Art of Theatrical Makeup
Author, Michael G. Westmore
Publisher, McGraw-Hill Book Company,
New York, 1966

RECOMMENDED COSMETICS

Allercreme
Almay
Clinique
Max Factor
Physicians Formula

*All names referred to in this chapter except for Pan-Cake are generic names; Pan-Cake is the trade name of Max Factor's water soluble foundation.

The form of a Noſe artificially made, both alone by it ſelf, and alſo with the upper lip covered with the hair of the Beard.

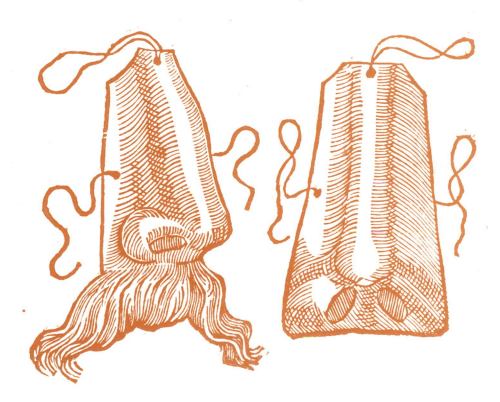

The Works of that Famous Chirurgeon: Ambrose Parey, 1678.

It is not so much what you say in a book that constitutes its value . . . (but) all you would like to say, which nourishes it secretly.

Gide

60

COSMETIC CLASSES

Irving Feller

Reconstructive operations of the face can improve the patient's function and appearance to a certain point. The skillful use of cosmetics can be very helpful to the patient who has burn scars. It is not sufficient to tell the patient to use cosmetics. Some may not be able to find the best cosmetician or may be reluctant to seek help on their own because of their feeling embarrassed about the scars.

Cosmetic classes are being developed at the Michigan Burn Center to provide the patient with the best products, professional cosmetologists and an environment to learn the appropriate cosmetics for their specific problem. The teachers are professional cosmetologists and patients who have learned to use cosmetics successfully. The latter are excellent teachers. They have learned to adapt the available products to provide the best cover for the burn scars, and communicate best with their fellow patients.

Patients are invited to attend the classes before they are discharged from the hospital during their acute admission and are continued on an outpatient basis.

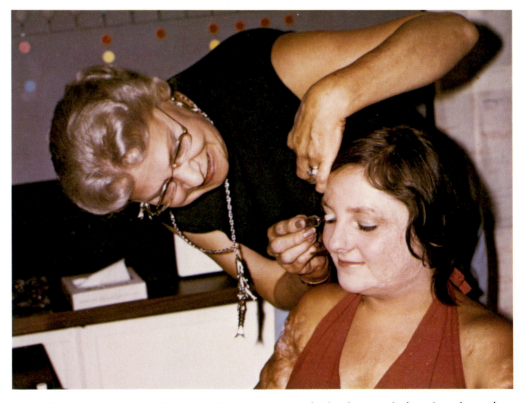

Fig. 1. The patient is instructed in the use of cosmetics by a professional cosmetologist and another patient who has gained expertise in using available products.

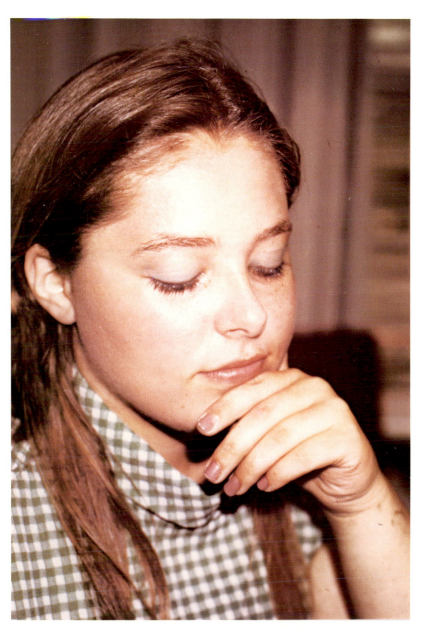

Fig. 2. There are many cosmetics on the market. Instructions given in the proper environment provide the patient knowledge of how to choose the best cosmetics and how to best apply them.

IX.

THE LIPS

PRINCIPLES OF TREATMENT

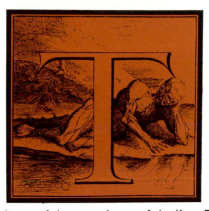

here is a difference between electrical burns and thermal burns of the lips. The former occurs almost exclusively in young children and there is usually deep destruction of muscle in a limited area. The thermal burns involve skin loss and scar contracture causing lip eversion and microstomia as the two main problems.

The principles in correction of lip eversion and microstomia are release of scar contracture with or without excision and adding tissue by a free autograft, split- or full-thickness, or a pedicle graft.

Thompson has described the essentials of treating electrical burn of the lips. There is a recent addition to the armamentarium of treating electrical burns of the commissure of the lips. This is the use of a tongue flap to the lower lip, two to three weeks post-burn. The rectangular tongue flap is raised from the smooth epithelium of the lateral anterior tongue tip and is based toward the dorsum. The flap should extend from the commissure to the medial extent of the burn defect. Muscle is included in the flap to provide bulk, and a deep traction suture of 3-0 chromic catgut is inserted. The child is fed a liquid and soft diet. Two weeks later the base of the flap is divided. A flap is not needed in the upper lip.

Irving Feller

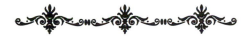

62

ELECTRIC BURNS TO THE MOUTH

Hugh G. Thomson

Electrical burns to the mouth are a common injury in the one-to-four-year age group. The destruction of soft tissue results both from the flash and from the current flowing through the tissues. The heat generated is proportional to the square of the current times the resistance ($H = I^2 R$). The extension cord at the male-female junction is the major causative agent and the oral commissure is the most commonly involved area (Figure 1). Because most houses are well insulated the current flows from the hot to the neutral lead using the moist lip as the regional conductor because it has lower resistance than any other route.

This injury creates a type of coagulative necrosis and regional endarteritis. The resultant excessive cicatrical contraction is quite unique and demonstrates extremely slow regression. These two factors will directly influence the timing of the reconstruction. For all electrical burns of the mouth supportive care is all that is initially necessary in the treatment

Fig. 1. Common mechanism of electrical burn injury.

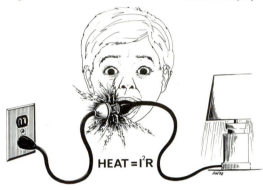

HEAT = I²R

program. It is essential to maintain good oral hygiene and adequate caloric intake, and to anticipate spontaneous rupture of the labial artery within 10 to 12 days.

The reconstructive phase should not be initiated before eight or more months. This permits the zone of soft tissue destruction to contract (Figure 2A), heal, and begin to mature prior to definitive surgical treatment (Figure 2B).

Fig. 2. A. Early result of the electrical burn involving red-white lip at one month.

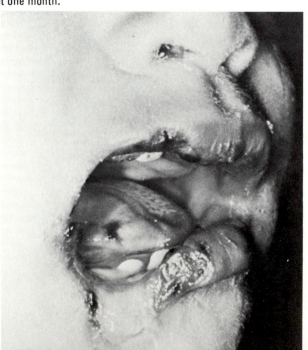

Fig. 2. B. Same patient after delayed wound healing, demonstrating contraction and commissure distortion six months later.

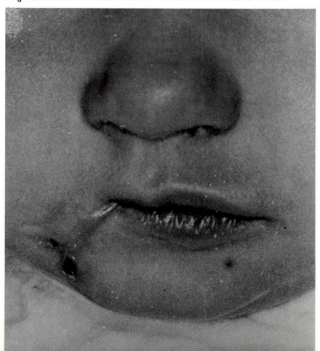

CONSERVATIVE TREATMENT

If only the red lip or red lip plus a very small portion of white lip is involved, a reasonable result can be anticipated (Figures 3 and 4). Allowing eight or more months to elapse will reveal which patients require specific surgical treatment.

Recently, Dr. R.G. Colcleugh has demonstrated the use of a fixed dental obturator, over a prolonged period, in more extensive white lip involvement of the oral commissure. His preliminary results strongly suggest this technique will decrease the need for reconstruction in many patients previously requiring

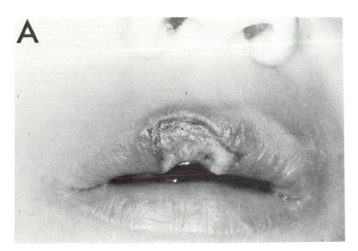
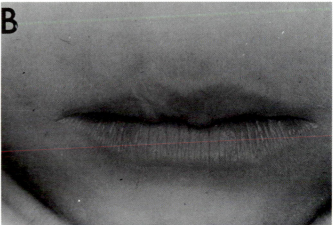

Fig. 3. A. Central red lip destruction. B. Complete healing with minimal distortion six months later.

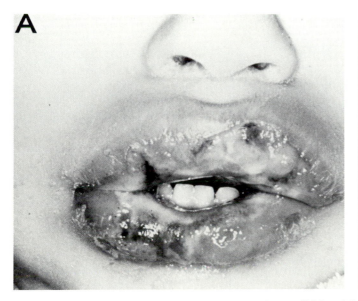
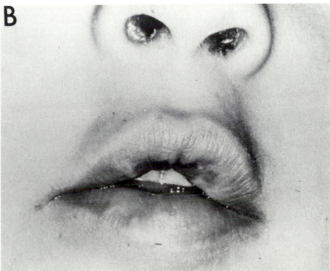

Fig. 4. A. Extensive red lip destruction, both superficial and deep. B. Complete healing with some distortion but much more acceptable appearance than one might originally anticipate.

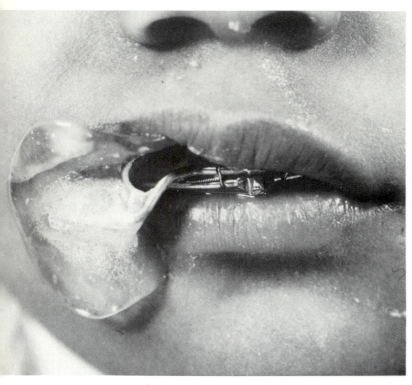

Fig. 5. Non-removable acrylic dental obturator holding the oral commissure open.

surgery. This has been the author's experience as well (Figure 5).

RECONSTRUCTION OF THE RED LIP

The primary concern in the initial phase of electrical burn reconstruction is the restoration or replacement of the destroyed red lip. The following techniques are a few of the many recognized and accepted methods.

Direct Advancement. If the oral commissure demonstrates a minor degree of scar contraction with a medial shift of the apex toward the midline, a simple excisional procedure is used (Figure 6). This consists of excising the erythematous scar in the zone of the previous commissure apex down to the mucosal lining (Figure 6B). The mucosal remnant is split and directly rotated up and down to meet its respective white lip component. It is better to err on the side of overcorrection because there is a tendency for recurrent contraction and a medial shift of the new apex after a period of one year.

Fig. 6. A. Isolated commissure contraction, anticipated angle and zone of excision outlined. **B.** Scar tissue just superficial to mucosa excised and incision made along dotted line. **C.** Mucosal flaps rotated up and down to meet white lip and suture.

A

B

C

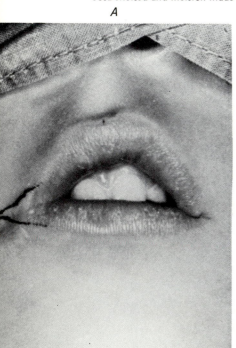

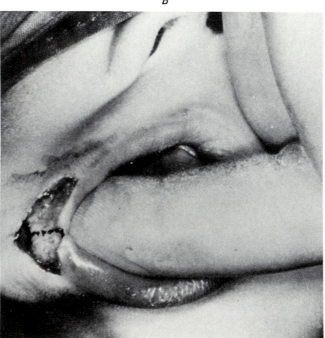

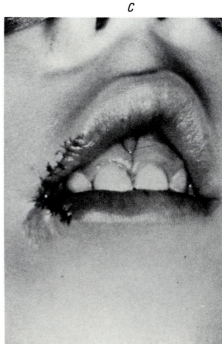

Rotation Advancement. With more extensive commissure destruction and resultant scar contraction, new mucous membrane must be brought into the corrected area, using local rotation advancement principles (Figure 7). A fan, Dieffenbach flap, or even an interpolated flap, may be used. In Figure 8 two interpolated flaps from adjacent mucous membranes are rotated down and up, respectively, and the mucosal donor sites are closed directly. This permits adequate excursion on opening the region of the commissure. The mucosal flap tends to assume a redder hue than normal adjacent mucosa.

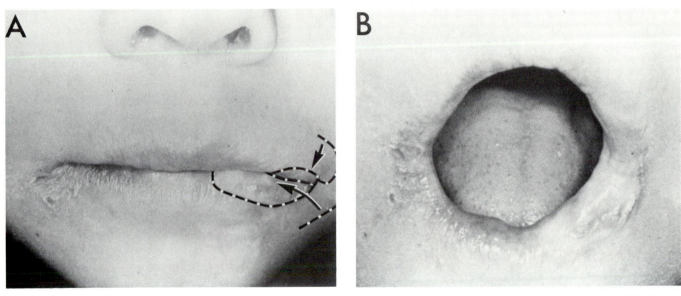

Fig. 7. A. Commissure shifted medially, dotted rotation advancement flaps on the upper and lower buccal gingival sulcus outlined.
B. Mouth open, demonstrating rotation flaps in position six months later with little webbing.

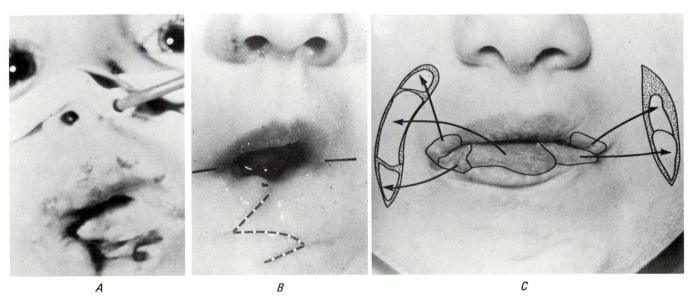

Fig. 8. A. Extensive red and white lip destruction, naso-gastric tube in place. **B.** At eight months a Z-plasty closure; revision of the lower lip (dotted line) is demonstrated. The commissures are to be opened (solid line). **C.** Commissure and upper and lower red lip areas covered with free mucosal grafts (donor sites outlined).

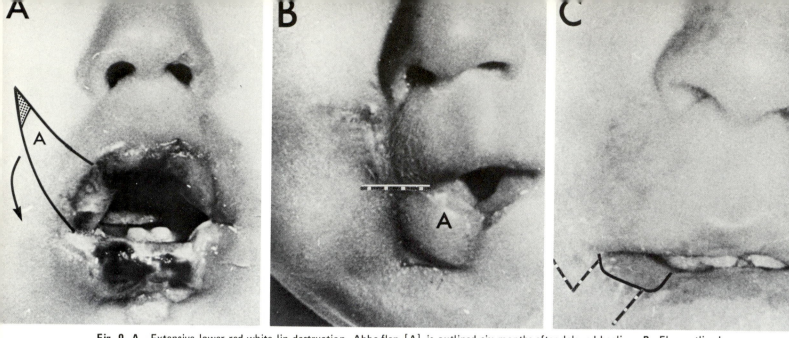

Fig. 9. A. Extensive lower red-white lip destruction, Abbe-flap [A] is outlined six months after delayed healing. B. Flap outlined (including white and red lip) rotated 180 degrees down into deficient lower lip [A]. Commissure must be opened (dotted line). C. After opening commissure the lower red lip deficiency is closed using a mucosal sickle flap (dotted and solid line).

Vascular Pedicle. If the destruction involves almost the entire upper or lower lip, consideration must be given to adding to the involved lip from the uninvolved, using an Abbe-Estlander flap based on an intact labial artery (Figure 9A and B). This by itself is merely an adjunct to the overall treatment program and can rarely provide complete correction (Figure 9C). It is, however, the most direct method of bringing local white and red lip tissue into the previously burned area.

RECONSTRUCTION OF THE WHITE LIP

The white lip reconstruction is commonly completed after the red lip replacement is well underway. It often consists of excising the red scar extending up into the white lip to provide a better definition between red and white lip zones. The created defect may be filled using any of the following methods.

Interpolated Flap. Skin pedicle flaps taken from the upper and/or lower portion of the nasolabial crease may be used to replace minor losses of white lip to provide better definition only after red lip reconstruction (Figure 10). This flap has a slight tendency to bulge with maturation.

Island Pedicle. A similar white lip defect may be replaced with a small island flap taken from a higher level on the nasolabial crease (Figure 11A).

Fig. 10. A. Red lip has been reconstructed, residual red scar on white lip gives vague definition. This is excised (solid line) and local flap from nasolabial crease rotated through 90 degrees.

Fig. 10. B. Flap is in place surrounded by ink and donor site closed directly.

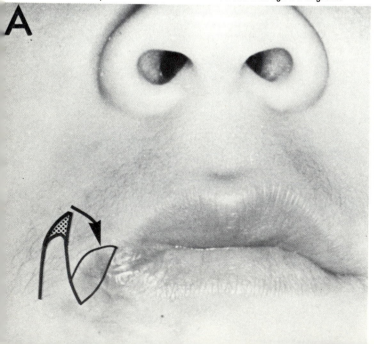

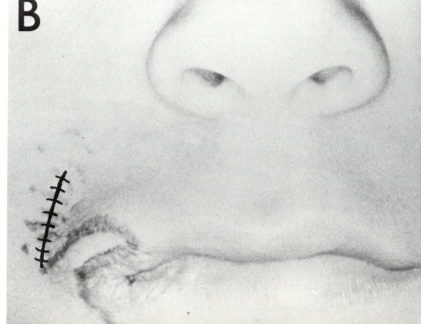

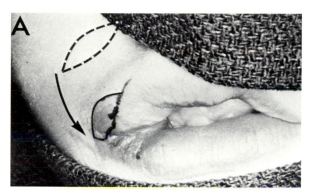

Fig. 11. A. Red lip reconstruction completed, erythematous, white lip scar is outlined for excision, island flap from high up on nasolabial crease is cut (dotted line).

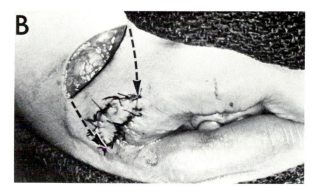

Fig. 11. B. Intermediate skin bridge is undermined and island pedicle shifted into excised defect on a subcutaneous pedicle.

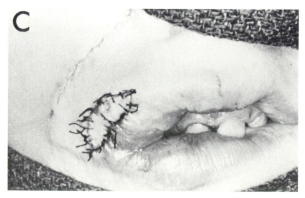

Fig. 11. C. Donor site is in a slightly different plane and closed directly with subcuticular suture.

This is tunneled on a subcutaneous bridge into the required site (Figure 11B and C). These techniques are equally advantageous.

Free Full-Thickness Graft Replacement. If the white lip destruction is too extensive to be covered with minor local skin shifts, free full-thickness skin grafts from the ear or neck should be used (Figure 12). This graft has greater advantages than a split-thickness graft because it is readily accessible in the operative region, and it provides blush-area skin.

Distant Pedicle Flap. If the extent of the burn destruction is very great, white lip addition must be obtained from a distance (Figure 13). Because this creates additional scarring, it should not be undertaken lightly. The transcervical region can be a useful

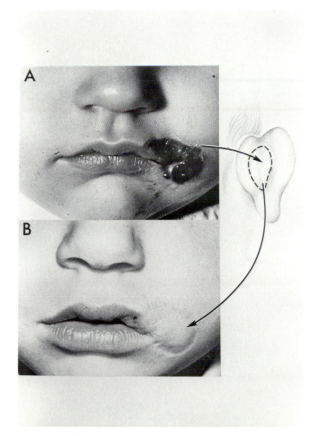

Fig. 12. A. Zone of white lip scar which has been excised. **B.** Free full-thickness skin graft taken from behind the ear. Result 12 months after transplant.

Fig. 13. A. Extensive burn which has had red and white lip replacement but lower lip is very tight, causing lingual collapse of lower centrals.

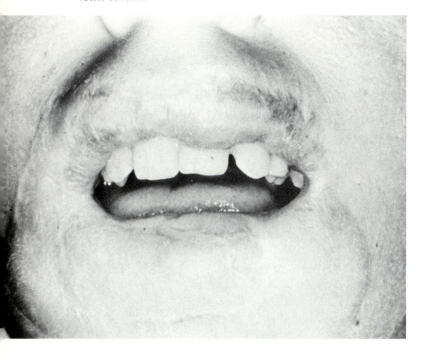

donor site, but this donor site usually provides an unsightly scar. If lining is required as well, a turnover of the distal flap can be created at the first delay. A vermillion can be obtained at a later date either by surgical tattooing or subsequent free mucosal graft replacement on the leading margin of the pedicle.

SUMMARY

The surgical treatment program of the oral electrical burn must be initiated with patience. Oral burns may require several operations and the combination of many reconstructive principles. While the surgeon can never achieve a pretrauma result, the dividends of surgery are proportional to the initial severity of the soft tissue destruction.

This chapter has not discussed alveolar ridge, dentition, tongue, or mandibular involvement. These sites are often involved but seldom create a problem for the patient or surgeon, unlike the damage in the red-white lip area.

Fig. 13. B. Transcervical pedicle is raised and the tip turned on itself to provide lip lining. Flap replaced in the form of a delay.

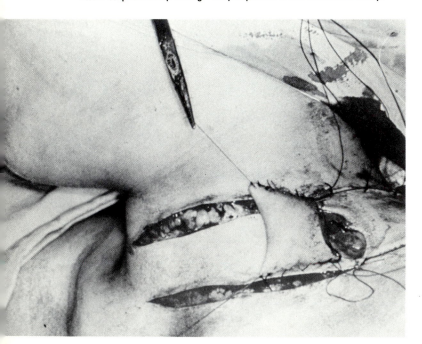

Fig. 13. C. At a later date flap is let into the deficient lower lip by tunneling underneath the chin skin through the sub-mental incision (arrow).

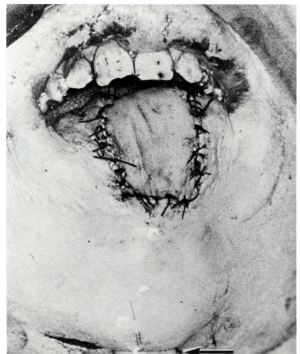

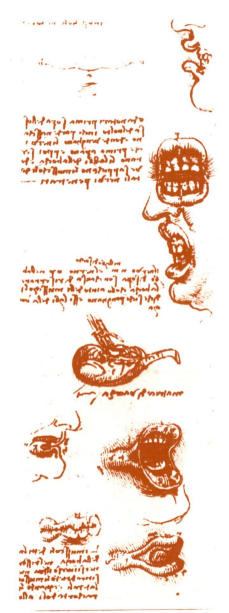

Leonardo da Vinci, 1452 – 1519.

63

CONTRACTION OF THE ORAL STOMA: MICROSTOMIA

Bent Sørensen

Contraction of the oral stoma (microstomia) may result from tissue loss, or from scar tissue contraction in skin, lip, or muscle. Isolated or multiple lesions may affect any or all of these structures, and lesions involving the angles of the mouth are particularly significant. Both the principle of treatment and the time chosen for treatment depend on the nature and site of the lesion, and, as always with burn patients, whether one is dealing with localized injury or with one area of an extensively burned patient.

Superficial partial-thickness burns may give rise to hypertrophic scars. Generally, treatment is expectant, consisting of daily massage and steroid dressings or cream. Compression of the thickened scar is not often possible, and surgical treatment is rarely indicated. Deep partial-thickness burns around the mouth usually heal spontaneously, reflecting the rich vascularity of the area. Healing proceeds despite frequent infection. Scar contraction is often marked, and microstomia results.

Severe contraction may follow full-thickness burns even though skin grafts were applied at an early stage.

The **time chosen for treatment** is important. Ideally the scar formation and contraction process should be complete. (This occurs approximately one year after the injury.) Reconstructive surgery can then be expected to be completed in one session. If microstomia is pronounced, or if dental treatment is required, it may be necessary to intervene earlier. In these circumstances, repeated surgery is often necessary.

The **basic principle of treatment** is the excision of all scar tissue and replacement by skin grafts or skin flaps, but some compromise, dictated by the eventual appearance of the patient, must often be made.

When dealing with a typical microstomia, all scar tissue must be removed from the angles of the mouth. The orbicularis oris muscle should not be spared if the cost is leaving scar tissue behind. If all scar tissue is not removed down to normal muscle, recurrence of microstomia is virtually certain. Even when the procedure is extensive, and the orbicularis oris has been totally transected, the other muscles in the vicinity allow near normal lip function. When both mouth angles are involved, correction should be undertaken at one session. This allows for better judgement of symmetry. Traditionally, defects are usually closed with a Y-V-plasty, but in my opinion the classical Z-plasty is better (Figure 1). The Z-plasty permits better removal of the scar tissue. Skin and lip tissue are usually interchanged in the Z-plasty, but in the vast majority of cases this is not evident. If the appearance is compromised, the mucosa and vermillion can be advanced outward.

Scar changes involving one lip, but not the commissural angles, are seen most frequently after electrical burns. The soft tissue is particularly prone to contraction, which may be so marked that malalignment of the teeth will occur.

Whatever the etiology, such burns are best treated by **the conservative** operative technique. The lip, and thus the visible scar, is left undisturbed, and instead the lip mucosa is used. This mucosa is present in abundance, and is richly vascular. It can be mobilized and used to cover very extensive defects without danger of loss. Should there be uncovered areas not involving scar tissue, epithelialization is spontaneous and rapid. We call the operation a sulcus-plasty and the technique is as follows: The mucosa in the bottom of the sulcus is incised laterally to the first molar tooth, then dissected from the musculature and sewn together in the middle to lengthen the lip. The

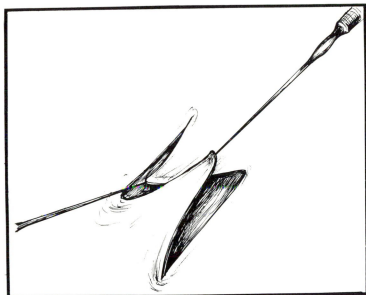

Fig. 1. **A.** Contracture of right mouth angles.

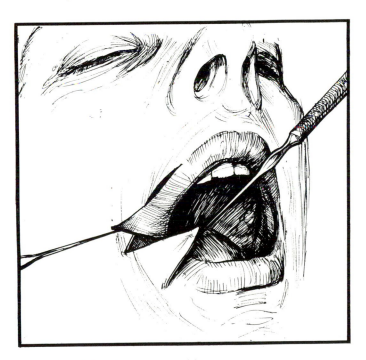

Fig. 1. **C.** Transposition of the Z-plasty flaps.

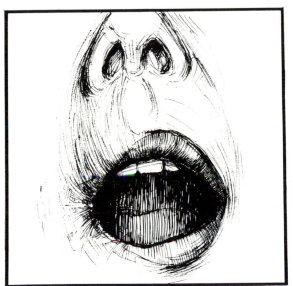

Fig. 1. **B.** Planned incisions for Z-plasty.

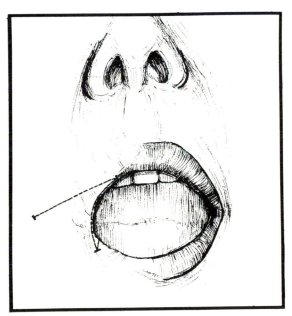

Fig. 1. **D.** Flaps in new position.

lip is freed from association with the teeth; fresh vascular tissue is available, and normal lip development continues. Supplementary orthodontic treatment may be necessary. The operation may be repeated if contraction recurs. When the child is full grown and the lip is of normal size, any embarrassing scar tissue can be removed.

In conclusion, I advise against the use of the larger plastic operations on the lip (Gillie's flaps, tube-pedicle grafts, etc.) in contraction of the oral stoma. **Smaller operations, repeated as necessary, give more satisfactory results and help preserve the patient's identity.**

64

LIP EVERSION DUE TO SCAR CONTRACTURE

David W. Furnas

Lip eversion occurs in all degrees, ranging from the minimum deformity of a partial-thickness burn to the grotesque mask resulting from the pernicious combination of an open hearth and a grand mal seizure. Usually the vermillion and mucosa are spared so that a wound contraction affects only the skin, causing the damaged segment of the lip to curl into an everted position. Gravity makes the lower lip especially vulnerable to eversion. A dense scar which extends laterally from the corner of the mouth may cause a cicatricial macrostomia as well as eversion, while a circumferential scar causes microstomia. Eversion of the upper lip usually involves small segments of the lip.

The tendency toward lip eversion may be greatly exaggerated by the force of neck and chin scars that transmit to the mouth. Application of an isoprene Texas-Shrine neck-chin-lower-lip splint in the immediate post-burn period reduces the amount of eversion of the lower lip. Application of an isoprene Texas-Shrine facial-pressure splint may also help reduce deformity of the upper lip. Splints are maintained constantly throughout the convalescent period.

PREOPERATIVE CONSIDERATIONS

Once wound closure and convalescence are complete and maximum benefit has been obtained from splinting, the eversion of the lip can be attacked surgically. Before proceeding with correction of the lip, however, all neighboring scars which contribute to the deformity must be recognized, and those of the neck in particular must be released (Figure 1, A through D). Sometimes release of neck contractures alone cures the lip eversion.

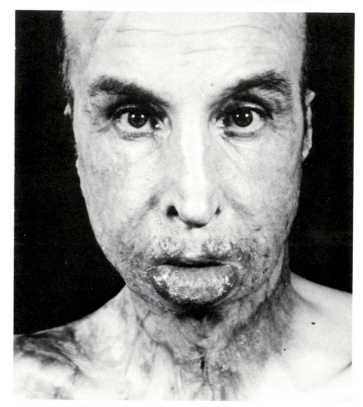

Fig. 1. A. Lip eversion, neck contracture, and exposed mandible due to gasoline explosion.

Fig. 1. B. Neck contracture and chin defect corrected with pedicle from chest.

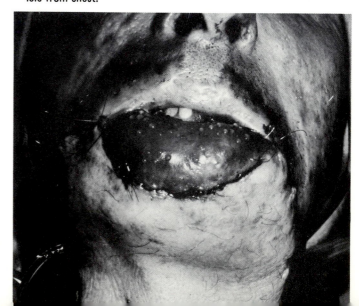

The depth of injury to the lips and surrounding tissue is estimated with a view to selecting the proper replacement procedure. Usually all of the oral musculature and most of the subcutaneous tissue are spared so that a full-thickness skin graft will be adequate. Extremely deep damage necessitates reconstruction with a skin flap. The width of the expected surgical deformity is estimated in order to judge whether a postauricular skin graft, the first choice, will be large enough to fill the defect without patchwork.

If the postauricular skin is damaged by burn scars, is insufficient in size, or is needed for eyelid repairs, supraclavicular skin is the next choice followed by infraclavicular skin. A donor site for a split-thickness skin graft must also be prepared in order to cover the original donor site because simple closure is sometimes impossible. A preliminary bacterial culture and sensitivity study of the mouth are made because of the likelihood of contamination by saliva. The patient is warned of the importance of absolute immobility of the lips in the postoperative period. A small feeding tube is inserted preoperatively.

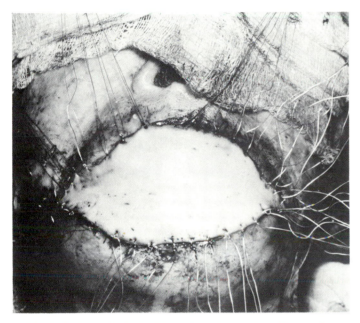

Fig. 1. C. Supraclavicular skin graft applied to release lip eversion at a later stage.

Fig. 1. D. Correction completed from combination of above pedicle and full-thickness graft.

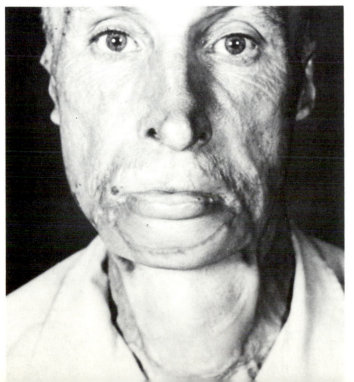

OPERATIVE PROCEDURE

An incision directly at the vermillion margin is extended from one angle of the mouth to the other, cutting through the skin down to the transverse fibers of the orbicularis oris (Figure 2A). The vermillion above and the skin below are undercut for a few millimeters, staying on the surface of the orbicularis muscle (Figure 2B). If release of the lip eversion is not complete, the incision is extended laterally from the angle of the mouth, millimeter by millimeter, until complete release is achieved (Figure 2C). Sometimes excision of some of the scarred skin of the lower lip is needed for complete release.

Hemostasis and Irrigation: Total hemostasis is secured with a needle point electrocautery. The open wound is irrigated copiously with Neosporin GU (Neomycin Sulfate – Polymyxin B Sulfate sterile irrigant).

Pattern: Translucent plastic drape material is laid on the defect (Figure 2D). While holding the vermillion in a slightly overcorrected position with skin hooks and pressing the pattern material well into the defect, the outline of the defect is traced with a marking pencil. The pattern is cut out and transferred to the donor site. Take care that the donor skin is in a relaxed position and that the pattern is right side up while the outline is marked out with the marking pencil.

227

Fig. 2. Operative procedure for eversion of the lip.

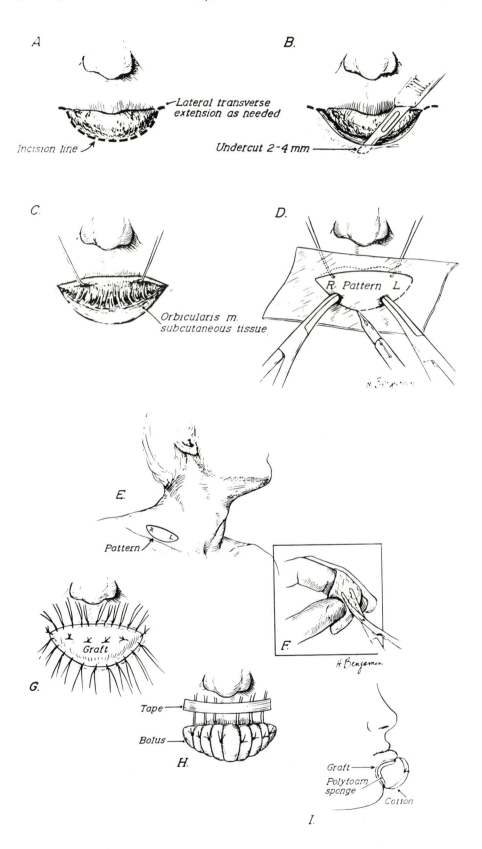

Procurement of the Graft: The graft is cut from the donor site (Figure 2E). Excess fat and dermis are cut away with a sharp pair of straight Mayo scissors (Figure 2F). Grafts from the clavicular region often need a considerable amount of dermis removed.

Application of the Graft: The graft is sutured to the recipient site with interrupted 5-0 nylon sutures (Figure 2G). The suture tails are left long and tied over a bolus formed of a thin layer of polyfoam sponge topped by absorbent cotton (Figures 2H and I). Mineral oil is applied to the graft to prevent adherence to the foam.

If the graft is quite large, it can be left open without a bolus; suction drains are applied with one or more lengths of fine polyethylene tubing having multiple perforations. These suction drains are brought out through separate small incisions in the intact skin and are attached to constant suction. The graft margin is sutured with a running 5-0 monofilament nylon suture, and a few quilting sutures are then placed. Separate sutures with long tails are placed at the upper border of the skin graft. These

are taped to the upper lip after the patient regains consciousness.

When proper correction has been performed, the lip appears floppy, somewhat thin, and overcorrected; however, this situation remedies itself in the postoperative period.

POSTOPERATIVE CARE

An antiemetic drug is given in the operating room and continued postoperatively. The suture tails are taped to the upper lip. If the patient gags excessively or is uncooperative, the feeding tube is dispensed with; otherwise tube feedings are used for the first week. If the graft has been left open, it must be watched closely for the collection of blood or serum so that evacuation can be instigated. Drainage tubes are usually removed by the third day, but seromas may form after their removal. If these tubes are left in for too long a period, a narrow strip of overlying graft is lost. The tieover dressing is removed in seven to ten days. The lip is supported with Micropore tape as the wounds mature.

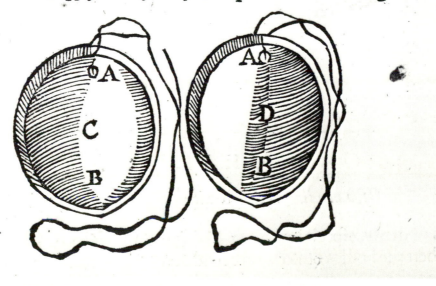

An Inſtrument made to ſupply the defeɛt of the Speech when the Tongue is cut off.

The Works of that Famous Chirurgeon: Ambrose Parey, 1678.

65

LIP EVERSION

Irving Feller

Eversion of the lips frequently occurs when the surrounding tissue is burned either deep partial-thickness or full-thickness. In the former, hypertrophic scar causes the eversion, while in the latter, the contracture that accompanies scar formation results in the eversion. Either the upper, lower, or both lips may be involved.

The repair of eversion of the lip is accomplished by releasing the contracture, excising excessive tissue if present, and applying thick or full-thickness autografts.

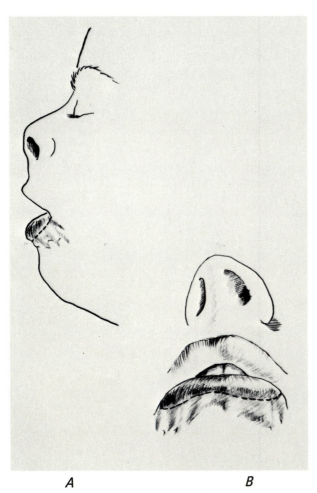

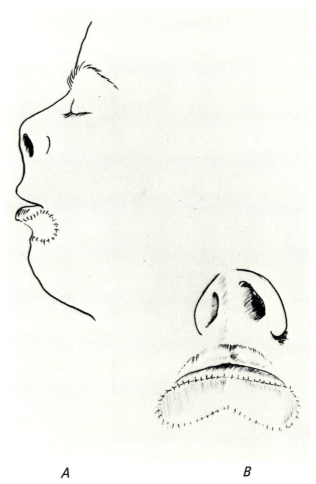

| *A* | *B* |

Fig. 1. Appearance of lower lip eversion with hypertrophic scarring. The dotted line indicates the area of hypertrophic scar to be excised. **A.** Lateral view. **B.** Anterior view.

Fig. 2. The autograft is fixed into position to cover the defect. It is necessary to overcompensate while correcting the defect as a certain amount of contracture will take place during the healing process. **A.** Lateral view. **B.** Anterior view.

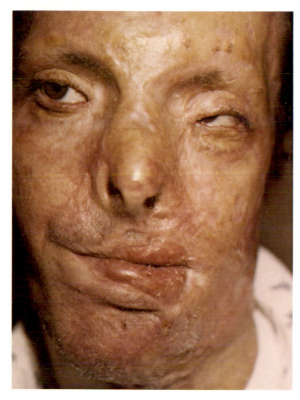

Fig. 3. A. This patient suffered full-thickness burns to the face in a truck accident. Eversion of the left side of both the upper and lower lip complicated his recovery. The upper and lower lips were repaired at different times, using the same technique at each operation.

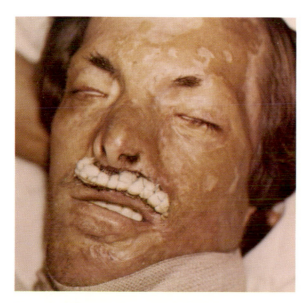

Fig. 3. B. The repair of the upper lip is shown.

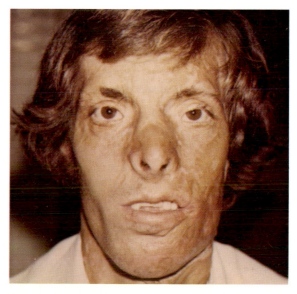

Fig. 3. C. One year after the reconstruction, both lips remained in good position.

X.

THE NECK

PRINCIPLES OF TREATMENT

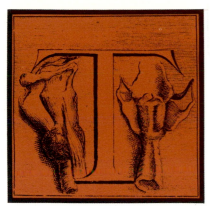

he principles of treatment of the burned neck are preventing or minimizing the contracture when possible, and correcting those that do occur early. Prevention of recurrence is then necessary.

Burns of the neck, both deep partial- and full-thickness, often result in contractures. Most of these contractures are anterior, but circumferential and posterior contractures do occur. Anterior contractures can become severe and occasional patients are seen with the chin fixed to the suprasternal notch.

The basic practices include early debriding, grafting, and splinting of the neck to avoid contractures. If the contracture has occurred, excision and/or release of the contracture with thick split grafting or Z-plasty is necessary. The use of splints during the postoperative period is very important.

Irving Feller

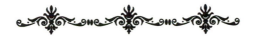

Someone said: "The dead writers are remote from us because we know so much more than they did."
Precisely, and they are that which we know.

T. S. Eliot

67

EARLY MANAGEMENT OF THE NECK

Irving Feller
Kathryn E. Richards

Basic wound care for the burned neck includes multiple dressing changes for early debridement, positioning the patient in the semi-Fowler's position to minimize edema and to prevent or limit deformity, and early grafting to cover the defect. Burns of the neck that are deep and circumferential require decompression escharotomy to avoid upper airway and venous obstruction (Figure 1). Wound care is similar to other parts of the body; however, splinting the neck before and after grafting is necessary to decrease contracture formation.

Early splinting of the burned neck can be carried out by applying a collar of ¾ inch foam plastic around the neck over a dressing held in place with an ace bandage. Care is taken to avoid constriction of the venous return and airway (Figure 2).

The constant position maintained by this dynamic elastic dressing inhibits contracture. Another method to keep the neck extended is to keep the patient's head on the mattress. Pillows should not be used. If contracture develops early, immediate release and split-thickness grafting followed by a neck splint is indicated (Figure 3).

When a tracheostomy is required, ideal care is not possible. However, it is necessary to debride the region around the stoma early to avoid purulent drainage into the trachea. Autografting should be done as early as possible to close the wound. Splints can be designed and built to accommodate the tracheostomy.

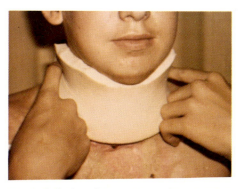

Fig. 2. Splinting of the neck to avoid contractures can begin during the acute period. **A.** A piece of flexible plastic foam is placed over the dressing.

Fig. 1. A relaxing escharotomy is often necessary for deep circumferential burns of the neck.

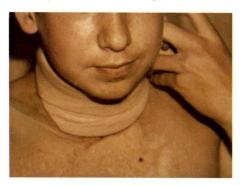

Fig. 2. B. Then an ace bandage is used to provide the necessary pressure and stiffness.

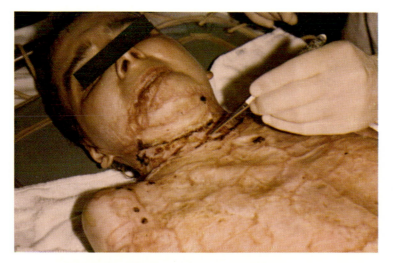

Fig. 3. When an early contracture of the neck appears during the first hospital admission, a release of the contracture with split-thickness grafting should be done. The patient continues to use a neck splint after discharge from the hospital.

68

RECONSTRUCTION OF THE NECK

John K. Barton

A case of severe burn involves, from the first moment, so many dangers to the patient, and calls for so much care and forethought upon the part of the surgeon, that the accident is rightly considered a most important one, and we find the subject has received the careful attention of the most celebrated surgeons. Should the patient have passed safely through the several stages, in each of which his life is threatened with danger from a different quarter, the prospect of deformity still remains, which often takes place in spite of every effort made to prevent it, and afterwards baffles every attempt to remove it, rendering the unhappy sufferers a burden to themselves and to others. These results of severe burns did not escape the attention of Dupuytren, who recounts cases of almost every conceivable kind of deformity thus produced which he had himself seen; and he further recommends for their treatment, when the cicatrix had fully contracted, an operation consisting of several parallel incisions through the cicatrix, and subsequently an apparatus to be applied, which, by means of springs, would keep up a constant separation of the edges of the wounds until they had been healed. Mr. James, of Exeter, recommended a somewhat different proceeding: he made an incision upon each side of the cicatrix, and then one across it, and dissected the two flaps thus formed from the parts beneath, afterwards keeping the parts separate by an apparatus, a description and figure of which, I believe, has been published by him, but I have not been able to find it. Earle and Sir B. Brodie followed a similar line of proceeding.

By these means many cases have been more or less successfully treated. But in many others, especially when the neck and face were the parts engaged, they have disappointed the expectations of both surgeon and patient,—the cicatrices being found to contract again in spite of every means taken to prevent them; and the deformity, which immediately after the operation had disappeared, returning as badly as before. Consequently, in addition to James' simple operation, it was proposed to fill up the wound, with a flap of healthy skin, taken from a suitable situation, and thus to prevent the possibility of recontraction. It has been found, however, that in a case where the cicatrix is large and the deformity very bad (the very cases which most call for relief), this plastic operation is quite inadmissible, inasmuch as the wound is so large, that a flap large enough to fill it up would invariably slough, which circumstance would render the case worse than if no attempt of the kind had been made. In consequence of the repeated failures of these means, surgeons very generally refuse to interfere in bad cases, especially when the contraction is in the neck, and the patients are consequently condemned to endure their deformity.

The causes of these unfavourable results from operations well planned and skilfully performed, will be found, I think, to arise from too much being expected from the operation, and too little attention being bestowed upon the subsequent process of extension or stretching; and that much more successful results will follow than have been hitherto obtained, by means of a careful and continued extension of the cicatrix, in some cases assisted by a cutting operation, such as has been mentioned,—in others, simply by subcutaneous section of the unyielding bands, and frequently not requiring any assistance from the knife whatever.

A consideration of the cause of these deformities favours this view of the treatment. The cause of the forcible contraction of the cicatrix which produces the deformity is the lymph which is shed in the repair of the ulcers left after the separation of the sloughs, which, following an invariable law, as soon as it becomes a part of the organized tissue, slowly but forcibly contracts. This law we may observe in many parts of the body; for instance, when the lymph is shed over the pleura, we find the walls of the thorax yielding to its contraction; and when poured out in the capsule of Glisson, we know with what a powerful grasp it compresses the liver. And in stricture of the urethra, it is the same substance which, shed upon or beneath the mucous membrane, produces such a train of evils by its tendency to close the canal; and tries the patience and skill of the surgeon, in overcoming its constant tendency to contract. Now, the treatment of stricture of the urethra has, for more than 200 years, occupied the attention of surgeons both in this country and on the Continent; and while there has been great diversity of opinion upon many points, I believe I am correct in saying that all the ablest surgeons who have written on the subject agree that, in the great majority of cases, dilatation alone is the safest and the most successful treatment that can be adopted; that in some the use of the knife may be required to obtain a passage, in the first instance, which then must be maintained by dilatation; and that the cases which admit an instrument at all, and will not yield to dilatation, are comparatively very few;—that, in fact, a cutting operation is only occasionally required, while careful and patient dilatation, is almost invariably sufficient, either in conjunction with operation or alone, to produce a successful issue. Now, the cause of the contraction in each case being identical, we may with great advantage use the experience which we have gained in the treatment of stricture of the urethra to guide us in the choice of means for overcoming the contraction of the cicatrices of burns, especially when cutting operations have so been freely tried; and when unassisted, or only partially assisted by extension, have failed to produce the desired result.

Whatever mode of treatment we adopt, our great object must be to obtain, if possible, the adsorption of the lymph, which is the contracting power; if this be removed, the case is cured. Now, no cutting operation will, of itself, produce this desirable object; on the contrary, it will cause the effusion of more lymph, which, being quite recent, will no doubt be far more amenable to extension than the old cartilaginous lymph; and so cutting may help. But the means which we must trust to, to gain the removal of the cicatrized tissue, is *extension;* and this, in some cases alone, in others aided by the knife, will, when perseveringly employed, produce the absorption of the tissues of the cicatrix, and so the permanent removal of the deformities dependent upon it.

Case

Isabella M'Owen, a healthy girl, fourteen years of age, from the County Meath, was admitted into the Adelaide Hospital, upon the 22nd of March, 1860. When about eight years of age, her clothes having caught fire, she was severely burnt about the right side of the neck and head. Her mother had endeavoured to prevent the contraction which she was told would follow, by placing a stiff leather collar round her neck when the ulcers were healing, and for some time afterwards; the contraction, however, went on increasing in spite of this, and, as the girl began to grow up, she became very much dissatisfied with her appearance, and urgently sought that something might be done for her relief. Her state upon admission is shown in the lithograph (Figure 1). The cicatrix, as

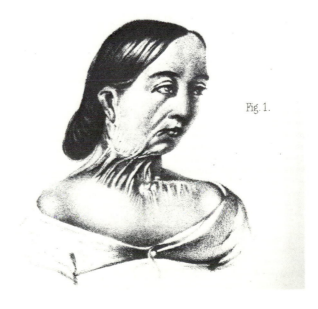

Fig. 1.

will be seen, occupied the whole of the right side of the neck, its densest and thickest part being close beneath the ramus of the jaw, extending from the lower part of the ear, which was involved in it, to the chin; from this central mass strong fibrous bands extended downwards below the clavicle, and as far forwards as the sternum; superiorly, the skin of the whole of that side of the face was drawn down to it; the angle of the mouth, and the external angle of the eye, being drawn downwards, the latter causing slight ectropion. The head was kept bent down to the right side, and when held straight caused increased distortion of the countenance; but by no effort could the patient turn her head to the left side.

The girl and her parents being very anxious to have something done to relieve her deformity, I determined to attempt it,—my colleagues having examined the case, and agreed with me, and having also had the advantage of Dr. Hutton's advice, who kindly gave me his opinion as to the best mode of proceeding.

Upon the morning of the 28th, as soon as the patient was well under the influence of chloroform, I proceeded to operate in the following manner;—An incision was first made along the posterior edge of the cicatrix, from the mastoid process to the acromion, then a second along the anterior or inner edge, from the chin to the sternum; thirdly, another incision was carried across the cicatrix just below its central mass, connecting the two former. The two flaps thus formed were then carefully dissected from their attachments to the parts beneath, which was a matter requiring both time and care, as the skin, platisma, and fascia were all matted together and to the muscles beneath, by the dense fibrous structure of the ciatrix. As soon as this had been satisfactorily accomplished, the deformity of the face was found to have disappeared, and a gaping wound remained, extending from the ramus of the jaw to the clavicle. No vessel required ligature. Lint wet in cold water was laid on the wound, and the patient removed to bed. Considerable constitutional irritation succeeded, which being followed by an attack of bronchitis, reduced the patient very much, and prevented me applying any instrument for keeping her head in proper position for some time, I

found some difficulty, also, in getting any instrument made which would fulfil the indication, viz, to keep the head in such a position that the cicatrization of the neck could not deform the face; at last I succeeded in getting an instrument mady by Read, which has answered so well, that I have had it figured (Figure 2), as, with modifications, I think it will be found applicable to all cases of contraction about the neck or face. It consists of a shoulder-piece (A, B) which, before the steel of which it is made was hardened, was fitted over the shoulder so as to sit closely and firmly; this was fixed in its place by two straps passing round the chest; from its upper side projected two steel slips, moving upon two others (X, X), which connected it with a firm cushion (C), which fitted against the ramus of the lower jaw, and was fixed firmly there by two straps, as seen in the figure. When the shoulder-peice and cushion were firmly strapped in their places, the head was forcibly drawn over to the left side, thus putting the parts between the jaw and the clavicle very much on the stretch; the two pairs of steel slips sliding upon one another; the screws (S) being then turned, the apparatus was fixed, and remained so the whole day: it was taken off at night, and reapplied, carefully, every morning. Recontraction was very rapidly taking place when this instrument was first applied; the bands of lymph in the cicatrix were extremely strong and unyielding, and the face was again being drawn into deformity; so that, from the first, the work this extending apparatus had to accomplish was to stretch the cicatrix, and thus cause its absorption. It became a matter of great interest to me to see if it could perform this; it was therefore carefully put on every day, for about three months. When about one month had elapsed, I saw some progress was slowly, but steadily, being made, to aid the process going on, I now divided, subcutaneously, two or three of the most resisting bands: this was decidedly of service, so I repeated this about every fortnight, until at the end of three months the thickness of the cicatrix was very much decreased; it was evident that the dense fibrous tissue was being removed, and that the steady extension, aided by the subcutaneous section of the bands, was producing an absorption of the lymph of the cicatrix; a corres-

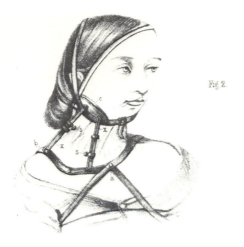

Fig. 2.

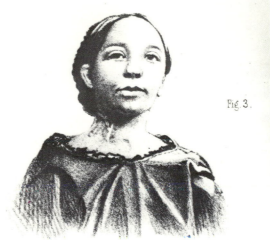

Fig. 3.

ponding improvement had taken place in the deformity of the face; the eye was quite free, while the corner of the mouth was very slightly pulled down; the head, too, could be turned to the left side with freedom, and the face turned round to the left side completely; but when this latter motion was performed, the mouth and cheek were still a good deal dragged. The patient now went to the country,—her mother having learned in the hospital, in a day or two, how to put on the instrument, and undertaking to apply it daily, and bring back the girl in November, which she did, having been absent about two months. Her neck remained very much in the same state when she returned as that in which it was when she left the hospital, but her general health was much improved. No doubt the apparatus was not kept on as regularly, nor applied as firmly, as it should have been; upon

her re-admission, however, it was again carefully put on, the most prominent bands in the cicatrix being again divided with the tenotomy knife, and a progressive improvement took place; the skin being soft and pliant, where it had been hard and puckered, the deformity of the face disappearing at the same time. All this, however, took place very gradually. She was still under treatment in March, 1861, when, on account of the death of a sister in the country, she suddenly left the hospital. Her parents did not wish anything further to be done, expressing themselves very much pleased with the improvement which had taken place, as a proof of which they again sent her up to town, at my request, to have a photograph taken, which has been lithographed in Figure 3, showing her present state.

Abstracted from:

THE DUBLIN

QUARTERLY JOURNAL

OF

MEDICAL SCIENCE.

AUGUST 1, 1861.

Editor's Note:

One hundred and seventeen years ago, Dr. Barton reported his method of treating neck contractures in the Dublin Quarterly Journal. This is presented here as a good example of the history of treatment of neck contracture. Pressure dressings after initial wound healing failed. Release of contracture without grafting but using splints was the method of the time. Subcutaneous cutting of the scar contracture was used intermittently to release the contracting scar bands as they formed. It is interesting to note that the only addition made to Dr. Barton's method is that we use autografts to close the defects, a method not known to him. It is also interesting that he did not recognize that the "bronchitis" may have been a complication of the anesthesia, a complication still a hazard today./I.F.

69

EXCISION OF SCAR CONTRACTURE OF THE NECK

Thomas D. Cronin

Until the late 1950's, the treatment of *complete* contractures of the anterior neck was haphazard, involving multiple operations with flaps, or repeated regrafting with split-thickness or free full-thickness skin grafts when contractures recurred. In 1957 and 1961, I demonstrated that after split-thickness skin grafting, prolonged *pressure*, exerted by a splint that *extended and molded* the contour of the neck, could prevent postoperative contracture. The anterior neck was once one of the most unsatisfactory areas in which to apply split-thickness skin graft. Now, with splinting pressure, it is the site of one of the most successful, wrinkle-free grafts.

OPERATIVE CONSIDERATIONS

Indications for Split-Thickness Grafting. Split-thickness skin grafting is indicated predominantly in complete neck contracture because of the resulting uniform appearance. The inelastic skin-grafted area in partial contractures is in marked contrast to the normal elastic skin. Repair with local flaps or Z-plasties is often preferable in partial contractures, augmented when necessary with split-thickness skin grafts.

Prevention of Scar Contractures. Ideally, scar contractures of the neck should be prevented rather than corrected. The neck should be kept extended; a pillow should not be used. In 1970, Barbara Willis of Texas Shrine Hospital advocated the use of isoprene splints molded to the neck early in the healing phase. **If a definitive thick-skin graft is to be used, it must be accomplished within the first four to five weeks— before contracture occurs.** *Definitive grafting should be attempted only when conditions are ideal.* If a satisfactorily clean wound cannot be obtained within

this time or the extent of the surrounding burn is so great that it interferes with the proper use of a splint, or the patient's general condition is poor, then it would be better to use a thin graft and temporarily accept contracture.

Timing of Operation. Surgery on patients requiring split-thickness skin graft coverage of the neck after scar excision should be performed as soon as the general condition of the patient will permit. If all the scar is to be excised, there is no need to wait for its maturation.

OPERATIVE TECHNIQUE

Excision of the Scar. Complete excision of the scar is indicated to minimize postoperative contracture. A scar extending over the chin or lower border of the mandible also should be excised; the splint can be made with an extension to press against these grafts. Inferiorly, excision should extend a little below the clavicles. If a heavy scar covers the upper chest, it is advisable to come back at another time, excise as much as possible, and apply split-thickness skin grafts. If this is not done, continued contracture of this scar may pull the newly applied neck skin graft towards the chest, impairing its efficiency in relieving the neck contracture. The vertical margins of the wound on each side of the neck are broken up by making one arm of a Z-plasty and transposing it. The other arm is formed from the skin graft when it is applied. If the chin-neck angle is still obtuse, it may be improved by doing a Z-plasty on the platysma muscle and its overlying subcutaneous tissue.

If the neck is still tight after the scar excision, overhead traction can be applied by placing a hook made from Kirschner wire under the symphysis of the mandible for as long as necessary until the skin grafts are applied. In 1970, Evans and others drilled a wire from side to side through the symphysis for this purpose.

Immediate application of the skin graft is almost never wise because 100 percent take of the graft is extremely important. Despite the greatest care, if the graft is applied immediately, small to large hematomas are prone to occur, causing skin loss.

The wound may be dressed with fine-mesh Furacin gauze or porcine skin grafts. With neck extended, a large fluffy dressing is applied and then wrapped with an elastic bandage. This dressing, plus padding behind the shoulders, keeps the neck extended. The dressing remains dry and unchanged until the skin graft is applied in about five days.

Graft Application. A five-day interval between scar excision and skin grafting seems to be optimal. By this time, a fine layer of granulation tissue has begun to form. Any spots of fat necrosis can be detected and curetted. With shorter periods, bleeding upon removal of the dressing may still be annoying. After five days epithelium begins to grow in from the edges of the wound and may need to be trimmed, again creating the possibility of hematoma formation. Further delay also increases the chance of infection.

The skin graft should be in one large piece if possible. The Padgett-Hood or Reese dermatomes are preferred because 4 by 8 inch grafts can be obtained. This is usually adequate for a young child. These dermatomes are also preferred because a thick (0.020 inch) graft is desired and can be more accurately obtained than with other dermatomes or knives. If more than one piece is required, the line of junction should be transverse. The grafts should be carefully sutured in a slightly stretched state, completing the second arm of a Z-plasty wherever a first arm has previously been made on the lateral edge of the wound. Scattered interrupted sutures may be left long to tie over a large bolster dressing of fluffed gauze or mechanic's waste, which is piled on a layer of gauze impregnated with Furacin (nitrofurazone) or an antibiotic ointment. A pressure dressing is preferred initially to ensure graft contact with all surface depressions and irregularities.

Free Full-Thickness Skin Grafts. Free full-thickness skin grafts have been advocated in the past by Blair in 1935, Kazanjian in 1936, and Blocker in 1941, but they are rarely used for large losses now because of the uncertainty of take, and the fact that the donor site would usually have to be grafted. In 1958, Brown and McDowell used full-thickness grafts after transverse incision of previously grafted necks to relieve postoperative contracture and accentuate the chin-neck line.

Local Flaps and Split-Thickness Grafting. In limited contractures, a combination of local flaps combined with split-thickness skin grafting may be used. In such cases an attempt would be made to shift the flap to the area of the chin-neck angle where contracture would be most likely, placing the graft on the lower neck on a flat area. Use of the split-thickness graft also requires the use of a splint.

POST GRAFT CARE

Following grafting, the neck is kept extended by placing folded towels or a small pillow under the shoulders and sandbag on each side of the head. The bolster dressing is **removed** on the first or second postoperative day to prevent localized loss of the skin graft over the larynx. The dressing fixes the graft in one position while the larynx moves under it, preventing adhesion. Because the graft is applied over a generally convex surface, a good contact with the wound occurs naturally so that it is not necessary to replace the initial dressing. Any accumulation of serum or blood is aspirated promptly. Any loss of skin of as much as 1cm should be regrafted to prevent scar contracture.

SPLINTING MATERIALS AND METHODS (CRONIN)

Impression for Splint. On the first or second postoperative day, the dressing is removed and the graft covered with a layer of Vaseline or Furacin gauze. Then an impression for the splint is taken. With the patient sitting up, a strip of heavy cardboard to cut against is placed on each side of the neck. A plaster cast is then applied around the slightly extended neck. The plaster should extend over the chin and border of the mandible, covering all skin-grafted areas. Below, it extends over the adjacent shoulder. After the cast has set, it is cut through on each side and removed.

Design. The splint is designed to accomplish three equally important things: extension of the neck, molding of the chin-neck angle, and application of even pressure to the grafted area.

The need for keeping the neck extended is obvious, but applying pressure to the graft and molding the chin-neck line are often overlooked. The use of ordinary four-post adjustable cervical braces fails two of the three essentials for a skin-grafted neck. Although it may keep the chin up, it does not mold the chin-neck angle which, therefore, bows across. It does not furnish pressure to the entire graft, which is most important in preventing hypertrophy of the scar and in producing a soft, smooth graft. Splints relying on pressure to the forehead are even less efficient, because the chin can be easily pulled down by scar.

In 1961, I gave the following description of my splint. A positive model is made from the negative cast by pouring in plaster around a heavy wooden post which is inserted in the center and used as a handle (Figure 1). The angle between the chin and neck is definitely deepened on the positive model, as are the depressions above and below the clavicles and manubrium sterni. Care is taken to avoid excessive smoothing off of bony prominences, such as the clavicles and the inferior border of the mandible, to prevent undue pressure by the splint at these points.

Construction. Construction of the splint is now begun by applying lightweight gray horsehide over the desired area, working it into all depressions. Next, a $1/8$ inch layer of wool felt is applied. The main support of the splint is made of $1/8$ inch thick Celastic. The Celastic is first soaked in XP 25 solvent for Celastic*, then carefully applied over the wool felt, working it into all depressions. In splints for adults, two layers may be used for added strength. In order

*Joseph Jones Co., 186 William St., New York, N.Y.

to mold the Celastic firmly to the contours of the model, depressions are accentuated with half-round rubber or felt and the entire splint is wrapped firmly with heavy elastic tape for 36 to 48 hours. After the elastic tape is removed, a lightweight horsehide cover is added to complete the buildup. The splint is made in two parts, front and back, with three buckles on each side and a tapered piece of leather between the two halves. The leather is attached to one half and slides beneath the edge of the other. There should be a distance of ½ inch to 1¼ inches between the two halves. If the grafted area extends into the cheek, the splint can be extended to cover it using a metal strut for reinforcement.

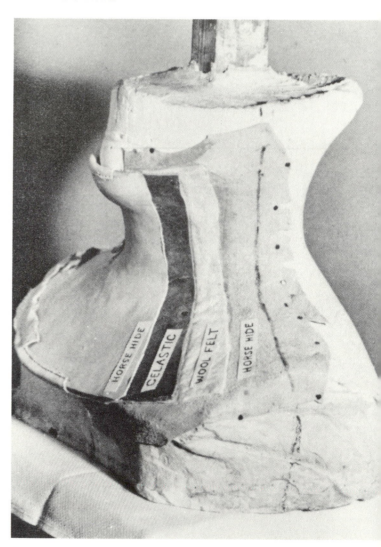

Fig. 1. Positive plaster model of neck, showing construction of splint.

Application. It is advisable to apply the splint sometime during the second week after grafting, even if there are small unhealed areas. By this time the graft has taken well and contracture will begin shortly (Figure 2). **The splint should be worn continuously, day and night, for a period of approximately six months,** or until the grafted area becomes soft and pliable and has no tendency to wrinkle (Figure 3). This may be determined by removing the splint for a day at a time and then for longer intervals if there is no wrinkling. If there is wrinkling and contracture, the splint is reapplied for another month.

SPLINTING MATERIALS AND METHODS (WILLIS)

Willis has described a simple method of constructing a splint that fulfills the three requirements using the following materials and equipment: orthoplast, 1 inch Velcro hook and pile, 1 inch webbing, 1 inch "D" rings, 1/8 inch polyvinylchloride (PVC) foam, medium and long rapid rivets (Tandy), Velcro adhesive, hot water and heat gun, scissors, hole punch, riveting machine (Rex Riveter), commercial spot remover, and needle and thread.

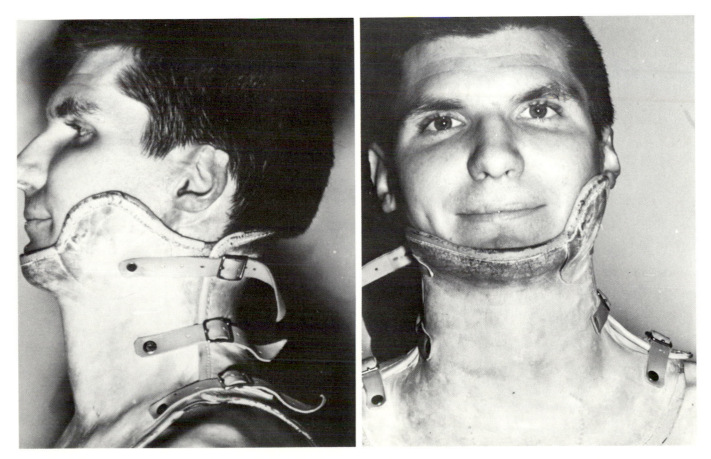

Fig. 2. The Cronin Neck Splint which extends and molds the contour of the neck. Note extension over cheek to apply pressure to a grafted area.

Fig. 3. A. and B. Contracture of neck following an early, thin split-skin graft for healing. **C. and D.** Appearance about three years later, following excision of old graft and scar and application of a thick split-skin graft. The patient has been wearing the described neck splint for six months.

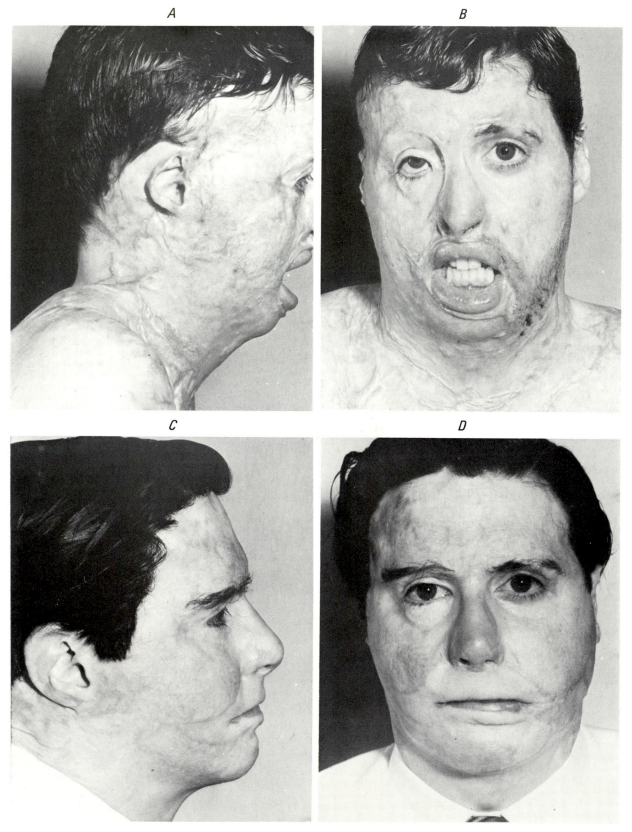

Construction. Figures 4, 5, 6, and 7 illustrate the construction of the Orthoplast neck splint.

1. Measure a length (A) from the mid-point of the chin to ½ inch to 1 inch below the sternoclavicular joint. Measure a length (B) from right trapezius (lateral upper fibers) around the jawline to the left trapezius (Figure 4).

2. Draw an ellipse using measurements A and B (Figure 5).

3. Trace pattern onto orthoplast, heat only enough to facilitate cutting. Cut out with scissors.

4. Heat plastic in very hot water, at least 57 degrees C. Do not use a heat gun as it will not give even all-over heat which will cause difficulty in shaping. Dry quickly with a towel and check that the temperature is bearable.

5. Position the splint by applying the plastic directly to the patient as follows: starting from the center, mold to the patient's chin and throat, easing and stretching on each side (Figure 6). Do not continue molding past the trapezius on either side. Gently flare edges for comfort. Cooling may be hastened by the application of an ice bag.

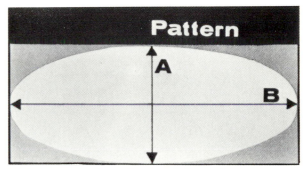

Fig. 5. Pattern for the Orthoplast anterior neck splint, using measurements A and B shown in Figure 4.

Fig. 6. Apply the heated Orthoplast to patient's neck and mold in place.

Fig. 4. Measurements for the Orthoplast anterior neck splint.

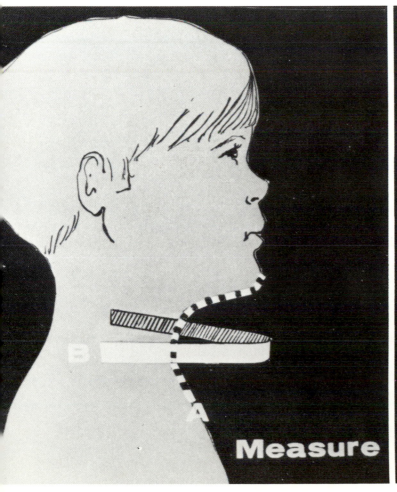

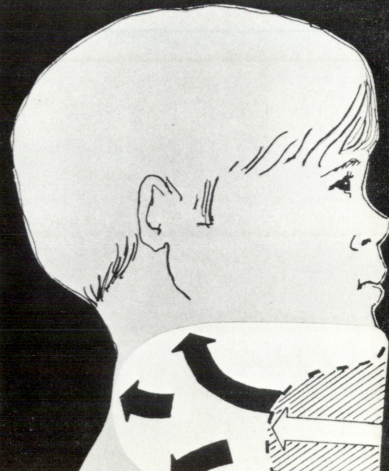

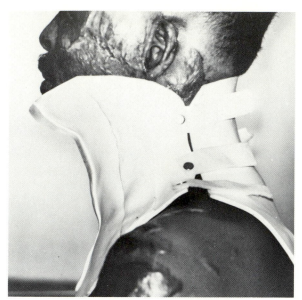

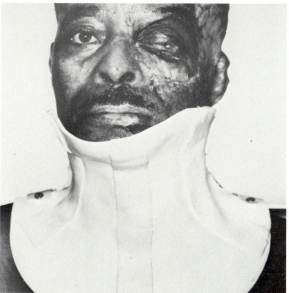

Fig. 8. Proper application of the Orthoplast splint.

6. Mark the position on either side for the attachment of fastening straps; mark the positions for reinforcing strips as follows: one on either side of the midline anteriorly and one on each side below the ear.

7. Reinforce the plastic. Cut ½ to 1 inch Orthoplast strips the length indicated in previous step. Clean the conformer with commercial spot remover in areas to be reinforced. Heat the reinforcing strips with hot water until of rubbery consistency. Do not apply heat to the prepared conformer. Brush one surface with commercial spot remover and apply this surface of the strip to the predetermined area on the conformer pressing firmly and evenly to bond the two surfaces together.

8. Attach a 2 inch loop of webbing and a "D" ring to one side of the brace using a long rapid rivet. Attach a combination pile-hook Velcro strap to the other side using a medium rapid rivet (Figure 7). Pad the straps with 2 inch wide strips of PVC foam, using Velcro adhesive. Figure 8 demonstrates proper application of the splints.

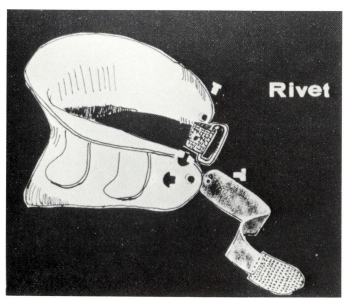

Fig. 7. Two-inch-wide webbing straps are riveted to the Orthoplast.

SUMMARY

Under ideal circumstances, complete full-thickness burns of the anterior neck may be skin grafted and fitted with a molded collar, thereby preventing development of a contracture. If there is any doubt of successfully accomplishing the above, it would be best to let the neck heal with or without thin grafts and do a definitive release later. The use of thick split-thickness skin grafts and prolonged (six months) *extension, molding,* and *pressure* with a splint contoured to the patient's neck is the preferred treatment for complete contractures of the neck. Thick split-thickness skin grafts may also be used in combination with local flaps and a splint.

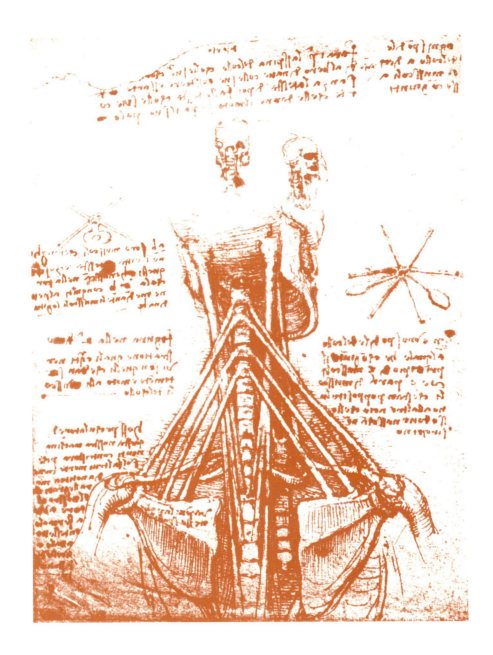

Leonardo da Vinci, 1452 – 1519.

Everyone calls "clear" those ideas which have the same degree of confusion as his own.

Proust

70

RELEASE OF SCAR CONTRACTURE OF THE NECK

Irving Feller

The basic problem in neck contractures is the lack of tissue which has resulted from the scar formation. The body's natural healing process has closed this wound by bringing together the chin and the chest.

An incision on the line crossing the middle of the defect will allow for maximum release of the contracture. The release may open an area up to nine inches wide in extreme cases. This area is then grafted with a thick split-thickness graft.

When the sutures are removed, a neck splint is applied and its continued use is necessary until there is no evidence of scar contracture formation. The time necessary to wear the splint varies from several months to a year, depending upon the patient. It is worn full-time until the tissue shows evidence of softening, and then part-time until not needed.

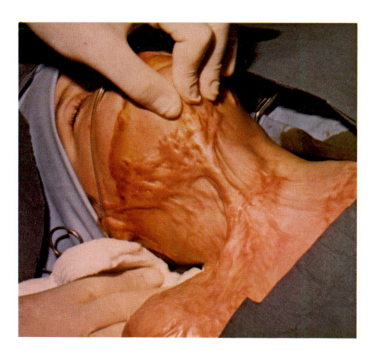

Fig. 1. This moderate scar crosses the neck causing the contracture.

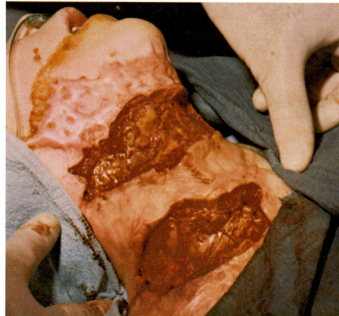

Fig. 2. Two horizontal incisions were made to release the contracture. Since no tissue was excised the open wounds demonstrate the area of contracture.

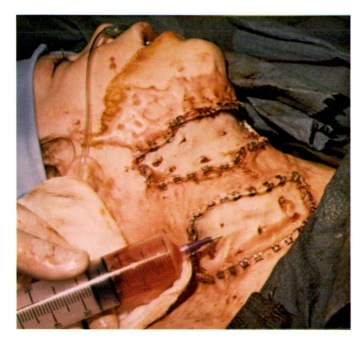

Fig. 3. Thick split-thickness skin grafts are used to cover the defect. The space below the graft is irrigated with a tissue culture solution before the dressing is applied. Splinting of the neck is important to avoid recurrence of the contracture.

71

Z-PLASTY OF SCAR CONTRACTURE OF THE NECK

David W. Furnas

Correction of three specific problems in the scarred, burned neck may be facilitated by use of the Z-plasty. It is ideally suited for breaking up and elongating a long, bridle-like, linear, vertical scar of the anterior surface of the neck. Unfortunately, this situation is far less common than diffuse scarring. It is occasionally useful for elongating a more diffusely distributed, nonpenetrating scar. However, the scarring must be light, the dermis-subcutaneous layers must have an intact blood supply, and the surrounding skin must have enough elasticity to permit rotation of the Z-plasty flaps. Where a deeply burned neck has been covered with skin pedicles, a Z-plasty is sometimes needed to break up and elongate linear pedicle junctures (Figure 1). Small Z-plasties are also occasionally useful in breaking up the junction between a skin graft and the surrounding skin.

DESIGN OF THE Z-PLASTY

Six design variables must be briefly considered in planning a Z-plasty (Figure 2).

Length of the three limbs of the "Z". The longer the limbs, the greater the releasing effect, but also the greater the tension needed for closure.

Tip angles of the two triangular flaps. Larger angles give more generous correction but require more tension for closure; angles which are too small jeopardize the blood supply of the tips.

Symmetry. Should the tip angles be equal or unequal? This is determined by neighboring geographical features.

Orientation. Should the incision describe a "Z" which rotates clockwise or reverse "Z" which rotates counter-clockwise?

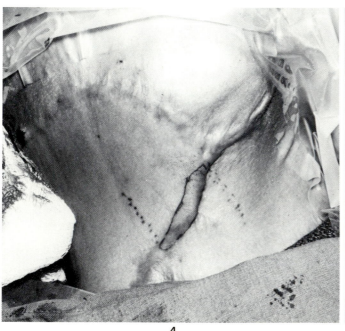
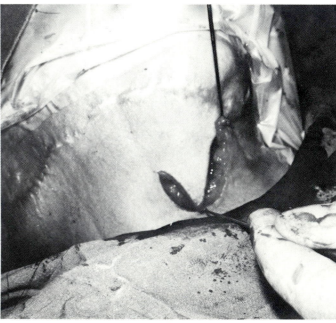

| A | B |

Fig. 1. Z-plasty. **A.** Linear contracture of the anterior surface of neck at the juncture of a skin pedicle placed for correction of a diffuse neck contracture. Incisions for the triangular flaps have been marked. **B.** The Z-plasty flaps are incised and elevated.

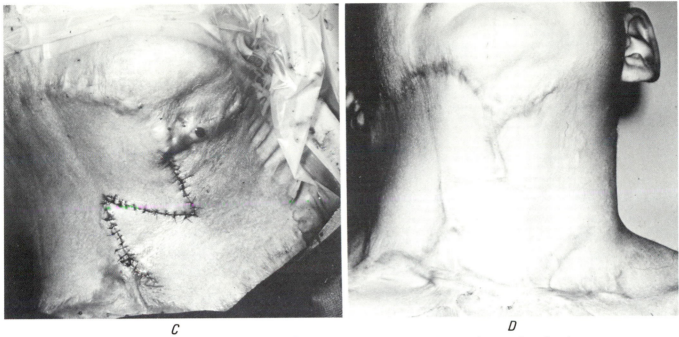

Fig. 1. **C.** The flaps are transposed and sutured. **D.** The patient has obtained appreciable gain in extension of neck.

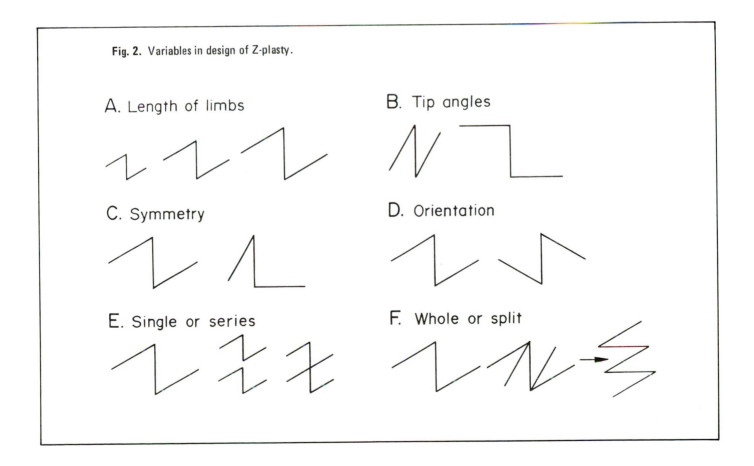

Fig. 2. Variables in design of Z-plasty.

A. Length of limbs

B. Tip angles

C. Symmetry

D. Orientation

E. Single or series

F. Whole or split

Single or serial Z-plasty. Will the correction be best accomplished by a pair of large triangular flaps with more efficient elongation but more tension for closure or by a series of smaller triangular flaps? A series can be constructed with interconnected Z-plasties or disconnected Z-plasties. The most common Z-plasty design for a bridle-like scar of the anterior neck is a symmetrical, single, large Z-plasty with tip angles of 60 degrees or slightly more.

Geographical features. Geographical features such as hair-bearing areas and skin-grafted areas must be accounted for in designing the Z-plasty. If the force of the contracted scar distorts the mouth, the Z-plasty is aligned for optimum release of the mouth. The neck is a compound curve. It is concave when viewed on saggital section, and convex when viewed on transverse section. Transposing a flap across the concavity is done with ease, while transposition across the convexity is difficult. A flap crossing a convex surface must stretch a relatively longer distance than a flap crossing a concave surface. (The flap over a concavity is like a race horse rounding a turn on the outside track position, while a flap over a convexity is like a horse which has leaped the fence and is crossing the infield directly to the other side.) The larger the flap and the farther the incisions extend laterally on the neck, the greater the problem of convexity becomes.

PLANNING THE Z-PLASTY

1. The central limb of the Z-plasty is placed directly upon the bridle-like part of the scar or, in a diffuse scar, central and parallel to the line of contraction.

2. The side limbs are then plotted at the chosen angles, making either a "Z" or a reverse "Z" pattern. The side limbs are about the same length as the central limb.

3. The tensions and directions of force of the skin are estimated by palpation, knowledge of anatomy, and intuition as planning is carried out. Remember that, in essence, skin is being moved from an area of adequate supply to an area of deficiency. Be satisfied that the supply source is adequate.

OPERATIVE PROCEDURE

The central limb is incised (Figure 3A). Particularly dense scar tissue is removed with the central limb incision, while soft pliable scar tissue is left in situ. The incision of each side limb is curved gently near the tip, so that the blood supply is enhanced by making the angle of the tip less acute. The triangular flaps are then elevated with or without the platysma. The neck wound is spread apart, releasing the contracture. If the platysma has been left in place, it can be incised transversely for further release.

The two flaps are interposed (Figure 3B), suction drainage tubes are inserted through stab wounds, and the tips of the flaps are sutured into place. If the tips fall short of their intended position, the side limbs are extended millimeter by millimeter, giving further release. This supplemental incision is more efficient if it is curved inward toward the base of the triangular flap, as in the back cut of a rotation flap. If the closure is still tight, the skin surrounding the Z-plasty is undermined. The subcutaneous-dermal layer is closed with inverted, clear monofilament nylon sutures. The first few sutures are placed diagonally so that when they are pulled up tight, they release tension on the tip of the flap, placing the stress proximally toward the base (Figure 3C). If the original plan proves inadequate and closure of the incisions cannot be completed, part of the defect will have to be closed with a skin graft. The upper two limbs are closed completely, if possible, so that the gap is restricted to the lower limb. The gap is then covered with a skin graft. (If the skin is this tight, correction with skin grafting alone is much preferred to a Z-plasty with supplementary skin grafting.) Final closure is performed with a running subcuticular nylon suture, and the incision lines are reinforced with Micropore tape. The sutures are removed in three weeks.

Fig. 3. Operative procedure for Z-plasty.

A. Incisions

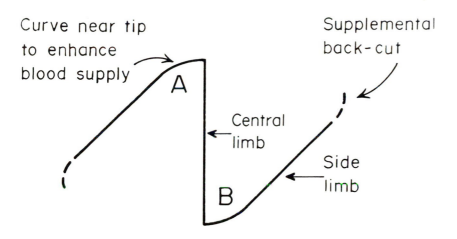

Curve near tip
to enhance
blood supply

A

Supplemental
back-cut

Central
limb

Side
limb

B

B. Transposition

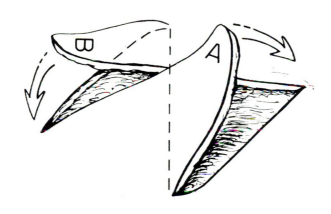

C. Sutures

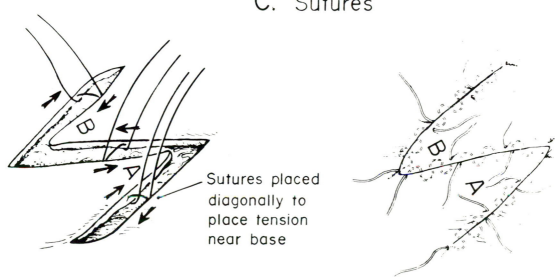

Sutures placed
diagonally to
place tension
near base

72

SPLINTING OF THE NECK

George H. Koepke

Flexion contractures of the neck may follow full-thickness loss of skin from the face, neck, and upper chest because the necessary care of a critically burned patient during the acute period may take precedence over the surgeon's attention to proper positioning of the head. Regardless of the type of bed used by the patient during the acute period, the patient should not be permitted to use a pillow under his head whenever there is full-thickness loss of skin from the chin, neck, or upper chest. Elevation of the head with a Gatch bed does not promote an anterior neck contracture, providing the patient is positioned so that the head portion of the bed is flexed at a point near the hips.

It would be desirable to immobilize and extend the neck immediately after the application of split-thickness skin grafts of the anterior surface. Unfortunately, hyperextension of the neck with a pillow or sand bag under the shoulders is quite uncomfortable and may interfere with the airway and with deglutition. There are several methods of keeping the neck in a neutral position. Each technique has its advantages and disadvantages. The simplest and most inexpensive is to cover the split-thickness skin grafts with surgical dressings and then to wrap the neck with a four to six inch elastic bandage. The moderate pressure provided by this elastic support may facilitate the take of the split-thickness skin grafts, help to maintain the contour of the anterior surface of the neck, and lessen any tendency to the formation of hypertropic scar tissue. An anterior neck contracture due to a bridle scar may be corrected satisfactorily with a simple Z-plasty and the postoperative application of an elastic bandage wrapped around the neck.

Of course an elastic bandage does not immobilize the neck as well as a four-post or Forrester collar.

The latter may be preferred for children and uncooperative adults who move the head and neck so much that they may loosen the grafts. Sometimes a surgeon will prefer to avoid any pressure on a split-thickness skin graft and will treat the wound by the "open method." In these instances, a four-post collar can be applied in the Operating Room, allowing later inspection of the split-thickness skin grafts without removal of the collar. Occasionally, four-post collars with a rigid yoke are stored and readily available to patients in a Burn Unit at a nominal rental fee.

Should the surface of the chin as well as the neck require split-thickness skin grafts, a four-post collar can be modified by substituting stanchions for the anterior two posts and by adding a forehead support as a substitute for the customary chin piece (Figure 1).

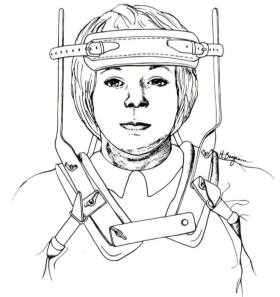

Fig. 1. To avoid pressure on fresh chin grafts, the chin piece of a four-post collar has been replaced by stanchions and a forehead support.

Some surgeons prefer to defer a splint until the split-thickness skin grafts have taken. They then utilize the pressure of a molded plastic or plaster collar to maintain the contour of the neck and chin. Others object to the occasional maceration that may be caused by the plaster or plastic and also to the occasional delay that is necessary from the time of grafting to the application of the plastic splint.

Lateral deviation of the head and neck is less common than flexion deformities and is seen among patients with full-thickness loss of skin from one side of the neck and the superior aspect of a shoulder. This deformity may lead to a scoliosis. For this reason, it is advisable to excise the scar, apply a split-thickness skin graft, and correct the lateral deviation by the postoperative application of a four-post collar modified by the addition of a pad that will support the side of the head (Figure 2). Instead of an orthosis, the same result may be achieved with a plaster Minerva jacket. The latter is a little less expensive, but is heavier and cannot be removed readily to bathe or inspect the wound.

Surgeons recognize the value of immobilization to facilitate the take of any graft; those working with collagen tissue have demonstrated that **collagen fibers become mature in approximately 50 days. After that time, collagen fibers cannot be stretched effectively.** In light of this, it seems most appropriate to maintain the head and neck in a neutral position whenever there is full-thickness loss of skin from the neck and to position the head opposite the anticipated deformity for at least four weeks following the application of split-thickness skin grafts.

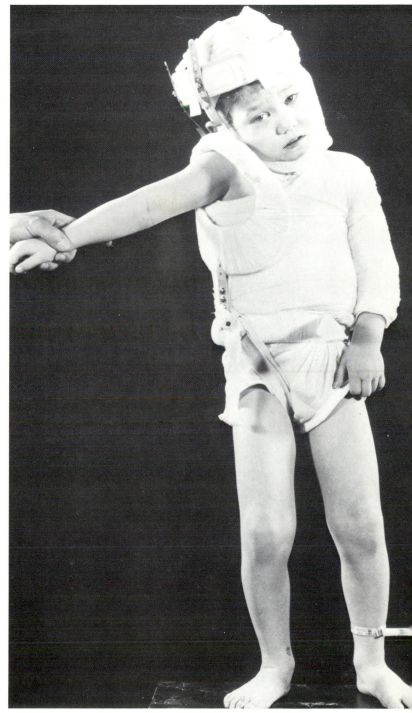

Fig. 2. Partial correction of severe lateral deviation of the head and neck with scoliosis.

XI.

THE TRUNK
AND
PERINEUM

PRINCIPLES OF TREATMENT

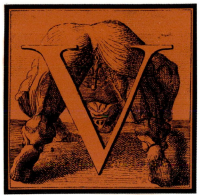

anity may be as incapacitating as the disabling and disfiguring scars and contractures of the trunk which include the breast, chest, abdomen, flanks, and perineum. Contractures of the breast in young females require release and grafting to accommodate breast tissue development. Contractures of the chest, abdomen, and flanks in growing children must be released and grafted to avoid deformity of the spine. Contractures of the perineum have to be corrected to allow for normal motion and body hygiene. Reconstruction of the penis and vulva may be necessary when these parts are scarred or destroyed.

Hypertrophic scar and occasionally keloids have to be excised and overgrafted. The need for these procedures must be individualized to meet the patient's needs without causing harm. Counselling of these individuals for good psychological acceptance of their injury and any residual disability or disfigurement is as essential as the reconstructive procedure.

Irving Feller

74

EARLY MANAGEMENT OF THE TRUNK AND PERINEUM

Irving Feller
Kathryn E. Richards

Immediately after the burn, releasing escharotomy may be necessary for circumferential wounds of the chest and abdomen to allow adequate respiration. General care for wounds of the trunk includes daily dressing changes, frequent shaving of hair, and body positioning to avoid decubiti for immobilized patients. Special care includes placing the patient on the abdomen for brief periods to allow full extension of the hips with precaution taken to prevent a decrease in chest excursion. Chest and abdominal dressings should be wrapped loosely and bolsters placed under the shoulders. Hair should be shaved at least two inches from the burn. Perineal and axillary hair should be shaved in all patients on admission and again once a week until all wounds are closed. If the perineum is severely burned, a urinary catheter is used and is changed once a week until all perineal burns are closed. A colostomy to direct the fecal stream has not been found to be necessary in most cases.

Grid escharatomy and enzymatic topical agents are used to hasten the debriding process so that early autografting or homografting can be done to close the open wound.

When the penis is severely burned and a foreskin remains, care should be taken to preserve the foreskin to be used as the pedicle graft to cover the shaft of the penis. When the foreskin is burned circumferentially, the outer layer may have suffered full-thickness loss and the inner layer may have been damaged and become edematous. If the edema is severe, a dorsal slit should be used to avoid constricting necrosis to the glans. The following color illustrations depict these principles of care.

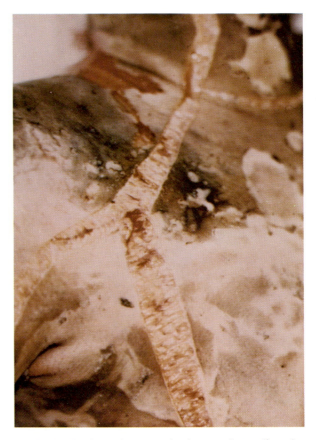

Fig. 1. A releasing escharotomy has been made to relieve the constriction of the chest in this patient with circumferential burns. Note how the simple linear incision has resulted in a wide defect.

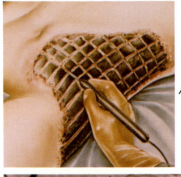

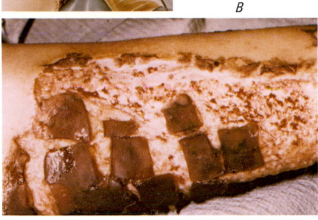

Fig. 2. **A.** This illustrates the technique of grid escharotomy. The grid of one-inch squares allow for more rapid debridement, **B.** which in turn leads to earlier skin cover.

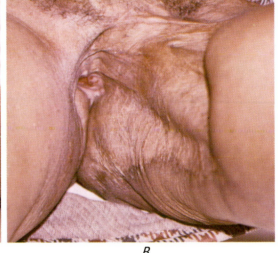

Fig. 3. Perineal burns increase the hazard of infection. All perineal hair should be shaved on admission and kept clean until the wound is closed. A urinary catheter should be used as a means of keeping the perineum clean in both males and females.

Fig. 4. **A.** Severe burns of the female perineum can also be manged by using the catheter and keeping the patient clean as is shown in this elderly woman's case. **B.** A bowel preparation and low residue diet were used during the grafting period. Colostomy is rarely needed to obtain good wound closure.

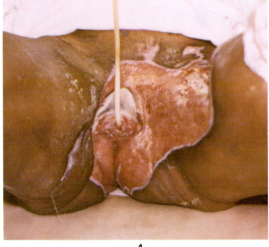

Fig. 5. When the penis is burned full-thickness and a foreskin is present and circumferentially edematous, a dorsal slit can protect both the glans and save the foreskin for reconstruction. **A.** The penis is shown after grafting revealing the edematous foreskin. **B.** The edema will subside and then the foreskin can be used to reconstruct the shaft of the penis if necessary or a circumcision can be done if it is not needed.

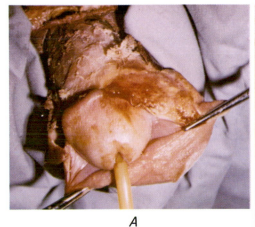

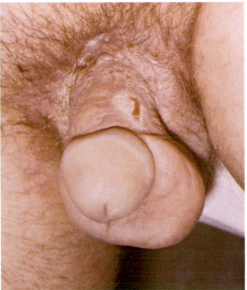

259

75

BREAST RECONSTRUCTION

Irving Feller

Fortunately the embryonic breast tissue is deep in the subcutaneous tissue in prepubertal girls and, therefore, escapes destruction even in full-thickness skin burns of the chest. When the patient reaches puberty, the breast tissue anlage responds to the normal stimulation and can be seen to grow. The forming breast tissue will bulge between the bands of burn scars. This is the time when the first release of the scar contracture should be carried out. A graft is placed in the defect created to allow for normal growth of the breast tissue. Timing is important, because the tight bands may inhibit the growth of the normal breast if the release is delayed. As the patient matures, further releases with grafts may be necessary to provide for full development of the breast.

Different circumstances resulting from the original injuries require that each patient receive individualized treatment. In some cases, only one breast is burned; in others, both have suffered full-thickness loss. Also, the areola may or may not have been destroyed.

It is usually easier to repair bilaterally damaged breasts as far as symmetry is concerned. When one normal breast is present it is important to approximate its shape when reconstructing its damaged counterpart.

When any part of the areola is identified, it should be preserved and used in the repair. If the areola has been destroyed and the patient so desires, tatooing on a circular graft from another part of the body can be used as a substitute.

In all cases, the patient must be counseled regarding the function of the breast should she become pregnant. With the program discussed above, our patients have had breast reconstruction followed by normal pregnancies and have had no problems. The following case study illustrates these principles.

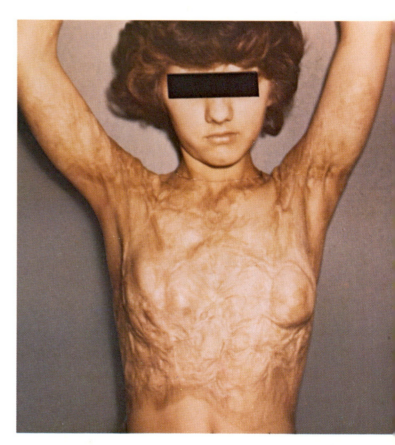

Fig. 1. This young girl was burned when she was 5-years-old. Her clothing caught fire causing full-thickness burns of the chest. She is shown at 12 years old; the forming breast tissue appears behind the contracture.

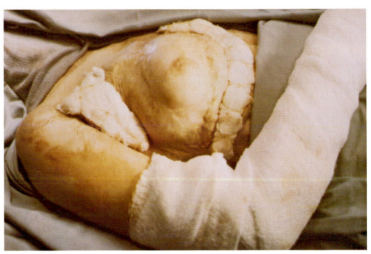

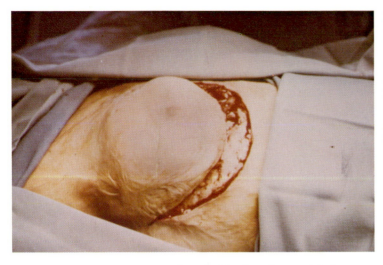

Fig. 2. At operation, a linear incision is made around the lower border of the breast. No tissue is removed and the size of the defect is the measure of the skin shortage.

Fig. 3. A thick split-thickness skin graft is used to cover the defect and a stent dressing is used to immobilize the graft.

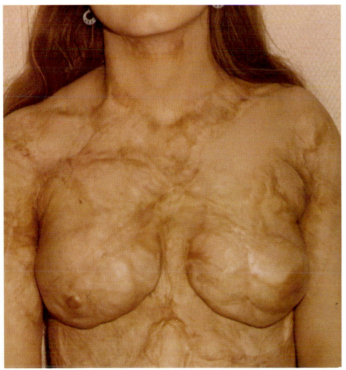

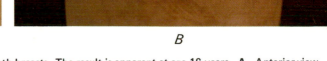

A   B

Fig. 4. Several similar procedures were required to reconstruct both breasts. The result is apparent at age 16 years. **A.** Anterior view. **B.** Profile.

76

BREAST PROSTHESIS

Denis C. Lee

Occasionally one or both breasts may be damaged from burns. Custom breast prostheses can be fabricated for burn patients suffering loss of a part or the entire breast.

A chest cast is taken of the patient using hydrocolloid impression material. The hydrocolloid is reinforced with plaster bandages and removed. This is then filled with plaster stone to give a duplication of the patient's chest.

The damaged areas are covered with clay and sculpted to match the patient's remaining breast or former shape if both breasts are missing.

Molds for the breast prostheses are then made over the clay. The clay is removed and a silicone skin matching the patient's skin color is placed into the mold and bonded together. The sac created is then filled with a glycerine gel. A special backing is applied so that the prosthesis may be adhered to the skin with doublesided colostomy tape. The nipple is then tinted to desired color.

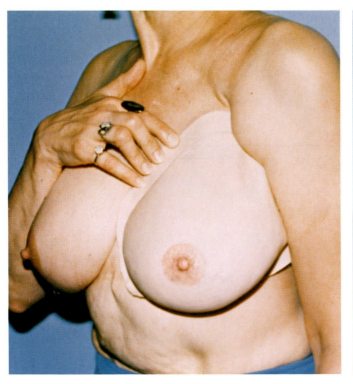

A

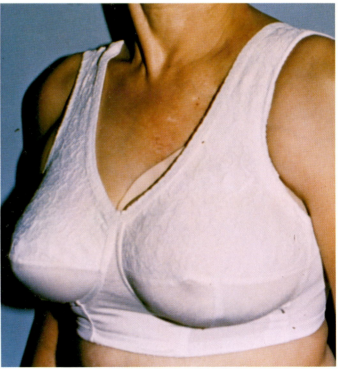

B

Fig. 1. A. External breast prosthesis in place. Prosthesis may be adhered with double sided tape. **B.** Prosthesis held in place with brassiere naturally provides patient with proper weight and allows her to wear most clothing.

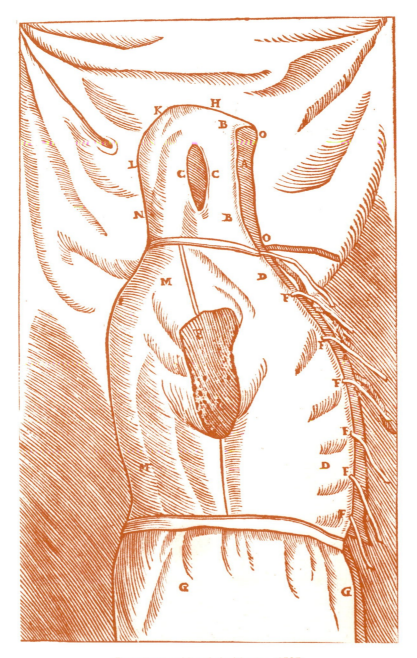

De curtorum chirurgia insitionem, 1597.

Wherever a doctor cannot do good, he must be kept from doing harm.

Hippocrates

77

SCOLIOSIS AND KYPHOSIS

E. Burke Evans

Abnormal curvatures of the spine which occur following severe burns are always extrinsically imposed. They occur frequently in children, rarely in adults. The causes thus far encountered are: (1) Scar contracture of the chest, trunk, groin, and axilla; (2) malposition of the hip secondary to dislocation, heterotopic bone formation, or ankylosis; and (3) lower extremity length discrepancy.

Any burn of the chest, axilla, abdomen, back, or groin may cause the patient to accommodate to the burn by bending the spine. The curve of accommodation may not be noticed until the patient stands, and by that time it may be difficult or impossible for the patient to achieve voluntary correction (Figure 1). However, as healing progresses and as the involved area becomes less painful to stress, most curves of accommodation disappear.

Occasionally, with progressive scar contracture a curve will persist until the contracture is surgically relieved (Figure 2A and B). If the contracture remains through a period of rapid growth for a child, structural change in the form of vertebral wedging may result (Figures 3A and B).

Symmetric or circumferential burns of the trunk do not tend to cause scoliosis. Burns of the back do not cause hyperextension of the spine and rarely cause restriction of flexion. Burns of the abdomen and chest, however, may cause flattening of the lumbar spine and exaggeration of the thoracic kyphosis.

Probably the most offensive burn is that which involves the upper chest and shoulders. Contracture of scars in this region causes protraction of the shoulders and exaggeration of the thoracic kyphosis (Figures 4A and B). Once this posture is established, it is difficult to correct even after repeated scar re-

Fig. 1. A four-year-old girl with full-thickness burns of the groin and right flank. This transient curve accommodated to the flank burn. After split-thickness graft the burn healed with minimum contracture and the curve disappeared.

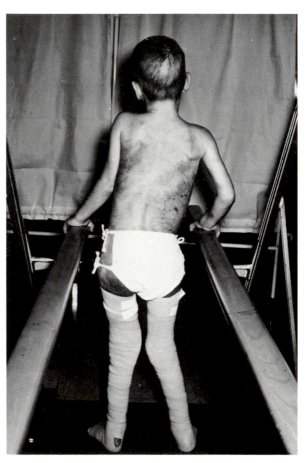

leases. The usual position in the usual bed helps to bring about the deformity. Burns of the neck in combination with burns of the chest may compound the problem by causing extreme flexion of the cervical spine.

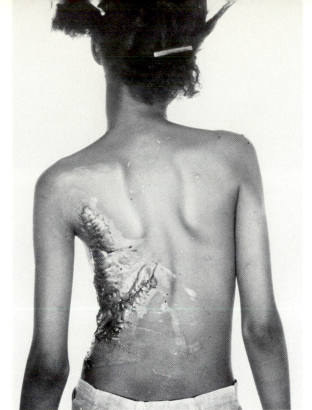

Fig. 2. A. Scar contracture caused a right low thoracic curve in this 11-year-old girl. **B.** After surgical release of the scar the scoliosis disappeared.

Burns of the groin and lower abdomen often lead to flexion contractures of the hip. If the contracture is bilateral, it may merely flatten the lumbar curve. If it is unilateral, it may cause pelvic obliquity and scoliosis.

Curves of accommodation are prevented by proper positioning during the acute phase. The trunk should be maintained in good alignment, with the iliac crests and shoulders level. The hips should be extended and symmetrically abducted. If the burn involved the upper chest and axillae, a towel roll should be placed posteriorly between the shoulders to discourage protraction. Arms should be symmetrically abducted at least 70 degrees and flexed approximately 35 to 40 degrees. A firm mattress is essential.

Fig. 3. The structural thoracolumbar curve in this 14-year-old girl resulted from a scar of nine years' duration. **A.** In this case surgical release of the scar did not correct the scoliosis. **B.** Roentgenogram illustrates the thoracolumbar curve.

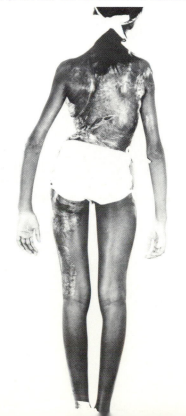
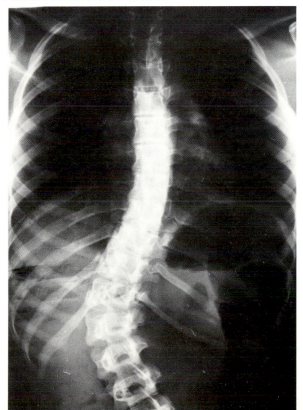

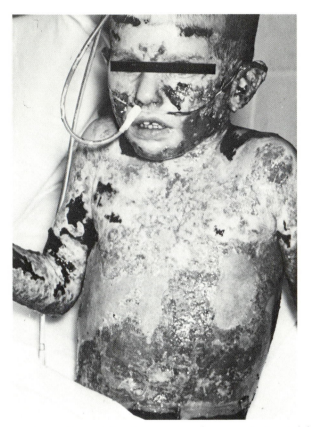
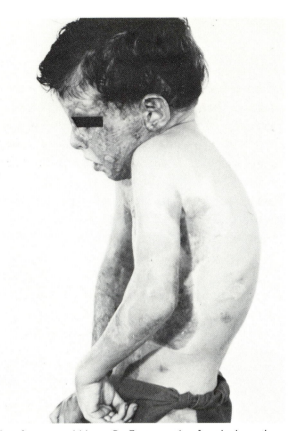

Fig. 4. A. Spotty full-thickness burns of chest, abdomen and shoulders in a four-year-old boy. **B.** Four months after the burn there was protraction and elevation of the shoulders and exaggeration of the thoracic kyphosis.

Fig. 4. C. After surgical release of the anterior scars and split-thickness grafting, a Milwaukee type brace with anterior shoulder pads was used to hold correction. **D.** One year after the burn, the kyphosis was less prominent but the shoulders remained protracted requiring further anterior surgical release. Adjustment and refittings of the brace were of little help as the brace had not been worn continuously.

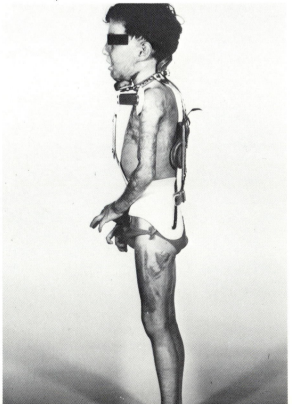
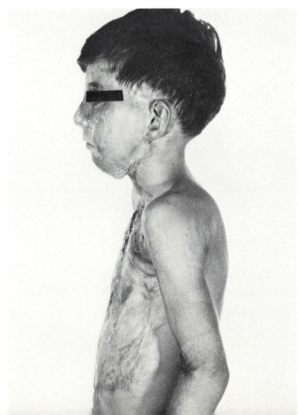

TREATMENT

All of the nonstructural curves occurring as a result of scar contracture either resolve spontaneously as the scar softens or when the contracture is surgically corrected. A structural curve persisting after scar release might require surgical correction and fusion, if it is severe enough. The author has observed one curve of this severity (Figure 3A and B). *Miller and McMillan have used Harrington rod correction and fixation in one case with a severe curve. They were unable to establish without question, however, that the curve resulted exclusively from the burn.

Resistant curves in young children may be treated with a Milwaukee brace. This type of bracing is especially useful for exaggerated thoracic kyphosis (Figure 4C).

Curves resulting from malposition of the hip correct spontaneously when the hip is properly aligned and the pelvic obliquity corrected. If the pelvic obliquity is secondary to bridging heterotopic bone, removal of the bone, after all skin lesions are mature and the abnormal bone appears radiographically to be mature, will usually result in sufficient mobilization of the hip to achieve correction. Displacement or dissolution of the hip will cause pelvic obliquity and secondary scoliosis (Figure 5). Curves resulting from loss of lower extremity length or arrested growth are corrected by appropriate shoe elevation.

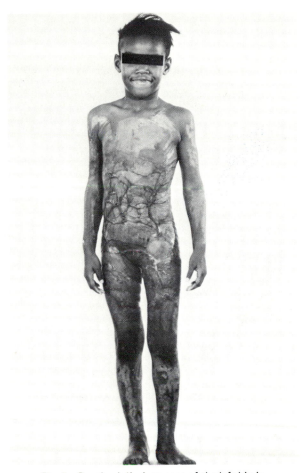

Fig. 5. Proximal displacement of the left hip in this six-year-old girl resulted in permanent extremity length discrepancy, pelvic obliquity and scoliosis. The pelvic obliquity and the scoliosis were partly corrected by a shoe lift on the short side.

---

*Edward H. Miller, M.D. and Bruce G. MacMillan, M.D., Shriners Burns Institute, Cincinnati, Ohio.

GENITAL BURNS

John C. Gaisford

Of the thousands of burns which occur in the United States each year, it is surprising how few are serious burns of the genitalia.

When burns of the genitalia are discussed, the penis and scrotum represent nearly all of the cases. The female genitalia, including even the most exposed areas, are rarely involved. The percentage of serious burns of the male genitalia is low because of the anatomical arrangement of the skin of the penis and scrotum. Because it is usually wrinkled, many islands of unburned skin often remain and spread during the healing phase.

EARLY CARE

In most cases a urethral catheter is necessary for fluid management. If, however, the patient does not require fluid therapy, a urethral catheter should be inserted when there is severe injury to the genitalia. The reason for this catheterization is that the urine is diverted making wound care easier and in the case of the male it serves as an internal splint when autografting.

The need for a dorsal slit (escharotomy) to release tension and preserve adequate blood supply is rare. However, it is justified if one feels the viability of the tissues is in danger.

Debriding is a prime procedure in preparing a burned area for skin grafting. However, one must be extremely conservative in debriding the penis or scrotum. As mentioned above, numerous tiny islands of viable epithelium usually remain from which serviceable skin will grow and coalesce to form a smooth, quite acceptable cover.

When the genitalia are so damaged that the skin is obviously lost, relatively prompt grafting with split-thickness skin should be considered. Usually it is not necessary to cover this area with a pedicle or full-thickness skin. Burying the testicles in the thigh areas can be technically difficult and impossible if the thighs are burned but split-thickness skin grafting of the entire genital area, scrotum, and/or penis with medium-thickness skin from whatever source is available is probably wiser anyhow.

Severe burns can and do lead to partial or total loss of the penis, which necessitates rather extensive reconstruction procedures.

Occasionally it will be necessary to perform a colostomy as the result of the scarring around the genital, perineal, and anal regions which diverts the fecal stream.

CASE REPORTS

Case 1 is a 12-year old girl who suffered 60 percent full-thickness burns involving the entire area over the vulva and perineum (Figure 1). This child

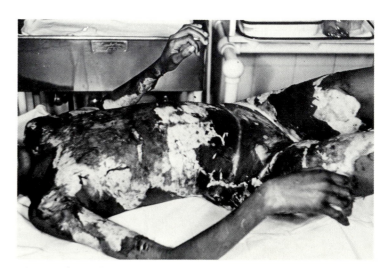

Fig. 1. (Case 1). Twelve-year-old girl with 60% full-thickness burns of the body.

survived and did quite well (Figure 2). She became pregnant at age 16 and had no complications referable to the free skin grafts covering her genital and perineal areas, but did have to have release of her expanding abdomen by the insertion of split-thickness skin grafts.

Case 2 is a man who lost considerable penile and scrotal skin as the result of a chemical burn (Figure 3). This problem was managed by prompt debridement, multiple dressing changes over a few days, followed by a Padgett dermatome graft of about 0.012 inches. The result was completely acceptable to both patient and surgeon.

While radiation burns of the penis have been rare on our service, one such case did appear. Case 3 (Figure 4) reveals the appearance of the genitalia of a man heavily irradiated for testicular cancer, with chronic ulceration, radiation cancers, and severe pain. Treatment consisted of amputation of the penis and local removal of the radiation-induced cancers (Figure 5).

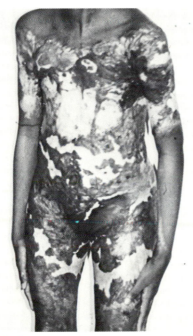

Fig. 2. (Case 1). Complete healing following extensive free skin grafting. No problems referable to the genitalia.

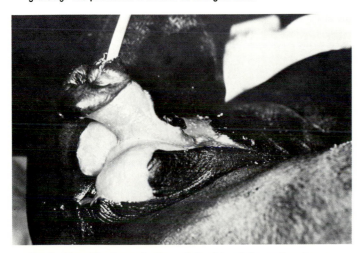

Fig. 3. (Case 2). Extensive loss of the skin of the penis and scrotum due to a chemical burn.

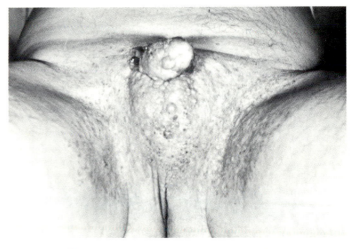

Fig. 4. (Case 3). Radiation dermatitis and radiation cancer of the penis and adjacent skin.

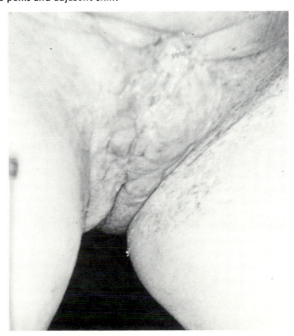

Fig. 5. (Case 3). Amputation of penis and adjacent skin cancers.

Although the male genitalia seems to be vulnerable to injury because of their location, many times adjacent areas are more severely injured. Case 4 represents such a situation (Figure 6). Both thighs, reaching several inches above the level of the penis, were charred, but the penis and scrotum were burned only in a spotty fashion. After two weeks the thighs were ready for skin grafting and the genitalia all but healed (Figure 7).

A catheter is probably inserted into the bladder of most burns of the genitalia in order to monitor the intravenous fluid requirements, but **how often does the surgeon think about the possibility of urethral damage, rupture, or obstruction as a result of the burn?** To repeat, we have never seen a ruptured urethra due to burns and have never had to perform a dorsal slit for edema of the penis due to an acute burn. In case 5 an acute, severe burn of the lower extremities and genitalia, a urethral catheter was inserted (Figure 8). No dorsal slit was considered and again, spontaneous healing of the genitalia was almost complete by the time the lower extremities were ready for primary skin grafting (Figure 9).

On more than one occasion, small boys have

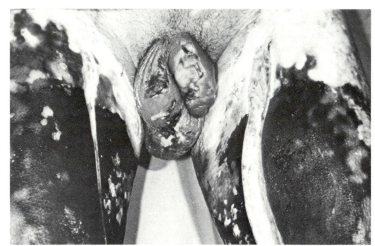

Fig. 8. (Case 5). Acute, severe burns of thighs and genitalia with loss of skin on the penis.

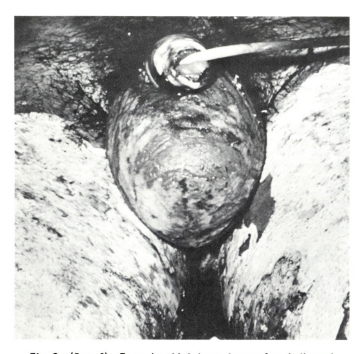

Fig. 6. (Case 4). Extensive third degree burns of genitalia and lower extremities.

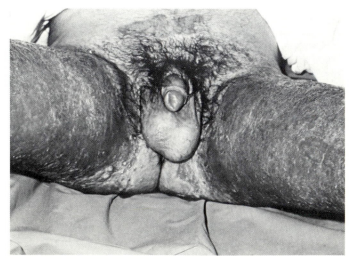

Fig. 7. (Case 4). Healing of genitalia and thighs just ready for skin grafting.

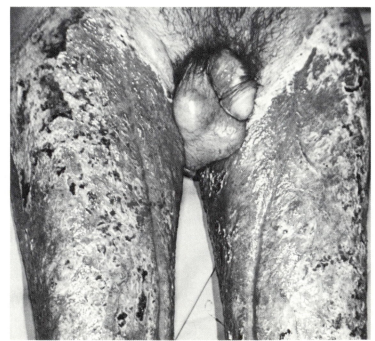

270 Fig. 9. (Case 5). No dorsal slit but uncomplicated penile healing.

lost all of their protruding genitals, which in several cases included both testicles. Case 6 (Figure 10) is an acute burn of the lower extremities, genitalia, and lower abdomen. When debridement was completed, the penis and scrotum were gone and only a hole was present for insertion of a catheter. Promptly, however, scarring about the perineum caused diversion of the fecal stream in such a fashion that this boy began to evacuate his rectum from behind his left knee. A colostomy was performed which permitted replacement of the perianal and perineal scar with good skin (Figure 11). The penis was

operated on three years later and the remains of the corpora dissected out of the suprapubic area (Figure 12) and covered with a Padgett dermatome skin graft (Figure 13). Dr. George Crikelair suggested through a personal communication that considerable penile length could be obtained during the reconstructive procedure by carefully dividing the suspensory ligament of the penis at its base. The final result here was satisfactory in that the boy could stand to void and had some penile length (Figure 14).

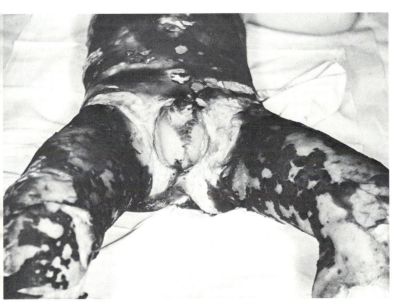

Fig. 10. (Case 6). Extensive full-thickness burns of abdominal wall, genitalia, and lower extremities.

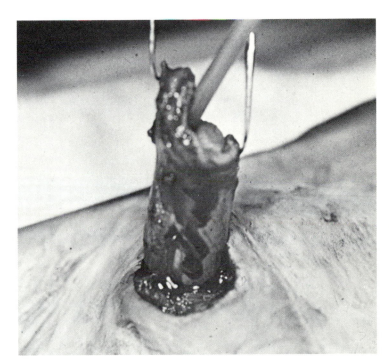

Fig. 12. (Case 6). Remains of penis dissected free, preliminary to grafting.

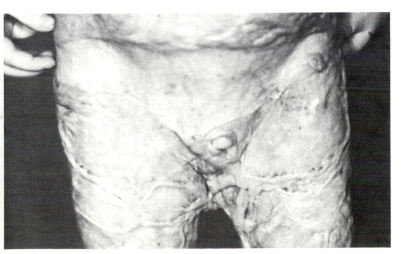

Fig. 11. (Case 6). Heavy scarring about the perineum, loss of genitalia, colostomy.

271

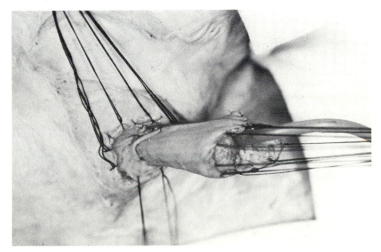

Fig. 13. (Case 6). Split-thickness skin graft wrapped around remains of penis.

Case 7 is almost identical (Figure 15). This patient was prepared for skin grafting in the usual way (Figure 16) and then covered with split-thickness skin (Figure 17). Later it became necessary to dissect out both testicles and the remains of the penis. The penis was grafted with a dermatome skin graft and a similar piece of skin formed a new scrotum. Figure 18 shows the penis ten years later and the pliability of the skin graft covering the testicles.

Neglected burns of the genital area can result in problems illustrated by Case 8 (Figure 19) and Case 9 (Figure 20). This type of old burn scar involvement is still too common and causes obvious unnecessary discomfort through tightness, chronic ulceration, and deformities. A victim of this unfortunate development can be markedly handicapped in performing his usual toilet and sexual functions.

SUMMARY

Burns of the genitalia can be minimal or very severe. In males, debridement should be performed in a meticulous, conservative fashion, recognizing that spontaneous repair in that area is frequently possible. Early skin grafting is advised with split-thickness skin grafts.

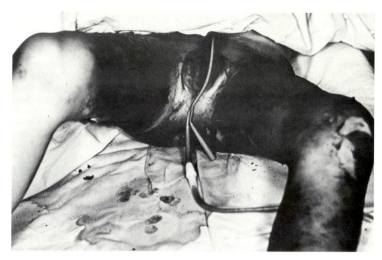

Fig. 15. (Case 7). Extensive full-thickness burns of genitalia.

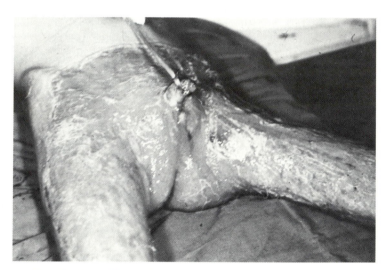

Fig. 16. (Case 7). Genital area, abdomen, and thighs prepared for skin grafting.

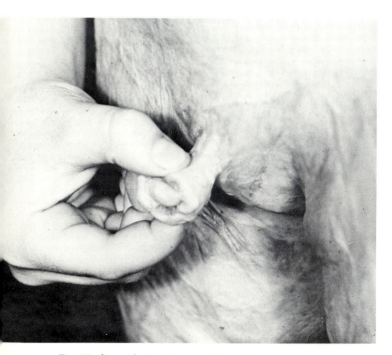

Fig. 14. (Case 6). Final result with some penile length and ability to stand to void.

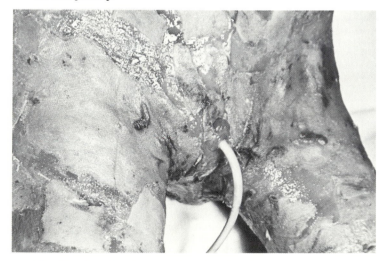

Fig. 17. (Case 7). Complete loss of penis and scrotum, catheter in urethra.

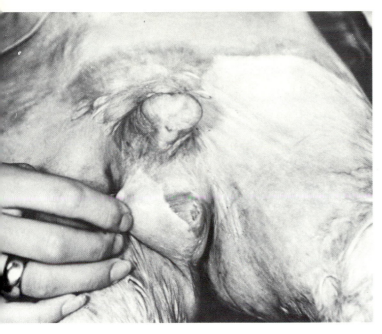

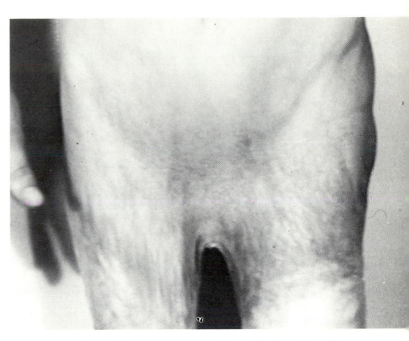

Fig. 18. (Case 7). Ten years after burn and repair, the penis is reasonably satisfactory and the scrotal skin is soft and pliable.

Fig. 19. (Case 8). Neglected burn patient with the male genitalia not even visible.

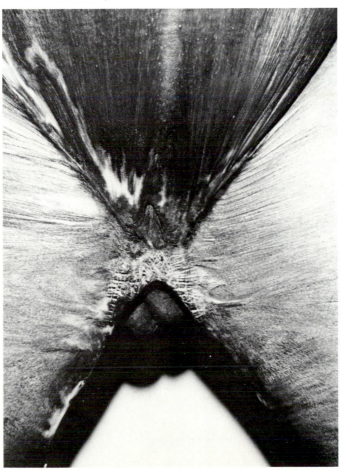

Fig. 20. (Case 8). Grossly neglected old burn in a man of 45, with the umbilicus over the pubis and the normal genitalia totally trapped in scar.

79

REPAIR OF THE PERINEUM

Irving Feller

Both deep partial and full-thickness burns of the perineum result in contractures that both interfere with normal motion and make body hygiene difficult. In males, horizontal contracture bands may appear above and below the penis. The repair is best accomplished by releasing the contracture and filling the defects with thick split-thickness grafts.

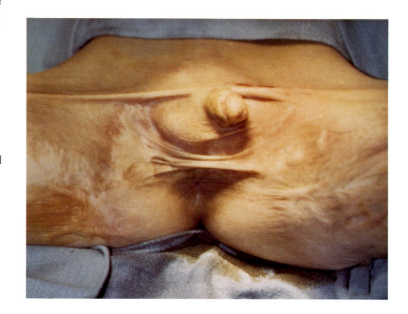

Fig. 1. Scar contractures are seen above the penis and between the scrotum and anus.

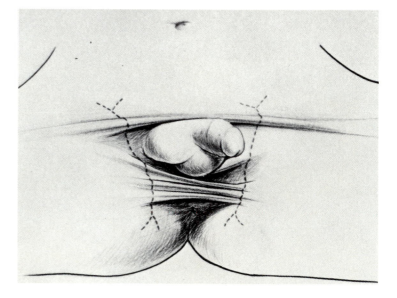

Fig. 2. The dotted lines indicate where the incision will be made to obtain maximum release of the contracture. The defect that is obtained with the double "Y" incision is a rectangle. The thick partial-thickness grafts are held in place with sutures or metal clips.

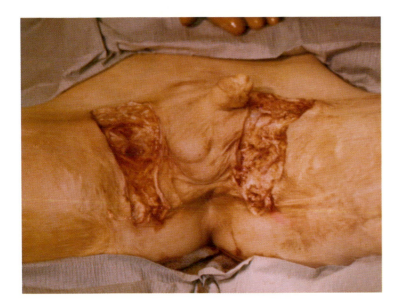

Fig. 3. The defect created after the scar contracture is released demonstrating the shortage of tissue.

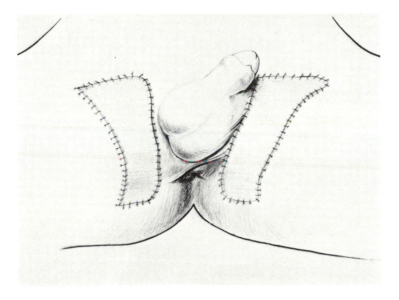

Fig. 4. The thick split-thickness grafts are sewn into place to cover defects.

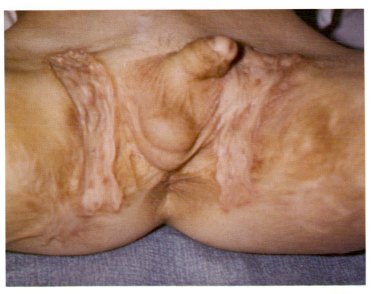

Fig. 5. The contracture has been corrected and the grafts are shown healing two weeks after the repair.

80

PENIS RECONSTRUCTION

Irving Feller

Thirteen percent of the 3000 patients treated at the Michigan Burn Center have had perineal burns. Fortunately, very few of the males suffered full-thickness loss of the penile skin; only one lost a major portion of his penis. The full-thickness skin loss was repaired by using split-thickness skin grafts and unburned foreskin. The latter makes an excellent full-thickness graft for covering denuded areas of the shaft of the penis.

The urinary catheter is used as an internal splint. The contractures are released and the split-thickness skin grafts applied to the defect. Occlusive dressings are used for the first 24 hours and are then removed to allow for better care of the grafts.

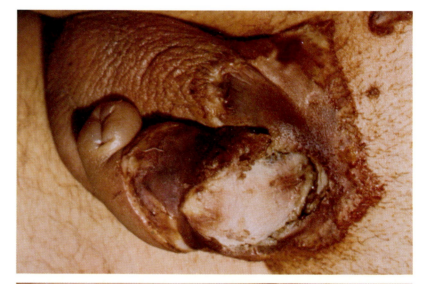

Fig. 1. This 25-year-old male patient suffered burns to his penis when a high tension wire fell on his truck.

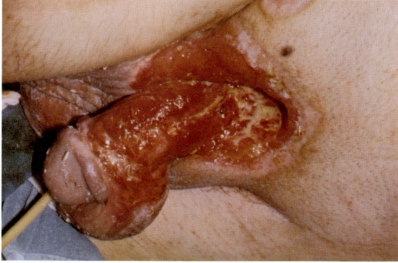

Fig. 2. Full-thickness skin loss occured which required split-thickness skin grafts for early care.

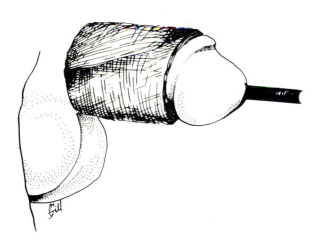

Fig. 3. The grafts are placed over the defect in the usual manner. An indwelling urinary catheter is kept in place to avoid obstruction of the urinary tract when a pressure dressing is used to immobilize the graft.

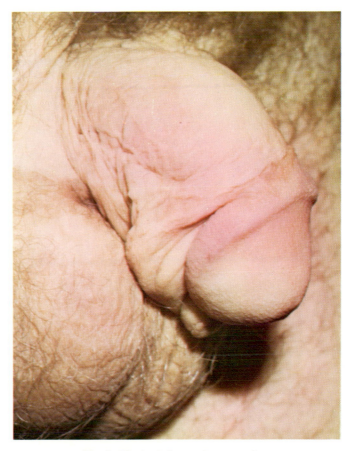

Fig. 4. The healed wound one year later.

XII.

THE AXILLA AND UPPER ARM

PRINCIPLES OF TREATMENT

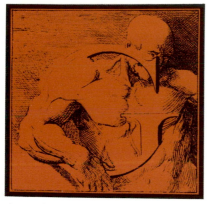

rafting with split-thickness skin after release of the axillary contracture is the usual method of repair. The shoulder joint is the most mobile joint in the body, and any burn or injury that limits the extensibility of skin of subcutaneous tissue around the joint limits its motion. Abduction is most severely restricted when burns scar the axillary area. One effect of bed rest is to limit shoulder activity, and the burn patient in bed with an axillary injury is even more unlikely to move his shoulder. Pain restricts motion, and periarticular fibrosis sets in.

The release of the axillary contracture is by operative incision of the contracted skin in a horizontal plane at the level of the depth of the pit of the axilla. A thick split-thickness skin graft is placed on this wound and held with a tie-over dressing. The upper extremity should then be splinted in 90 to 100 degrees of abduction with pre-made abduction splint as described by George Koepke in the chapter on Physical Measures in Axillary Burn Management, or a plaster slab fashioned in the Operating Room also described in this section. Overhead pulley exercises to provide and maintain full abduction are also essential. They should be started after the skin graft has healed and continued for at least three months postoperatively.

Z-plasties are very effective in releasing contracture bands with reasonably good skin on both sides of the burn. Similarly, local skin flaps are rarely indicated, and then only if the skin to be used in the flap has not been burned.

The upper arm can be resurfaced with split-thickness skin grafts.

William C. Grabb

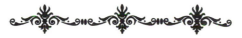

82

EARLY MANAGEMENT OF THE AXILLA, ARM, ELBOW, AND HAND

Irving Feller

Kathryn E. Richards

General care of wounds of the upper extremity includes dressing changes and cleansing of wounds at least twice a day, active and passive exercises, and splinting when necessary.

During the early edema period, arms should be elevated in such a way as to facilitate adequate venous and lymphatic drainage, taking care to avoid constricting pressure at wrist and elbow. Frequent daily exercise actively and passively of all joints should be carried out (Figure 1). The patient should be encouraged to move all joints as many times a day as possible. The positioning of the shoulders should be in abduction; elbows should be alternately placed in flexion then extension, repositioning about every two to four hours.

Splinting and early grafting of the hands is important. One proven method of positioning of the hands is in slight extension at the wrist, 90 degrees flexion at metacarpals two, three, four, and five; 180 degrees extension at metacarpal one and extension of all interphalangeal joints (Figure 2). Palmar burns do not occur as often as extensor surface burns, but when they do exist the contractures can be more severe.

Deep burns of the extensor surface of the hands result in destruction of the skin, tendons, joints, and bone. Gradual debridement is indicated until all dead tissue is removed, care being taken to conserve all living tissue. Amputation should not be undertaken until all considerations for reconstruction have been made.

Special consideration in wound care to deep burns of the upper extremity includes releasing escharotomies to improve circulation when circumferential burns exist proximal to a non-burned or superficially burned hand. Exposed bone or tendons should be kept moist with frequent saline soaks. When deep electrical burns of the extremities occur, fasciotomy as well as releasing escharotomies may be required. Anticoagulation therapy should also be considered for the several days following deep electrical burns. Enzyme topical therapy appears to be helpful in loosening tight eschars.

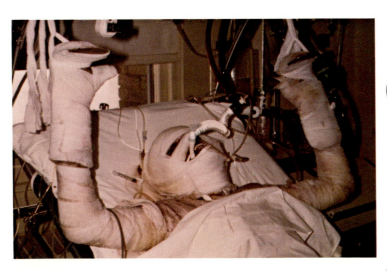

Fig. 1. During the first few days post-burn elevation of the upper extremities above the level of the heart will facilitate venous and lymphatic drainage.

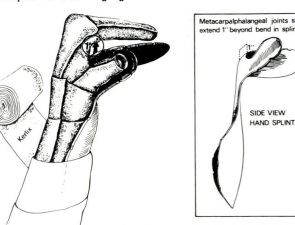

Metacarpalphalangeal joints should extend 1" beyond bend in splint.

SIDE VIEW
HAND SPLINT

Fig. 2. Placing and maintaining the hand in a position of slight extension of the wrist, 90 degrees flexion of metacarpals 2, 3, 4, and 5; 180 degrees extension of metacarpal 1, and extension of all interphalangeal joints is a proven method of assisting in functional control in the hand.

The Erector of the Hand.

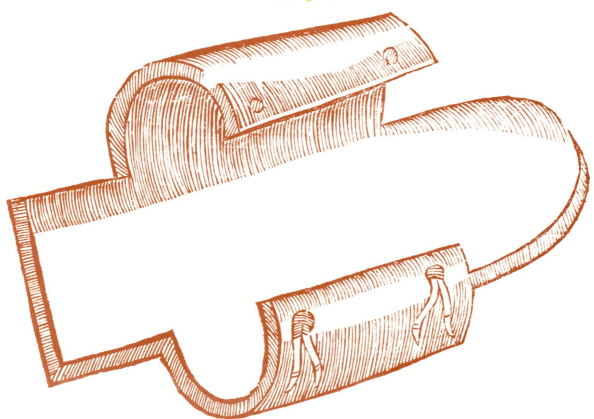

The Works of that Famous Chirurgeon: Ambrose Parey, 1678.

To accept good advice is but to increase one's own ability.
Goethe

83

EXCISION AND REPAIR
OF THE AXILLA

Shattuck W. Hartwell, Jr.

EXCISION OF BURN SCAR CONTRACTURES AND SKIN GRAFTING

The principal restraining areas in the healed axillary burn are in the anterior and posterior folds. The concavity of the apical axillary skin is such that it is usually spared severe injury. Dermal appendages in the axillary skin lie deep, and the apocrine ducts and hair follicles in this area contribute to epithelialization, making most burns superficial in the pit of the axilla. Full-thickness skin loss with secondary scarring is most common in the anterior and posterior folds. Primary resurfacing with flaps is rarely if ever indicated. Skin grafts and local healing are the rule. Limited abduction of the shoulder may ensue, and this is a handicap. Its correction should be carried out as soon as the patient's general condition and rehabilitation program permit. If skin grafts have been applied to resurface axillary burns, enough time must elapse so that a program of physical medicine will give the utmost range of motion while the skin softens and matures. It must be emphasized that physical medicine can never overcome bridling scars and extensive fibrosis. As soon as the extent of fibrosis is recognized and epithelial healing has matured, restricting scar tissue must be excised and the areas resurfaced.

Skin grafts employed to release axillary contractures are usually large and must be planned so that the margins do not lie in the line of contracture. A suspending device to hold up the arm during the operation is useful (Figure 1). Bilateral axillary contractures are common, and it is wise to repair only one at a time. This permits the patient to help himself with at least one arm in the immediate postoperative period. When a skin graft is employed, a shoulder spica is used not only to dress the wound but also to provide bulk on the lateral side of the chest and on the medial side of the arm. A plaster-of-paris abduction splint can then be fashioned over the dressing to maintain a position of 90 degrees (Figure 2). After each dressing change a new plaster-of-paris slab will be necessary, because the old one never fits the new dressing very well. When epithelialization is complete or the take of the graft is nearly 100 percent, it is no longer necessary to use a splint.

SPLINTING AND PHYSICAL MEDICINE

An immediate postoperative splinting program is important, helping to ensure the acceptance of the skin graft and to provide the patient with some comfort. Manipulation of the shoulder under anesthesia results in considerable pain if the shoulder is moved to any extent immediately after the operation. Smaller skin grafts and most Z-plasty releases of axillary contractures do not require a rigid splint as a part of the dressing, but a program of physical exercise is always necessary to regain a range of motion.

When a skin graft is used and epithelialization is complete, range of motion exercises may be instituted. A good program of physical rehabilitation will recapture much of the lost motion in young patients. Severe periarticular fibrosis may decrease the ultimate range of motion in older patients, no matter how completely resurfaced the periarticular skin may be.

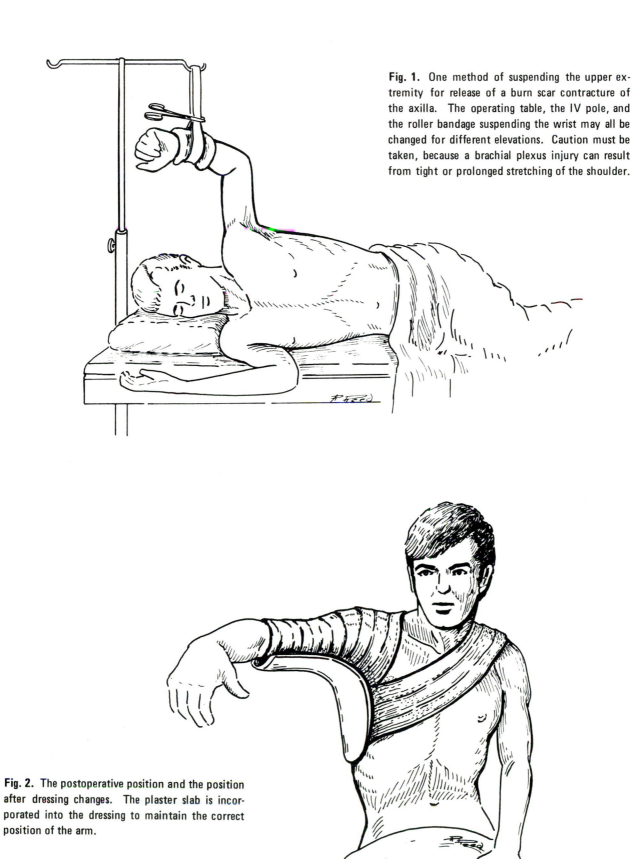

Fig. 1. One method of suspending the upper extremity for release of a burn scar contracture of the axilla. The operating table, the IV pole, and the roller bandage suspending the wrist may all be changed for different elevations. Caution must be taken, because a brachial plexus injury can result from tight or prolonged stretching of the shoulder.

Fig. 2. The postoperative position and the position after dressing changes. The plaster slab is incorporated into the dressing to maintain the correct position of the arm.

84

Z-PLASTY AND LOCAL FLAP
OF THE AXILLA

L.O. Vasconez
M.J.Jurkiewicz

Three fundamental methods are available for the correction of axillary scar contractures: the application of a split-thickness skin graft to replace the burned skin; the Z-plasty procedure; and the rotation, advancement, and transposition of adjacent skin flaps. Each procedure has its indications and advantages, but in many cases the best result will be obtained by combining two of these methods. The aim of this surgery should be to correct the burn scar contracture and to restore function, particularly abduction and elevation of the arm, in a single operation. Even small contractures can be functionally significant when one considers that the shoulder has the greatest range of motion of any joint.

Most surgeons involved in the care of burn patients are aware of the importance of preventing contractures of the hand and elbow, yet readily accept axillary contractures. This is probably related to the difficulty of preventing them without the use of skeletal traction, which in itself presents difficulties and considerable discomfort to the patient. Moreover, once incurred, axillary contractures can be corrected satisfactorily by one of the methods described above.

The use of split-thickness skin grafts to repair an axillary contracture is described in another chapter. This chapter will describe the Z-plasty technique and the use of local flaps.

Z-PLASTY FOR THE CORRECTION OF AXILLARY CONTRACTURES

Use of the Z-plasty for correction of axillary contractures requires that suitably constructed triangular flaps of skin be transposed from adjacent areas to release a contracting band. In the axilla, a vertical contracting band can be lengthened by transposing flaps from its lateral aspect. The Z incision is used most suitably in the presence of a web, and preferably where the surrounding skin is of normal texture. This web should be limited to either the anterior or the posterior axillary line.

OPERATIVE PROCEDURE: SINGLE Z-PLASTY

The long axis of the Z-plasty should be placed along the axillary contracting band, and ideally should extend the full length of the contracture, even though it requires large flaps which cannot always be outlined and raised safely. The scarred band should be excised if it is thick and rigid; otherwise it may be used in making triangular flaps (Figure 1). Next, one must decide where the flaps should be. This is best done by drawing an equilateral triangle on each side of the contracture. From the resulting parallelogram the more suitable set of limbs should be selected according to the following criteria:
(1) Which flap is less scarred especially along the base, and will have the better blood supply?
(2) Which flap will least distort the normal anatomy? If possible, one should avoid transposing the specialized axillary skin, which contains hair and apocrine and sweat glands, to an outside and visible location.

All three limbs of the Z-plasty must be equal so that the triangular flaps can be transposed without difficulty. The angle of the limbs with the central band should be 60 degrees. This provides a theoretical 75 percent increase in length of the contracting bands. With a smaller angle, the percentage increase in length will decrease. An angle of much less than

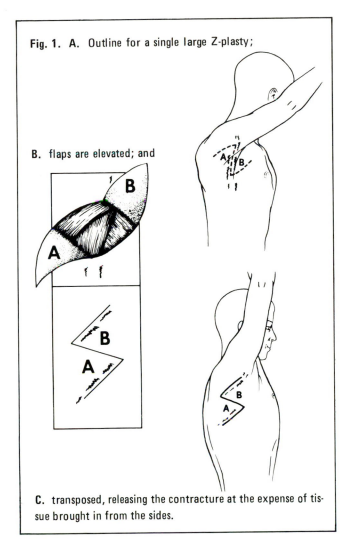

Fig. 1. A. Outline for a single large Z-plasty;

B. flaps are elevated; and

C. transposed, releasing the contracture at the expense of tissue brought in from the sides.

MULTIPLE Z-PLASTIES

An alternative to the use of a large Z-plasty is the creation of multiple small Z's (Figure 2). The line of contracture can be regarded as a series of contracted segments, and a small Z can be constructed for each segment. The smaller Z-plasties distribute tension more evenly, allowing the transposition of small quantities of tissue all the way down the line of the contracture.

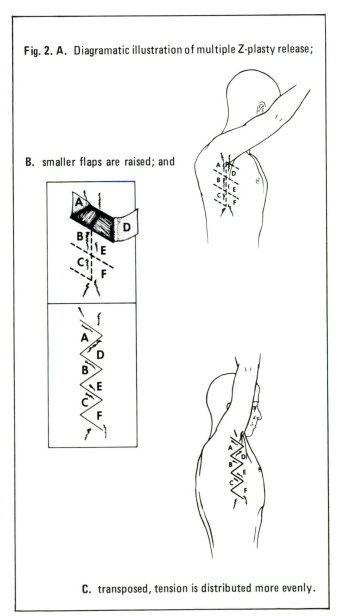

Fig. 2. A. Diagramatic illustration of multiple Z-plasty release;

B. smaller flaps are raised; and

C. transposed, tension is distributed more evenly.

60 degrees would defeat the object of the Z-plasty, however, since the smaller angle would produce less gain in length. Theoretically, angles of up to and beyond 90 degrees could be used with steady increase in amount of lengthening. However, the amount of tissue available for transposition is limited, and as the angle is increased beyond 60 degrees, sufficient tension is produced so that adequate flaps cannot be readily transposed.

Fairly thick flaps should be made to ensure a good blood supply and the tips should be rounded off to avoid necrosis. If the Z-plasty is properly planned, the flaps should fall into their new transposed position without tension once the contracture is released.

Z-PLASTY AND SKIN GRAFT

Many times a single Z-plasty or a series of smaller Z's may not completely correct the axillary contracture. In these cases, a combined method must be used. This entails using a Z-plasty in the central part of the axillary web and completing the release by transverse incisions at the superior and inferior ends of the contracting band (Figure 3). The raw surfaces that are created can be covered with split-thickness skin grafts.

All flaps should be handled as atraumatically as possible with skin hooks. Hemostasis must be meticulous, and fine sutures of nylon should be used. A light conforming dressing is applied, and the shoulder is immobilized with a sling and swath for about five days. After this time progressive active motion of the shoulder, especially exercises of abduction and elevation, are encouraged. Sutures are not removed before the tenth postoperative day.

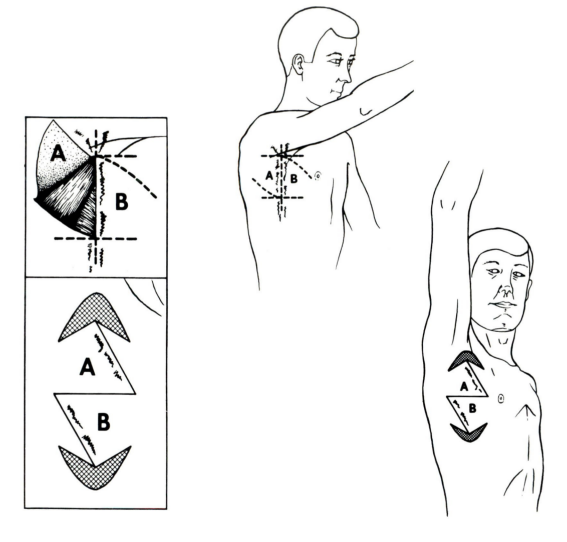

Fig. 3. A Z-plasty is outlined in the center of the contracting band, and for complete release of the contracture, free split-thickness skin grafts are required above and below the Z.

LOCAL FLAPS FOR THE CORRECTION OF AXILLARY CONTRACTURES

Correcting axillary contractures using local flaps is confined to cases where a flap of normal skin and fat can be designed for transfer into the apex of the axilla. This condition limits the use of this technique to only a few select cases. However, one should attempt to mobilize local flaps into the axilla whenever possible and to use skin grafts on the chest wall where donor site contracture of the wound will not result in a functional disability.

OPERATIVE PROCEDURE

The first step consists of releasing the axillary contracture by a transverse incision which should extend beyond the mid-lateral line both anteriorly and posteriorly. The defect that is present can be covered by transposition of a local flap. An example of a flap that could be designed is shown in Figure 4. There a posteriorly based flap is outlined in the direction of the intercostal vessels. A thick flap that extends down to the intercostal muscle fascia is elevated. By preliminary planning with a pattern a flap is outlined that is sufficiently longer than the defect so that it can rotate on its far axis and still reach the apex of the axilla without tension. Meticulous hemostasis is imperative. The secondary defect is covered with a split-thickness skin graft.

A flap can also be designed based anteriorly and superiorly on the acromiothoracic vessels. However, one should be careful not to include the nipple and areola in such a flap.

When a flap is transposed, suction catheters should be used postoperatively for three to five days so that the flaps can be closely apposed to the concavity of the axilla.

In some patients, especially males, where the secondary deformity would not be as important, the surgeon may use the rather popular deltopectoral flap. This flap can be extended up to the lateral deltoid area, elevated and transposed into the axilla, providing good elasticity and freedom of movement of that shoulder (Figure 5). This flap is based on the

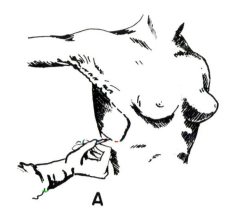

Fig. 4. A. Diagram of flap of normal tissue outlined on the chest wall.

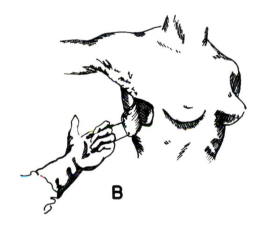

Fig. 4. B. Flap is elevated.

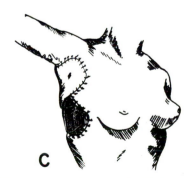

Fig. 4. C. Flap is transposed to apex of axilla to provide good elastic skin. The secondary defect is covered with a split-thickness skin graft. In some patients, particularly women, this defect can be closeed primarily after undermining the wound edges and excising a triangle of skin at the anterior-inferior end of the defect.

perforating branches of the internal mammary arteries and can be elevated safely in one stage. One precaution is that the flap should be elevated with the deltoid and pectoral fascia since the perforating vessels are just above the fascia and are very likely to be injured if the fascia is left behind.

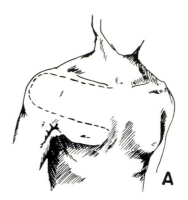

Fig. 5. A. The deltopectoral flap outlined along the lower border of the clavicle to the lateral deltoid area;

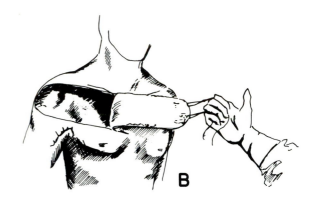

Fig. 5. B. the flap is elevated in one stage with the deltoid and pectoral fascia; and

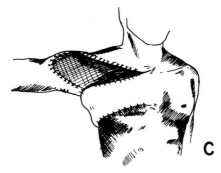

Fig. 5. C. transposed to the axilla. The defect on the anterior chest and deltoid area is covered with a split-thickness skin graft.

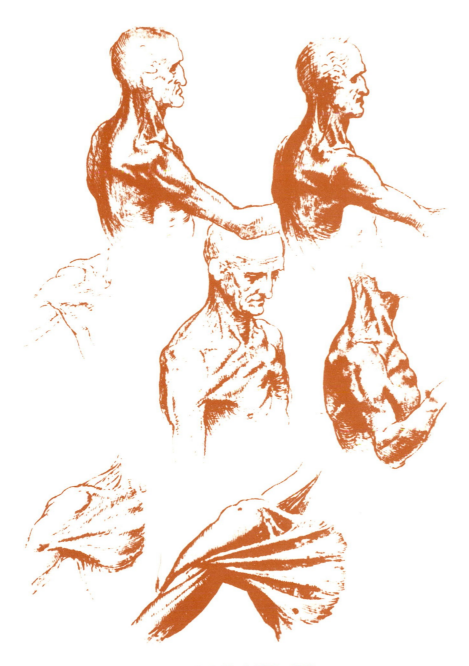

Leonardo da Vinci, 1452 – 1519.

I am afraid humility to genius is as an extinguisher to a candle.
Shernstone

85

PHYSICAL MEASURES IN CARE OF THE AXILLA

George H. Koepke

Full-thickness skin loss from the arm and axilla may result in disabling contractures of the shoulders and elbows. These contractures can be lessened if simple prophylactic measures are taken during the emergent and acute periods of treatment. Proper positioning of body segments during the initial treatment regimen will shorten the period of rehabilitation.

Although the child may have full range of shoulder and elbow motion when discharged from the hospital, with skeletal growth, an axillary web may develop because the scar will not grow as fast as bone. As a result, the axilla may appear to become progressively lower. The most effective means of correcting the deformity is to excise the scar and replace the skin deficit with a split-thickness skin graft that is large enough to keep the shoulder in a corrected position. It should be maintained in abduction for at least four weeks following the application of the split-thickness skin graft. (Figure 1 illustrates one of several types of adjustable abduction splints that can be adapted to the patient's individual needs.) Should the scar involve the anterior axillary contracture, the shoulder should be held in abduction and external rotation. If the entire axilla is involved, the arm can be abducted to 90 degrees and the position of midrotation. The splint can be stocked in three sizes and can be made readily available to a patient on a rental basis. This postreconstruction splint will permit the patient to become ambulatory on the day following surgery and will insure shoulder immobilization to facilitate the take of fresh split-thickness skin grafts. After the grafts are mature, improvised overhead pulley exercises are an excellent means of maintaining the rheologic properties of soft tissues.

Antecubital contractures should be excised and

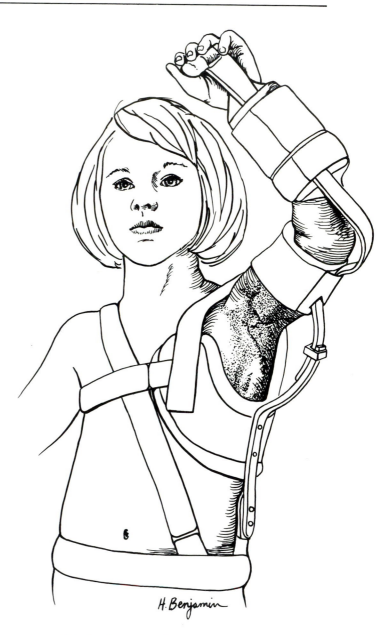

Fig. 1. An adjustable shoulder abduction and external rotation splint.

the elbow splinted effectively in extension after split-thickness skin grafting by means of a simple posterior plaster mold that is worn for approximately two weeks. An alternative method is to provide a three point anterior aluminum splint as shown in Figure 2. Active and passive exercises should include movements that provide full supination of the forearm as well as flexion and extension of the elbow.

These simple procedures coordinated with good surgical care will lessen the time and expense of rehabilitating the patient with extensive burns of the arms and axilla.

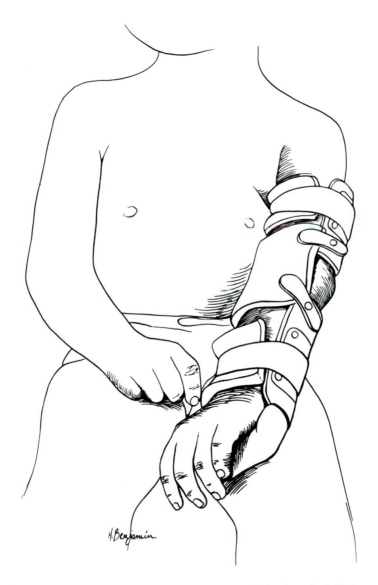

Fig. 2. Three point splint to maintain elbow extension and to facilitate "take" of antecubital graft.

XIII.

THE ELBOW AND ANTECUBITAL SPACE

PRINCIPLES OF TREATMENT

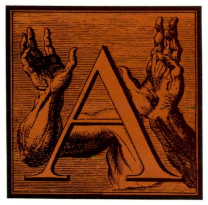

ge groupings are an important consideration in the treatment of flexion contracture at the elbow. Children, prior to the age of puberty, are the easiest group to treat, and usually only require release of the contracture and split-thickness skin grafting. Adults may have a more complex deformity caused by heterotopic bone. The heterotopic bone may immobilize the joint and require surgical excision.

The skin contractures in the antecubital space are incised transversely, the forearm is extended and the defect covered with a thick split-thickness graft, followed by splinting in extension. After the skin graft is well healed, the splint should be removed twice a day and the elbow put actively and passively through a range of motion.

In adults, it is important to avoid forced mobilization of the elbow joint under general anesthesia because of the danger of injury to the ulnar nerve. Chapters by Colson and Janvier and by Smith and Fisher in this section provide information on the orthopedic procedures for treatment of elbow joint stiffness.

William C. Grabb

87

HETEROTOPIC BONE FORMATION OF THE ELBOW

David P. Fisher
William S. Smith

Treating the stiff elbow in the burn patient depends entirely upon the pathologic anatomy of the involved elbow. Two main types of stiffness are recognized. The most common is associated with heterotopic bone formation. In the less common type, heterotopic bone is frequently present but the elbow is stiff because of intra-articular damage from pyarthrosis, thermal effects on the articular cartilage, or prolonged immobilization from either of these.

The formation of heterotopic bone adjacent to joints in amounts significant enough to limit joint function occurs after approximately 2 percent of all major burns and most frequently involves the elbow. In many instances, the heterotopic bone is deposited in an elbow adjacent to the burn, but frequently it develops in an elbow or other joint remote from the burn site. This phenomenon seems to be related to the magnitude of the physiologic insult. It seldom develops in patients with burns of less than 20 percent full-thickness. Evans noted that he had not observed this formation of heterotopic bone in patients who were confined to bed for any time less than two months.

The process of heterotopic bone formation about the elbow begins with the deposition of an amorphous calcium mass which most frequently occurs in the posteromedial aspect along the border of the triceps tendon. The calcification may be absorbed completely within the first three to six months after the burn. In children up to the age of puberty, total absorption is almost always the rule. For reasons that can be only speculative at this time, the process continues to a stage of mature bone in some cases.

The block of heterotopic bone in the elbow is invariably confluent with the distal posteromedial aspect of the distal humerus (Figure 1). It is approx-

imately 4cm long and 1.5cm thick. Its course is oblique from the medial aspect of the humerus to the olecranon process, where it forms a stop or block to extension. From the distal part of the heterotopic bone to its counterpart on the olecranon, there is a thick bridge of cicatrix, forming an additional block to flexion of the elbow. In our experience, the bridge

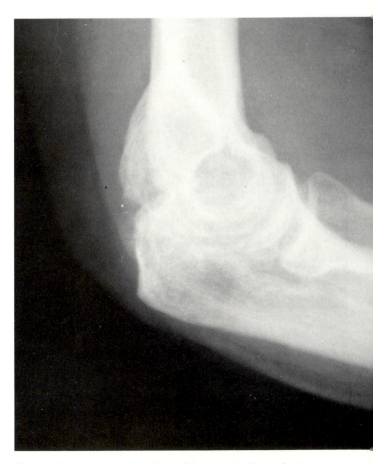

Fig. 1. Appearance and location of heterotopic bone about the elbow in a patient with severe burns. Note that the cartilage space of the elbow joint is well preserved and that there is an absence of heterotopic bone anteriorly.

from the heterotopic bone to the olecranon is almost always fibrous tissue and is seldom osseous. The heterotopic bone is **not part of the triceps tendon**, but is extrinsic to it.

TREATMENT OF HETEROTOPIC BONE

In our experience, exposure for the removal of heterotopic bone at the elbow is accomplished by a midline triceps-splitting incision, exposing the ulnar nerve and reflecting a major part of the triceps tendon, but carefully preserving continuity of the triceps insertion and the periosteal tube of the proximal ulna. The heterotopic bone and cicatrical bridge to the olecranon are readily exposed. The bony bridge is osteotomized, as is the proximal 0.5cm at the tip of the olecranon (Figure 2). At this point, if joint stiffness remains, a medial and lateral capsulectomy is performed. The split triceps is reapproximated and wound closure is accomplished with ease. Severe burn scars over the distal aspect of the ulna have not interfered with healing in our experience.

Active elbow motion is begun on the third postoperative day and progressively increased thereafter. Improvement in the range of motion has continued up to six months. Six patients with heterotopic bone formation alone were treated in this manner. These patients had an average range of motion of 20 degrees prior to the time of operation and gained an average of 65 degrees after the operation.

ANKYLOSED ELBOW

When loss of the elbow motion is the consequence of loss of articular cartilage (pyarthrosis, deep thermal effects), the surgical management is quite different. The **ankylosed elbow with extensive intra-articular involvement** may be recognized by three general characteristics: the cartilage space of the elbow joint is either diminished or there is little or no motion and heterotopic bone, as described above, is frequently present and sometimes is also found on the anterior and lateral aspect of the joints (Figure 3). Here, excision of the distal end of the humerus is the main point in surgical management.

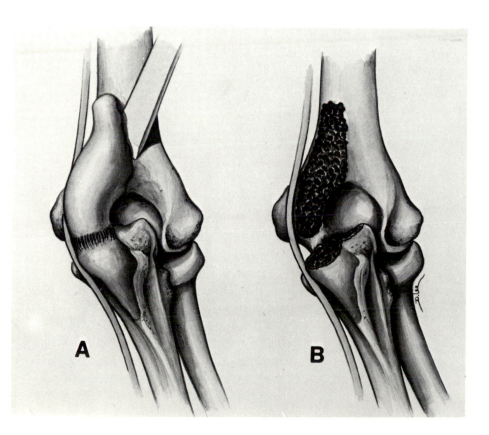

Fig. 2. A. Schematic representation of heterotopic bone being removed from posterior aspect of the elbow. Note the bridge of scar at junction of heterotopic bone and olecranon. The ulnar nerve is shown in close proximity to the heterotopic bone. **B.** Appearance of posterior aspect of elbow after excision of heterotopic bone and olecranonoplasty.

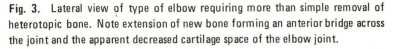

Fig. 3. Lateral view of type of elbow requiring more than simple removal of heterotopic bone. Note extension of new bone forming an anterior bridge across the joint and the apparent decreased cartilage space of the elbow joint.

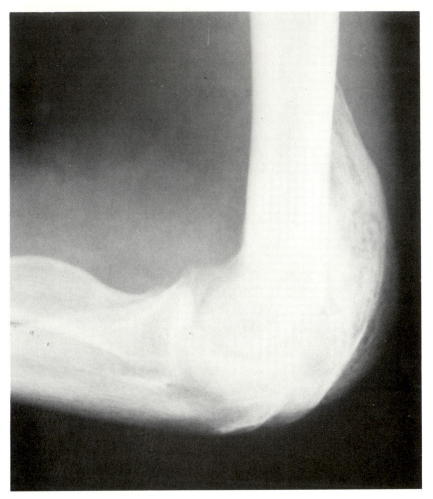

The surgical exposure for treatment of the ankylosed elbow with intra-articular adhesions is identical to that used above. The ulnar nerve is first exposed, mobilized, and protected. The insertion of the triceps is sharply dissected off the ulna, using a scalpel. Continuing with the scalpel, the origins of the wrist flexors and extensors are removed from the condyles, as are the collateral ligaments. The intra-articular adhesions are sharply incised. Occasionally, a curved osteotome must be used to facilitate mobility of the joint. After the condyles are cleared, a sharp periosteal elevator can be used with caution to lift the periosteum off the front of the humerus along with overlying brachialis muscle. In the event that the ankylosed joint must be osteotomized, use of retractors anteriorly easily protects nerves and vessels. The radial head is excised. If the articular surface has been severely damaged, we remove approximately 1.5 to 2.5cm of the distal humerus (Figure 4), round off the end, and then deepen the olecranon fossa. The elbow will appear to be quite frail. At this point there are bleeding surfaces at the ends of the humerus and the proximal ulna. If the freshly cut surfaces are placed in apposition, ankylosis might well be the result. We prefer to distract the joint by using a threaded Steinmann pin (Figure 4). Another alternative is to apply overhead skeletal traction, using a Kirschner wire through the olecranon. Bleeding from the cut suface of the ulna is controlled by a thin layer of beeswax. Soft tissue bleeding is meticulously controlled after release of the tourniquet. We have not interposed fascia lata in this group. The joint should

Fig. 4. Schematic drawing of before and after appearance of elbow with excisional arthroplasty and method of maintenance of distraction of the cut bone ends.

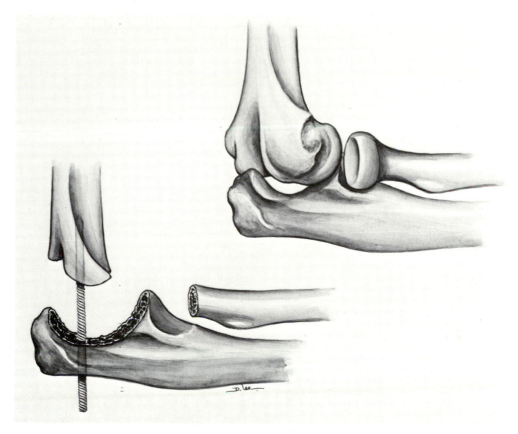

be distracted by at least 2cm at the conclusion of the operation. Closure is then effected in the midline posteriorly and a cast is applied.

The pin is left in place for three weeks. The patients continued to gain strength about the elbow for over a one-year period. Instability is more of a problem to the surgeon than it is to the patient, who is generally pleased to trade some stability for much greater mobility. Our patients have returned to fairly heavy labor. Seven burned patients with elbows meeting the above criteria were treated by this method. Preoperatively, they had an average range of motion of 7 degrees. The average gain after surgery was 88 degrees.

The spectacular success of total joint replacement of the hip, and to a lesser extent of the knee

and hands, leads us to believe that the future appears promising for the elbow and shoulder replacements. However, at present, the state of the art regarding elbow joints is such that very few can seriously recommend any of the total elbows currently available. The constrained elbow joint appears to have met its demise by virtue of the inevitability of loosening of the components at the bone cement interface. Whether a non-constrained resurfacing type of joint with a minimum of foreign material will prove to be successful is a matter for conjecture at this time.

There is very little question but that function of the stiff elbow, secondary to burns can be significantly improved by the surgical measures outlined.

88

CONTRACTURE RELEASE OF THE ELBOW AND WRIST

Pierre Colson
Helénè Janvier

Burns of an upper limb, whether healed by spontaneous epithelialization or by skin grafting, often result in stiffness and flexion contracture of the elbow. The elbow can move but the range of motion is reduced both in flexion and in extension.

Although useful movement of the upper limb does not require more than a mobility of the elbow from 30 degrees in flexion to 120 degrees in extension, it remains desirable to attain more. When the entire upper limb is burned, the shoulder or the wrist cannot be relied upon to act as a substitute. The functional value of the hand then depends mostly upon the mobility of the elbow.

Any of the tissues from the skin to the joint may account for joint stiffness, either separately or with others. Consequently methods of obtaining elbow release are many. Only two methods of treatment involving the skin and the joint will be described here. The first deals with the hypertrophic scar which often is stretched like a web between the arm and the forearm. The second deals with the retracted ligaments in the vicinity of the ulnar nerve.

USE OF LOCAL SKIN FLAPS

The use of a skin flap following the release of an elbow contracture is indicated only in adult patients. Children do not suffer joint lesions; therefore, after total excision of the scar, full extension of the elbow can be more easily achieved. In children, good results are regularly obtained by skin grafting, as long as the arm is splinted in extension for three months. This splint should be removed once or twice a day to put the elbow through a full range of motion.

When the complete resection of the burn scar at the elbow does not permit full extension of the elbow, we prefer to swing a large flap of good skin from the anterolateral aspect of the forearm to cover the fold of the elbow and then rely on the appropriate exercises to improve the amplitude of the movements. The flap constitutes a reserve of elastic tissues that will then permit an increased range of elbow motion.

The use of a skin flap applies to localized burns only, for there must be enough healthy skin on the anterolateral aspect of the forearm to provide a large flap. Burned skin should not be used because of its impaired blood supply. When there is no local skin of good quality, unburned skin from the thoracico-abdominal wall is preferred. This procedure applies only to wide scars, because the efficient and attractively simple Z-plasty may be used for a narrow scar contracture.

In our series of 17 burn patients with elbow contractures, only one did not recover satisfactorily by this method of treatment. The use of a local flap at the elbow to increase mobility is essentially functional; it should rarely be used for esthetic purposes.

Operative Technique. The flap should be situated with its base on either side of the elbow, so that its proximal end is on the arm and its distal end on the forearm. The skin of the flap must not be extensively scarred or consist of skin grafts. The flap should be long enough to cross over the anterior aspect of the elbow, so that its tip covers the epicondyle or epitrochlea. It is helpful to use a cloth or paper pattern in the planning of the flap. In order to avoid necrosis of the flap, great care should be taken not to sever the veins while undermining. The incision of the scar contracture should slant toward the forearm (Figures 1 thru 5).

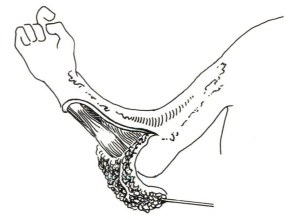

Fig. 1. A skin flap for the release of a burn scar contracture of the antecubital skin is taken from the anterolateral aspect of the forearm. A pattern of cloth or paper is helpful in designing this flap.

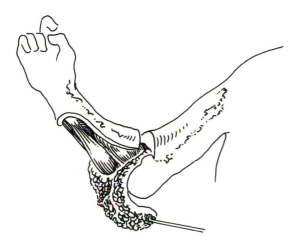

Fig. 2. Incision of the scar of the antecubital region.

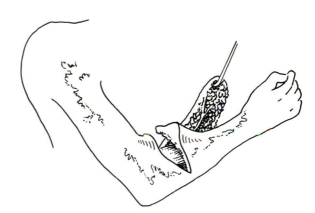

Fig. 3. Lateral view of this incision to demonstrate that it is slanted toward the forearm.

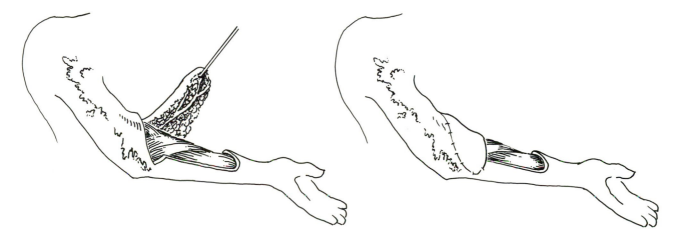

Fig. 4. The thick scar tissues are excised and the flap rotated into the defect.

Fig. 5. The flap is long enough to cross over the epicondyle. The flap donor site is resurfaced by split-thickness skin grafts.

SELECTIVE CAPSULECTOMY

In cases where the stiffness of the elbow can be observed even when there is no skin retraction and where roentgenograms reveal neither osteoarticular lesions nor exostosis, the surgeon needs to determine the exact cause and localization of the stiffness of the joint.

In the severely burned patient lying in bed for a long time, the epitrochlea rests on the bed. A necrotic process often develops at this point, which is followed by cicatrization leaving a deep scar adhering to the bone (Figure 6). This superficial lesion is of the greatest clinical interest because it reveals the existence of deeper alterations. Ischemia, followed by infection, affects the joint. The articular capsule and ligaments retract, imprisoning the ulnar nerve in a fibrous tunnel, which is often calcified.

Operative Technique. There are three things to be accomplished in the capsulectomy. One of these is to transpose the ulnar nerve. Freeing the nerve is often difficult, and fasciculate dissection is necessary to preserve the collateral roots (Figure 7). This transposition fulfills a double purpose. It exposes the capsule and lateral ligaments which are to be resected (Figure 8) and it protects the nerve from being stretched when the postoperative mobilization begins. The retracted ligaments must then be resected. This operative stage seems to be greatly simplified when the epitrochlea is first separated with a bone chisel.

Fig. 6. Patient with deep scar adhering to the epitrochlea.

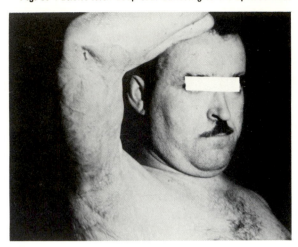

Along with the epitrochlea, the ligaments are then removed (Figure 9). At this point the freedom of the elbow should be checked. It is our observation that the removal of the epitrochlea does not usually lead to joint laxity. It will facilitate the healing of the surgical wound, though, by relieving wound tension. Covering the open joint with a local or distant skin flap, important to the preservation of joint mobility, concludes the procedure (Figure 10).

Forced mobilization of the elbow under general anesthesia should be avoided because it may lead to ulnar palsy. Although there may be a lack of progress in joint mobilization following capsulectomy, any temptation to forcibly mobilize the elbow should be avoided (Figure 11). (Also see case study Figure 12.)

Fig. 7. Dissection of the ulnar nerve preliminary to capsulectomy at the elbow joint.

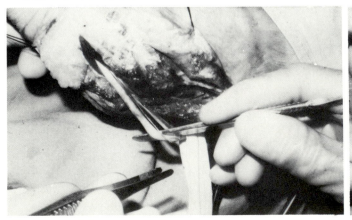

Fig. 8. Dissection of capsule ligaments of the elbow joint.

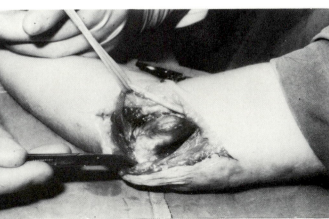

Fig. 9. Resection of epitrochlea and of lateral ligaments of the elbow joint.

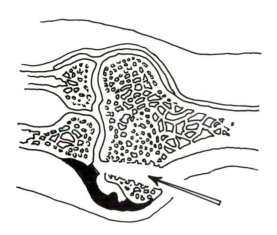 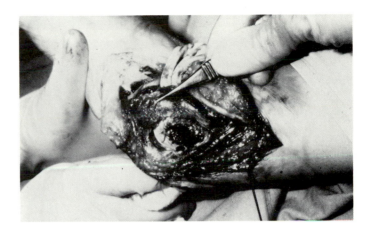

Fig. 10. A local skin flap is used to cover the open joint, with a skin graft being applied to the flap donor site.

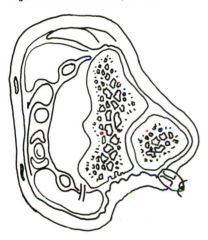 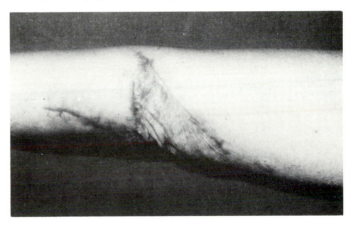

Fig. 11. This patient now has a full range of motion following capsulectomy of the elbow joint. Prior to operation she had only 35 degrees of motion at this joint.

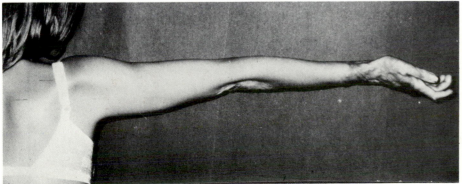 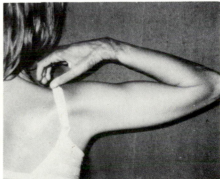

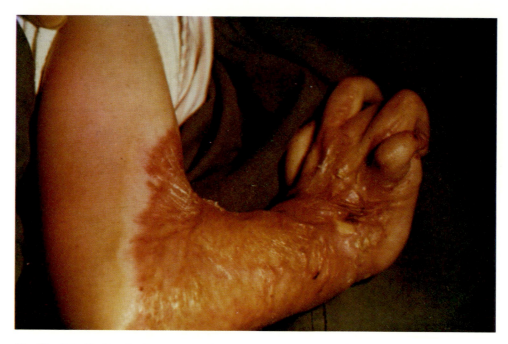

Fig. 12. Case Study. **A.** Severe contracture of antecubital space and retracted ligaments at the wrist when patient first seen in 1965.

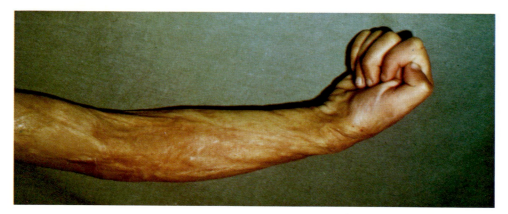

Fig. 12. B. In 1969, after release with local flaps at elbow and wrist the patient has regained normal growth of the arm and hand.

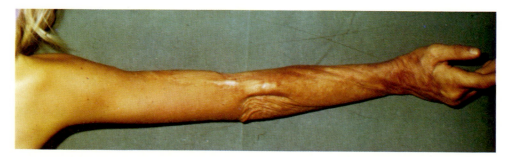

Fig. 12. C. 1975, the child now has near full range of motion of both wrist and elbow.

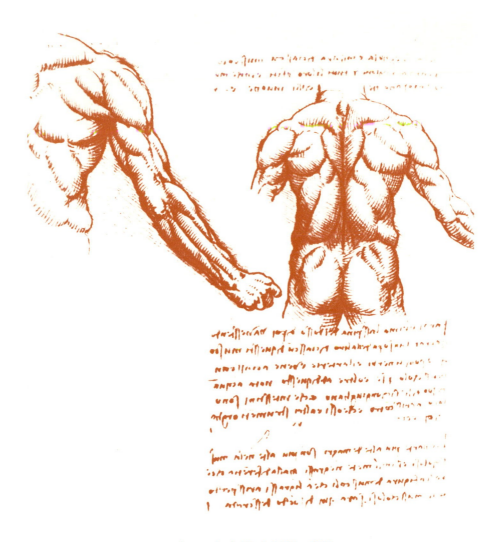

Leonardo da Vinci, 1452 – 1519.

XIV.
THE FOREARM, WRIST, AND HAND

PRINCIPLES OF TREATMENT

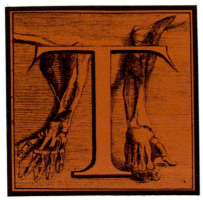

The early return of function of the hand should hold top priority in the rehabilitation of the burn patient. It is essential to splint the hand with the metacarpal joints in extreme flexion and abduction, interphalangeal joints extended, and thumb abducted (see chapter entitled Hand Splinting). This counteracts the forces pulling the hand and wrist in the opposite directions.

Primary early excision of the full-thickness burn of the hand is emphasized in a chapter of the same title by Krizek. Early return of function allows the patient to assist in his own care and provides a psychologic lift.

Dorsal hand burns are quite common. Almost all can be resurfaced with split-thickness skin grafts placed on paratenon, or even short segments of bare tendon. The determination of whether the paratenon and the tendon are viable is discussed at length in the chapter entitled Managing Exposed Tendon in the Forearm and Hand by Madden. Occasionally a skin flap from the contralateral chest wall will be indicated to cover heat-damaged tendon. Even heat-denatured tendons will be replaced by newly synthesized scar collagen beneath a skin flap. The extensor tendons fortunately have only a short gliding distance, but unfortunately if they have to be debrided they usually cannot be successfully replaced with tendon grafts.

Information on amputation of the fingers and hands, as well as finger and hand prostheses, is also included.

William C. Grabb

90

DAMAGED WRIST

George E. Omer, Jr.

Function of the wrist is intimately associated with the hand. The extrinsic muscle-tendon units of the hand cross the multiarticulated carpus, producing reciprocal positions of the wrist and metacarpophalangeal joints. The volar and dorsal carpal ligaments are anchored to a central bone core and form rigid tubes crowded with tendons, blood vessels, and nerves. Vascular obstruction in these carpal tunnels produces distal ischemia. Destruction of tendons or nerves at the wrist robs the hand of movement and sensibility. Management of the burned wrist should be planned to restore optimal function to the hand.

Hands are the most common site of burns, but the volar surface of the wrist rarely sustains full-thickness injury unless the burn is an electrical, chemical, or direct-contact thermal injury. The dorsal surface of the wrist has thin skin and the burn is often full-thickness, even though the injury appears to be superficial. Circumferential carpal burns produce an immediate, inelastic eschar with rigid compression, but all burns of the wrist result in reactive contracture and imperil distal vascular circulation. Immediate carpal joint involvement is most likely in a localized deep injury, such as an electrical burn, but secondary infection usually results from skin or vascular deficiency.

The significant bony and musculoskeletal deformities observed in thermal burns are largely sequential to pain. The patient immobilizes the entire injured extremity in an analgesic position, resulting in flexion of the wrist. The flexed wrist is a reciprocal position with extension of the metacarpophalangeal joints, flattening of the transverse palmar arches, and abduction-extension of the thumb. The burn wound will continue to contract and the wrist will remain flexed until it is opposed by correcting forces.

EARLY CARE

Often local burn wound care must be performed after the patient's general condition is stabilized. However, one immediate procedure should be performed on the burned wrist even when there are massive associated injuries. The wrist should be placed in 5 to 20 degrees of extension. This can be done on an emergency basis by fitting the forearm and hand on an aluminum universal (Mason-Allen) splint, secured with elastic bandages. The basic functional position of extended wrist, cupped palm, flexed fingers, and abducted thumb is obtained. The injured extremity is then suspended in a stockinet-loop sling from an intravenous stand. Elevation will improve venous and lymphatic drainage and decrease brawny edema. **If the patient maintains the wrist joint in painful flexion for as short a period as 12 hours, a contracture deformity will result.**

Local wound care begins by cleansing the surface of the burned extremity. A circumferential inelastic eschar should be released by a volar longitudinal serpentine incision similar to an elective release of the carpal tunnel. If the injury involves deep volar tissues, such as an electrical burn, the volar carpal ligament and deep fascia must be released. Overlying skin should be incised along the entire length of the fasciotomy. The skin-fascia incision need not be undermined, but is allowed to retract fully to prevent tension. Homografts or heterografts are excellent temporary dressings over the fasciotomy-exposed tissues.

Isolated full-thickness burns of the wrist's volar surface should be excised at the time of initial treatment to avoid secondary infection of tendons, nerves, and bone. Initial debridement of tendons and other deep structures should be minimal, even in the electrical injury. Replacement of the full-thickness skin is not indicated until the extent of the wound can be determined, but the exposed vessels, tendons, and nerves must be covered immediately. A heavy split-thickness homograft will provide excellent temporary cover for tendons and nerves and a healthy platform for the splint and occlusive dressings usually used to maintain wrist extension.

Partial-thickness burns of the dorsum of the wrist are usually associated with burns involving a significant area of the entire body. We have treated these burns most often with topical antibacterial agents and meticulous skin care. The wound must be closely observed for maceration. Eschar can be removed by surgical debridement or changes of wet dressings three or four times daily. Motion should not be forbidden because debridement exposes tendons. Homografts and definitive autografts are applied to granulation tissue to reduce pain and allow easier active motion.

Primary excision can be used in a localized dorsal wrist burn. If possible, the subcutaneous layer should be left intact and covered with an immediate homograft or heterograft. Mesh grafts are not indicated over a joint surface. If both sides of the wrist are involved by full-thickness burn, only one surface should be excised and grafted at a time. We prefer to do the volar side first, and the dorsal side three to seven days later. Primary excision promotes earlier closure, decreases secondary deep infection, reduces contracture, and allows use of circular dressings with splints to prevent deformity.

Ankylosis of the carpal joint occurs when there is direct exposure to the burn or following secondary infection. The exposed joint should be irrigated and debrided as necessary. If autograft coverage is not convenient, a homograft or heterograft should be applied to prevent drying and to combat infection. Homograft coverage should be changed frequently and all necrotic cartilage removed. Unless an early definitive autograft can be applied, the initially exposed carpal joint usually will progress to spontaneous ankylosis. We have not observed periarticular calcification or heterotopic bone formation in the wrist.

Fixed wrist contractures can be prevented by proper positioning, supportive splints, and motion. Supportive splints are used in treating most burned wrists and hands. Prevention of fixed wrist flexion is essential in preventing hand deformity. The wrist should be positioned in 5 to 20 degrees of extension. Plaster-of-paris, aluminum, or plastics can be utilized for static splints, which are adequate for the localized wrist burn. Supportive splints should be applied at night and during all periods of inactivity while under active treatment. **Nighttime extension of the wrist should be maintained for at least 12 months after surgery and even longer in children.** Metacarpal skeletal suspension can be used for circumferential grafting of the upper extremity. The hand injury may require skeletal traction for dynamic splinting. The wrist is the anchor area for some skeletal traction splints, and when the wrist is burned, such splints are a source of potential septic complication.

Every burned wrist and hand should have early motion, preferably beginning immediately after the injury. Only a few degrees of joint motion will decrease stiffness and limit shortening of ligaments or other capsular structures. Exercise maintains muscle tone, reduces edema, and prevents stuck tendons. The patient should understand the need for maintenance of the functional position, supportive splints, and exercise. The surgeon should explain that the burn wound will contract until it meets an opposing force provided by exercise or splinting. Exercise can be active, passive, or isometric. Active motion should be performed at regular intervals throughout the day. Water will provide buoyant motion that is less painful. The hands should never be in a dependent position but in front of the patient where he can observe the movement. Isometric exercises for flexion and extension of the wrist can be performed in a supportive splint. Some patients, because of associated injuries or age, cannot cooperate in an active motion program. Passive exercise can be judiciously used in these patients to maintain range of motion. The wrist should be moist or lubricated. Limited motion is allowed the day after skin grafting and is increased daily until optimal activity is achieved. Until the surgeon and his staff are convinced that the burned wrist has achieved maximal active motion, therapy should be as frequent as necessary.

A fracture or dislocation of the carpal joint complicates the early motion program. Kirschner wires are the preferable method for internal fixation. If the carpal fractures are stable after reduction, active finger motion can be performed; but isometric wrist exercises are best with a supportive splint.

LATE COMPLICATIONS

The carpal joint is the basic joint of the hand. The motion and congruity of this joint determines much of its mobility. Reconstruction of the wrist-hand area following a burn injury should consider the status of the carpal joint as well as the residual sensibility and motor potential of the hand. The wrist should be reconstructed before the hand. No wrist motors are indicated when there is bony ankylosis of the carpal joint. A single central extensor and a single flexor are required to provide controlled motion, while other extrinsic muscle-tendon units can be utilized in the restoration of digit motion. In our experience, elective incisions through healed partial-

thickness burns that were treated with topical antibacterial agents often result in local sepsis.

SUMMARY

Management of the burn-damaged wrist should be planned to restore optimal function to the wrist-hand unit. The wrist never should be allowed to assume the flexed position secondary to pain or contracture. The prognosis of the burned wrist is directly related to wound healing time. We often excise the wrist burn to prevent secondary sepsis of nerves, tendons, and bones, and provide a healthy skin platform for supportive splints. Fixed wrist contracture can be prevented by proper positioning, supportive splints, or motion. Active motion should be instituted immediately into the therapy program, complemented by isometric and passive exercises. The factors that significantly affect wrist function are the depth of injury, the presence of infection, associated injuries, and the patient's age and ability to cooperate. Functional potential of the wrist is the first consideration in the reconstruction of the wrist-hand unit after healing.

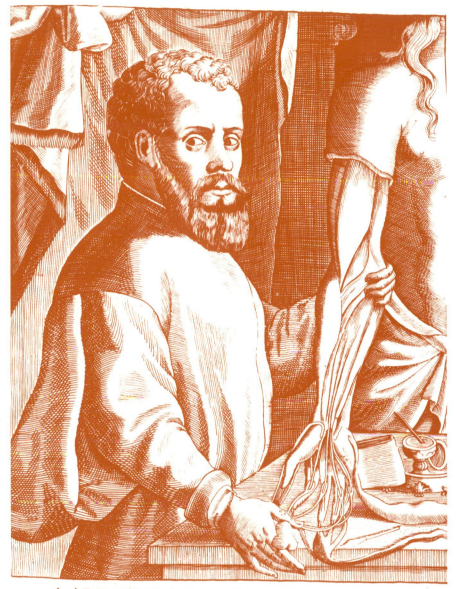

ANDREAE   VESALII . ÆTA. 28

Anatomia viri in hoc genere princip, 1617.

He cures most in whom most have faith.

Galen

91

EXPOSED TENDONS OF THE WRIST

John W. Madden

Injured tendons in the forearm and hand may affect gliding function, passive mobility of joints, healing of wounds, and function of muscle units. To achieve maximal functional results when tendons are exposed, problems in each area must be anticipated and therapy designed to minimize potential complications. Proper management requires a thorough understanding of the biology of wound healing, the architecture of tendons, and the physiology of muscle function. Based on these concepts, three clinical judgments provide a rational scheme of treatment.

THE PROBLEMS

Tendon Gliding. Following any tendon injury, wound healing and scar formation produce adhesions which limit tendon gliding. The magnitude and the precise location of the injury determine the nature of the tenodesis, but all injured tendons lose some ability to glide. The functional impairment created by tenodesis, however, depends entirely on gliding requirements. Physiologically, there are two distinct types of tendons in the forearm and hand. Although all tendons glide relative to fixed structures to perform their normal physiological function, the relationship of gliding distance to normal function varies widely. For example, with the wrist in a fixed position, only 20 percent as much gliding is required for full extension as for full finger flexion. Finger flexors must glide long distances regardless of wrist position, while long gliding distances are less important in other tendons. Scar remodeling can improve gliding with time, but normal gliding distances are rare following significant tendon injury. Therefore, a rational therapeutic plan must consider the gliding requirements of the specific tendon and the magnitude of the anticipated tenodesis.

Joint Function. In addition to influencing active motor function, tenodesis of any tendon affects the passive mobility of distal joints. The primary goal in managing any hand injury is to preserve joint mobility. Passive mobility can only be maintained by establishing motion quickly. Because tenodesing tendons in certain positions can prevent full passive motion of distal joints, tendon injury may lead to permanent joint stiffness. For example, tenodesing a finger extensor with the MCP joint in extension prevents passive flexion and, ultimately, collateral ligament remodeling creates MCP joint stiffness. An extensor tenodesis with MCP and IP joints in flexion, however, allows passive mobility and preserves motion. Thus the therapeutic program must minimize permanent joint stiffness by maintaining proper joint position during periods of immobility.

Wound Healing. Exposed tendons may affect the establishment of early passive motion in another way. Because pain and edema are the primary deterrents to early motion, hand wounds must be closed quickly. If an exposed tendon dies, the devitalized tissue becomes a foreign body. Although normal wound healing processes will ultimately reject an infected, devitalized tendon, the process is prolonged. Rapid wound healing requires the early debridement of the infected tissues. Death of the tendon, however, need not be a deterrent to primary wound healing. Experimental evidence in animals and man indicates that even heat-denatured tendons, if placed in normal tissue, re-establish a blood supply and become invaded by fibroblasts. Gradually, denatured collagen is replaced by newly synthesized scar tissue. Although gliding properties of the "reconstituted tendon" are far from normal, scar remodeling can provide a small amount of relative gliding. Therefore, therapeutic measures should salvage devitalized structures when feasible, but once infection occurs, debridement must be performed quickly.

Muscle Function. Finally, exposed tendons may have a profound effect on the physiology of muscle function. If a discontinuity in the musculo-tendonous unit develops and the muscle retracts, permanent changes in muscle function occur. Fascial remodeling and internal changes in the muscle architecture prevent normal extension and contraction. Once continuity in the musculo-tendonous unit is lost, the muscle may lose its physiological function permanently. Thus the preservation of muscle function

following tendon exposure requires maintaining musculo-tendonous continuity.

THE THERAPEUTIC JUDGMENTS

A therapeutic plan minimizing problems with tendon gliding, joint stiffness, wound healing, and muscle function requires three clinical judgments: Is the tendon exposed or just visible? Is the internal blood supply of the tendon intact? Is the tendon infected or only contaminated?

All tendons are surrounded by a thin, specialized vascular network, the paratenon, which supplies nutrition to the tendon (Figures 1 and 2). Although the tendon is easily visible through the paratenon,

Fig. 1. Cross-section thru tendon demonstrating the surrounding paratenon.

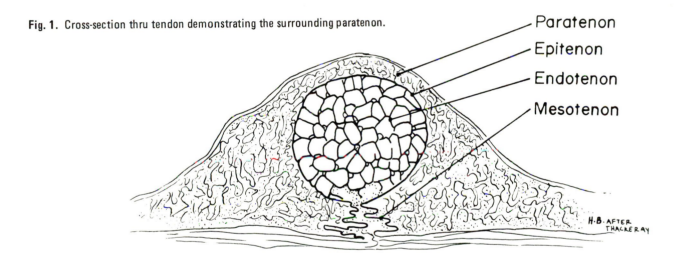

Paratenon
Epitenon
Endotenon
Mesotenon

H.B. AFTER THACKERAY

Fig. 2. Tendon of Palmeris Longus with attached mesotenon.

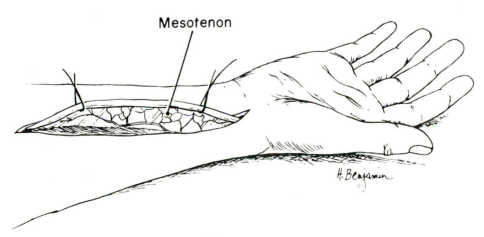

Mesotenon

H. Benjamin

gliding occurs at the interface between paratenon and tendon substance. The first step in deciding how to manage an exposed tendon is **to determine if the fine vessels in the paratenon are intact.** Careful inspection (in the proper light, using magnification if necessary) will reveal the presence or absence of fine surface vessels. If the paratenon is intact, the tendon should be covered as quickly as possible with a split-thickness skin graft. With viable paratenon and immediate split-thickness skin coverage, gliding can be re-established satisfactorily even in finger flexors. Because exposed paratenon can be destroyed by dehydration and the application of antiseptic chemicals, viable paratenon must be protected until permanent coverage can be established.

If the paratenon is damaged, a second judgment must be made. Within the substance of the tendon, small blood vessels, connected segmentally to the paratenon, supply nutrition to the tendon substance. Although this longitudinal blood supply is marginal, **short segments of tendon can survive on the longitudinal blood supply alone.** If the paratenon is viable over most of the exposed tendon but small areas of shiny, white tendon are exposed, the internal blood supply is usually intact and will support a skin graft. Exposed areas of tendon substance are even more susceptible to dehydration than exposed paratenon. Recent evidence supports the concept that any covering supplying a continually moist environment prevents dehydration and provides a chance for salvage. Dressing grafts (autografts, homografts, or heterografts) or wet dressings constantly applied can prevent dehydration until appropriate coverage is established.

If the internal blood supply of the tendon remains intact, the physiological function of the tendon determines therapy. **Tendons requiring only moderate amounts of gliding should be covered with split-thickness skin** as soon as possible. Although the skin graft becomes adherent to the tendon, enough gliding will be re-established as the scar remodels to allow adequate physiological function. All joints should be maintained in a position consistent with early passive mobilization. Thus, if injured finger extensor tendons are preserved, MCP and IP joints

should be maintained in flexion; if flexors or extensors of the wrist are exposed, the wrist should be maintained in a natural position. Passive range-of-motion exercises should be started as soon as possible, but between intervals of therapy, joints should be maintained in a protected position. **Tendons requiring long gliding distance for full function must be treated differently.** The tenodesis created by direct application of split-thickness skin to the tendon surface will not provide enough motion for physiological function. Thus, if the internal blood supply to a finger flexor is present, the exposed tendon should be covered by a **pedicle flap.** Subsequent remodeling usually permits enough gliding for adequate function.

If the exposed tendon is dry, dehydrated, and the surface dull, the internal blood supply has been destroyed and therapy depends upon the presence or absence of clinical infection. Direct inspection and the history of exposure help to determine whether an exposed tendon has an established clinical infection or is merely contaminated. During primary excision, although the wound surface may be contaminated, the final field represents a surgically clean wound. Injured tendons rarely, if ever, have established bacterial infections within hours of injury. In contrast, even the most carefully managed wound can support a heavy bacterial growth, and tendons without an internal blood supply exposed during the course of delayed debridement should be considered clinically infected. When suppuration is grossly visible around an exposed tendon, when the white, glistening surface of the normal tendon is replaced by a yellowish-gray surface, or when the tendon bundles are fragmenting, tendons are infected.

Once absence of clinical infection has been established, the physiological type of the exposed tendon becomes the important consideration. Tendons that function with minimum gliding should be preserved regardless of their inherent blood supply. Immediate coverage by a pedicle flap can preserve the longitudinal architecture and, ultimately, physiological gliding will be re-established. Again, the key to this therapeutic plan is maintaining all joints in a position consistent with early passive mobilization. With successful pedicle coverage, even heat-denatured tendons will be replaced by newly synthesized scar collagen and active motion can be restored. Tendons requiring long gliding distances, particularly finger flexors, must be treated differently. In the palm, nonviable flexor tendons should be excised and the wounds covered with split-thickness skin as rapidly as possible. Preserving nonviable flexors in the palm creates a severe tenodesis, limits small joint motion, and may produce permanent muscle dysfunction. If passive joint mobility is maintained, active motion can be re-established by resurfacing the defect at a later time with an abdominal pedicle flap and subsequent flexor tendon grafting. If the bed seems appropriate following excision, the defect can be closed primarily with a pedicle flap, eliminating one stage of the repair. In contrast to the palm, an attempt should be made to preserve nonviable finger flexors exposed at the wrist. Loss of continuity in the tendon at this level produces maximal retraction and permanent muscle dysfunction. Exposed wrist flexors should be covered with a pedicle flap preserving the longitudinal architecture of the tendon. Even if the ultimate tenodesis prevents full flexion, subsequent tendon grafting or tenolysis can restore active motor function. As the pedicle flap heals, the wrist and fingers should be maintained in extension during the intervals between passive exercise. If a significant tenodesis occurs, flexing the wrist allows full range of passive motion in the distal joints.

Once an exposed tendon becomes grossly infected, the infected portion must be debrided quickly. Wound healing will occur after the infected tissue has been removed. In excising any infected tendon, care should be taken to remove the structure well away from the wound margins, preventing tenodesis in an undesirable position. Passive range-of-motion exercises to the distal joints should be started quickly and the wound surface covered with skin grafts when feasible. If passive joint mobility can be maintained, subsequent surgical procedures can restore active motion.

Every man, however wise, needs the advice of some sagacious friend in the affairs of life.

Plautus

92

ELECTRICAL BURNS OF PERIPHERAL NERVES

William C. Grabb

Contact with a high-voltage (high-tension) electrical source that is conducted through the body to a ground is the usual etiology of electrical burns severe enough to cause damage to peripheral nerves. The nerves involved in the upper extremity are usually the median and/or the ulnar nerve.

Electric current passes through the body as though it were passing through a structureless gel, always choosing the shortest path from contact to contact without deflection by anatomical landmarks. Animal experimentation has repeatedly disproved the old fallacy that electric current is conducted at greater distances along the nerve fibers and blood vessels. Rather, the entire body is a colloidal system which is in isotonic equilibrium. These colloids are in the sol state in blood and the gel state in most solid tissues. To the electric current, the body as a whole is a uniform mass, and the **heat** of the electric burn destroys tissue at and beneath the entrance contact point en bloc. Contact with a high-tension wire provides the voltage to the human body, especially at the point of contact that provides the resistance, so that the **large amounts of heat generated cause a true burn.** It is as though the body were the resistance wire in a large toaster.

Most functional loss of peripheral nerve is the result of this immediate thermal destruction of the nerve at the contact site. A secondary fibrosis around partially damaged nerves may also contribute to further loss of function.

TREATMENT

The functional results of treating these high-tension electrical burns of peripheral nerves are not good.

INITIAL TREATMENT

Early debridement of the necrotic tissue (one or three days post-burn) is uniformly agreed upon as a requirement for proper treatment. Necrotic tissue will have a brownish or tan color and will not bleed. General or regional block anesthesia without a tourniquet is employed. Other tissue will exhibit a spectrum of degrees of injury. Marginally injured deep tissue may be saved, especially if it is immediately covered with a skin flap. Although we know of no reports of use of the intravenous fluorescein test to ascertain skin and muscle viability, this test could be employed. Twenty cc's of 5 percent sodium fluorescein (available in most hospital pharmacies as Fluorescite or Funduscein) can be given slowly intravenously. Then the questionable tissue is exposed to an ultraviolet light (Wood's light) in a darkened room. Evidence of yellow fluorescence should indicate that the tissue is viable.

There is a controversy in the literature as to the advisability of **a second debridement** three to five days later to excise tissue originally of questionable viability. Perhaps immediate skin flap coverage would have allowed the marginally injured tissue to survive. At any rate, following the second (or even the third) debridement a **direct skin flap** from the contralateral anterior chest or the groin is placed on the debrided burn wound. My choice of flap coverage is usually the U-shaped Willie White skin flap based laterally on the anterior chest wall. Its base is about 5cm wide and its length about 10cm long, with one side of the flap extended laterally to the same distance from the base as the width of the base of the flap. This flap can be turned 90 degrees, either superiorly or inferiorly depending on which side of the flap is lengthened. The flap is sutured to the hand or arm, and the flap donor site closed primarily. Remember that a split-thickness skin graft will provide satisfactory wound coverage in a superficial electrical burn.

Amputation of completely necrotic fingers or hands is obviously indicated in extreme cases.

LATE TREATMENT

Sural nerve cable grafts are indicated in almost all instances where a peripheral nerve has been destroyed. This should be carried out four to six months post-burn. The sural nerve has a length prior to branching of from 14 to 35cm, the usual length being 30cm. Three or four nerve segments will approximate the caliber of the median nerve in the forearm.

Under magnification, and with a tourniquet on the extremity, the burned nerve ends should be cut back until viable axons without scar tissue are found. The nerve gaps should be sutured in loosely with number 8-0 or 10-0 nylon perineural sutures. Adjacent joints should be splinted for three weeks post-operatively. There are no long-term results of nerve grafting in electrical burns, but usually we are thinking in terms of return of protective sensation in almost all cases. Younger patients will have better results than older patients.

The restoration of supination following deep electrical burns at the wrist has been reported by Schmidt and Jaffe (1970). This is accomplished by excision of the fibrotic pronator quadratus muscle and possibly oblique resection of about 1.5cm of the distal ulna. Immobilization in extreme supination is maintained by a large Kirschner wire across the radius and ulna for three weeks.

Everyone has talent at twenty-five. The difficulty is to have it at fifty.

Degas

315

93

PRIMARY EXCISION OF THE HAND

Thomas J. Krizek

Primary excision refers to total removal of all areas involved in the burn, irrespective of the timing of the procedure. Well-localized, obvious full-thickness injuries in an otherwise healthy patient may be treated by immediate excision and skin grafting. More often, delay is indicated because of the patient's other burns and unstable condition, or the difficulty in accurately assessing the depth of the injury to the hand.

Routine use of topical antibacterial agents in the care of burn patients has particularly influenced the care of the burned hand. Effective control of potential infection gives the surgeon an increased margin of time in which he can safely perform total primary excision and definitive closure. In contrast, many cases of deep partial-thickness burns with multiple epithelial islands may heal spontaneously. This may occur, however, at the expense of unstable epithelium and, because of the nature of this healing, wound contracture.

In no other area of the body is poor healing so incompatible with form and function as in the hand. The hand should be considered the primary area for grafting, even in the patient with large total body surface areas of burn. Early return of function in the hand preserves the patient's hope for successful rehabilitation and gives a psychological boost by allowing him to help himself and to participate in his own care.

DIAGNOSIS

Accurate assessment of depth of damage of burned tissue is difficult. The degree of injury is determined by the nature of the burning agent and time of exposure and is influenced by the water content of the skin, pigmentation, skin thickness, and the presence of dirt, oil or grease on the surface. The same dry, anesthetic eschar may cover an area of full-thickness burn or a deep partial-thickness wound. Although burns of the palm are less common than burns of the dorsum, they most frequently result from contact with hot objects and tend to be very deep. The palm skin is usually protected from injury by flash or flames because the dorsum is reflexly thrown up to protect the face, by far the most common circumstance of burning. Because the skin of the dorsum is thinner, the relative depth of the burn is often greater. When first seen, some wounds are clearly full-thickness or at least very deep partial-thickness injuries. In other wounds the depth becomes obvious after several days of observation. A large number of wounds, however, can be accurately diagnosed only in retrospect, as eschar separation begins and healing potential is observed. In general, burns which heal spontaneously within two weeks are so sufficiently superficial that the healed wound has functional epithelium and there will be no contraction.

Timing. Timing of the burn excision is related to the confidence with which the diagnosis of injury depth can be made. As soon as a wound can be identified as a full-thickness or deep partial-thickness injury, excision and skin grafting are indicated. The timing may be classified as immediate, early and delayed.

Immediate Excision. Immediate excision may be carried out within 24 to 48 hours after injury in patients whose general condition permits and whose wounds are sufficiently localized and identifiably deep (Figure 1).

Fig. 1. A. Localized, deep burn of the palm, 48 hours after contact injury. **B.** Excision of wound and primary grafting. **C.** Healed, without contracture.

A   B   C

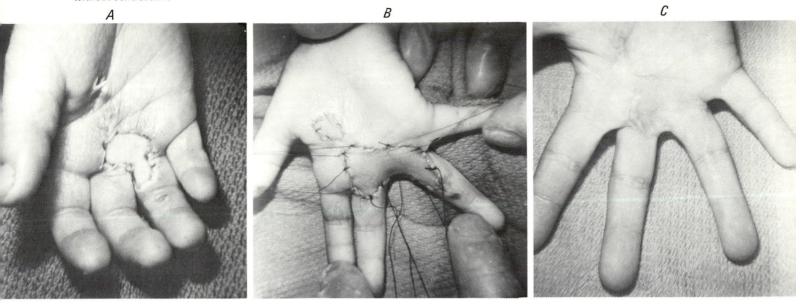

Fig. 2. A. Obviously deep flame burn of the dorsum of the hand seen at five days, the day of excision. **B.** Entire burn wound excised to level of healthy bed. **C. and D.** Six months after primary excision and grafting.

A   B   C

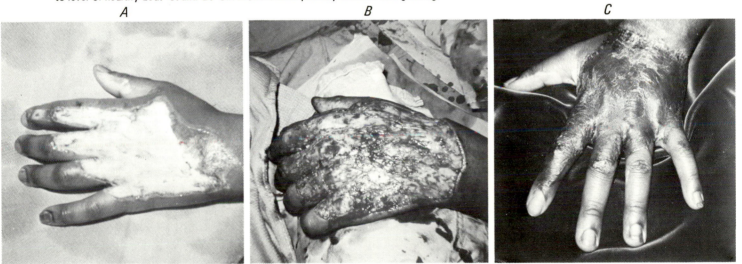

D

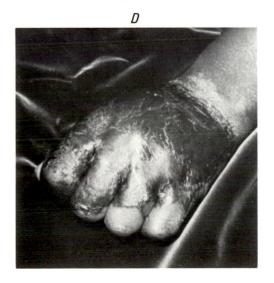

Early Excision. Early excision is performed within three to seven days on wounds where the depth of injury is not immediately obvious or in those patients whose condition was not sufficiently stable to allow surgery (Figure 2).

Delayed Primary Excision. Delayed excision refers to excision and grafting more than one week after injury. Topical antibacterial agents can maintain sufficient bacterial control that excision and definitive grafting are feasible even several weeks after injury (Figure 3). Most wounds which are not healed spontaneously within two weeks should be treated by delayed excision and grafting.

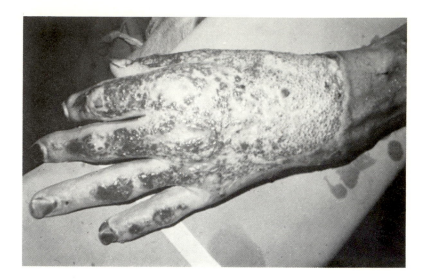

Fig. 3. A. Burn of the dorsum at 20 days. Multiple epithelial islands suggest that spontaneous healing would eventually occur. Topical antibacterials rendered this wound essentially bacteria-free.

Fig. 3. B. and C. The wound totally excised and grafted. Metacarpalphalangeal flexion maintained with skeletal fixation. The proximal interphalangeal joints extended by rubber band traction. The thumb-index web space maintained by abducting the thumb.

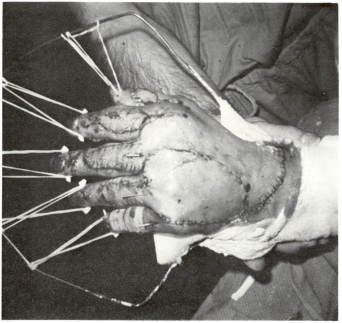 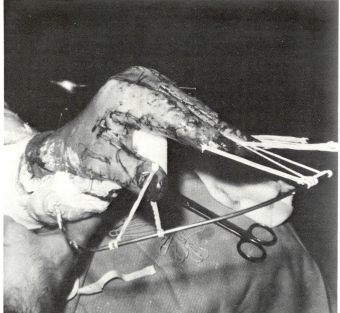

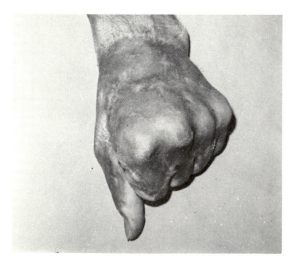

Fig. 3. D. The healed wound, with full range of motion.

TECHNIQUES

Anesthesia. Total resurfacing of the burned hand in an adult requires over 100 square inches of skin. Such large areas of donor skin can best be removed under general anesthetic. Even in small burns, the need for tourniquet control dictates the need for at least regional anesthesia.

Tourniquet. Identification of delicate underlying structures requires the use of a tourniquet. Careful hemostatic control, however, is necessary after removal of the tourniquet, before application of the grafts. Bleeding is rarely so troublesome that delayed grafting is required.

The Excision. The entire burned area should be removed. Granulating areas, often with islands of viable epithelium, should be totally sacrificed to the level of healthy underlying tissue. Such wounds are usually surrounded by a margin of healing, covered by new epithelium which hides a rim of contracting tissue. Application of a skin graft to the center of this wound will not prevent further contraction (Figure 4). Tourniquet control of the excision is indicated. Obvious blood vessels are identified, clamped, and either cauterized or ligated. Hemostasis is then completed after releasing the tourniquet. Wounds (such as those caused by electrical burns) which destroy the underlying tendons or their sheaths are not suitable for skin grafting, either primarily or later, and should have pedicle flap coverage.

The Skin Graft. A medium-thickness graft is indicated. This may be 0.012 to 0.014 inches when taken from the anterior thigh of an adult male. However, in a young child or an elderly patient a graft this deep might well be full-thickness. The thickness, therefore, must be determined relative to the characteristics of the donor site. A drum-type dermatome (Padgett or Reese) provides a nice, uniform sheet of skin. The mesh graft has little, if any, role in the management of burned hands. The graft is fitted to the defect and sutured marginally. Small "darts" should be placed in larger wounds to avoid long, straight, suture lines, particularly at flexion and extension creases. Small triangular extensions of the graft are fitted into the darts. The graft also should

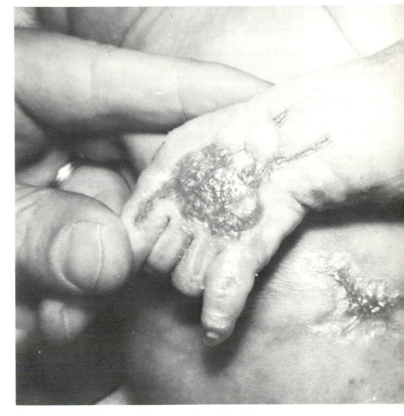

Fig. 4. A. Burn of the dorsum of the hand in an infant three weeks after burning. A healthy granulating bed is surrounded by a margin of healed, but contracting tissue.

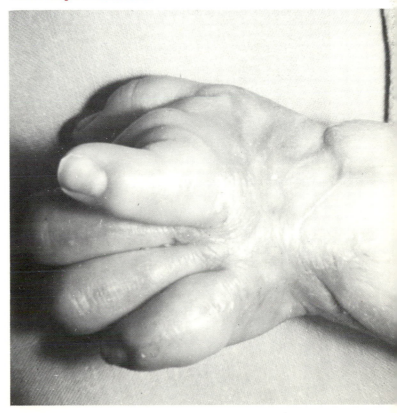

Fig. 4. B. A graft, successfully placed on the bed has not prevented the ravages of contracture.

be inserted deeply into web spaces when they are involved in the wound, making sure the entire web is covered with a single sheet of skin. The graft should be cut to fit the defect which should not be stretched to conform to the graft. Long, straight suture lines will contract and are to be avoided. A stent dressing (tie-over bolus) may be useful in the palm where contouring can be achieved and positioning accomplished over the dressing. However, with the fingers positioned properly, the convex surfaces of the dorsum make application of such a dressing difficult.

The Dressing and Positioning. The unsplinted burned hand will assume a position of metacarpophalangeal joint hyperextension, proximal interphalangeal joint flexion, and thumb-index adduction. To prevent this deformity, the hand should be placed in a "position of advantage" from which *motion* is most easily regained and which protects against the tendency to the above deformity. Such positioning maintains the length and tone of the metacarpophalangeal collateral ligaments and prevents contracture of the accessory collateral ligaments of the proximal interphalangeal joints. A closed dressing technique is suitable for palm skin grafts. For burns of the dorsum, we use a volar splint with wrist slightly extended. Skeletal traction via small Kirschner wires through the distal phalanx, attached by rubber band traction to a "hay-rake" outrigger, hold the PIP joints in extension. The pins may be placed either transversely through the distal phalanx or vertically, taking care to avoid injury to the nail bed. Flexed

over the end of the splint, the MP joints are maintained in 90 degree flexion by Kirschner wire skeletal fixation across the joint. The thumb-index web space is maintained by traction. No dressing is applied. Postoperatively, small blebs are evacuated by aspiration of small incisions.

Postoperative Care. The extremity is maintained in some elevation. If the fingers themselves have not been grafted, active and passive range of motion is maintained daily. If the rubber band traction is not too snugly applied, motion can be maintained within the "hay-rake" itself. Exercises are begun within four to five days in grafted areas and both active and passive exercises are continued until all motion is regained.

SUMMARY

Full-thickness and deep partial-thickness burns of the hands lend themselves well to excision of the entire wound and skin grafting. From a functional point of view, such wounds should be given priority for grafting. Topical antibacterial control of infection has prolonged indefinitely the time when those wounds may be primarily excised and grafted. Granulating and partially healed wounds may be excised and skin grafts safely applied, even more than two weeks after injury. A deep burn heals without grafting at the expense of deformity. Failure to excise the wound before applying the graft may also result in deformity.

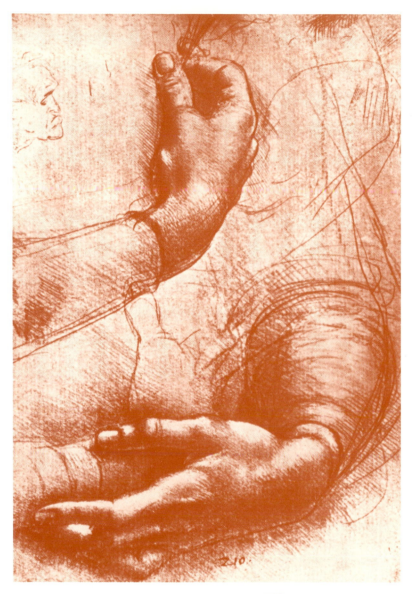

Leonardo da Vinci, 1452 – 1519.

94

RELEASE OF INTERDIGITAL WEB CONTRACTURES

Robert W. Beasley

The vast majority of interdigital web contractures are caused by thermal-flash type burns. Typically the victim of this injury has reflexively covered his face with his hands so their dorsal surfaces bear the brunt of the injury. There are two basic categories of interdigital contractures to be considered: those between fingers and that between the thumb and index finger resulting in an adduction contracture of the thumb.

INTERDIGITAL WEB CONTRACTURES

Interdigital contractures (Figure 1A) typically result from dorsal burns. A web develops between the proximal phalanges of the fingers while the normal volar skin fold usually is not disturbed. The greater the tissue loss, the tighter and more distal the web contracture will be. The contracture not only limits separation of the fingers, but in combination with scar tissue on the dorsum of the hand also flattens the transverse arch significantly.

When a conspicuous web has developed, the tissue deficiency is surprisingly large. One may be tempted to undertake correction with some form of the versatile Z-plasty, but this will be satisfactory only for the most minor web contracture. Occasionally diamond-shaped excision of the scar and the web followed by tissue replacement with a diamond-shaped skin graft is useful, but the results are inferior to reconstruction with a local flap. Fortunately, in most cases at least one of the opposing sides of the involved fingers has escaped significant injury and is available as donor site for a transposition flap (Figure 1B). The flap is based proximally on the normal volar skin fold and rotated 180 degrees into the defect created by longitudinally incising the transverse interdigital contracture. The donor site on the side of the finger is repaired with a hair-free skin graft, usually taken from the inguinal fold. The volar margin of the grafted donor site runs obliquely from the normal palmar web at the base of the finger up to the pivot point of the proximal interphalangeal joint to avoid a troublesome longitudinal volar scar on the proximal phalanx. The flap should be as large as available donor tissue permits and may safely have a length-to-width ratio of 2:1, provided the flap is not sutured in place under tension. The interdigital webs of all fingers can usually be repaired at the same operation by this method which results in an excellent correction (Figure 1C).

ADDUCTION CONTRACTURES OF THE THUMB

Contracture of the web between the thumb and index finger severely impairs hand function by limiting the size of objects that can be readily handled (Figure 2A). Very mild contractures can be satisfactorily improved by one or more Z-plasties, but this approach to significant contractures creates a deep cleft rather than restoring the normal web. Release of the severely contracted thumb results in a gaping space. Tissues for restoration of the web must be folded on themselves to create a thin web. This requires a distant flap with its own blood supply and precludes use of a graft. Innumerable designs of flaps are possible, but generally the best choice is a superiorly based contralateral epigastric flap (Figure 2B). The flap donor site is closed directly. The simplest effective way to maintain divergence of the first and second metacarpals is with a threaded Kirschner wire drilled through the second and into the first. The flap is carried over the dorsal surface of the denuded first metacarpal and its tip set well into the palm as a

Fig. 1. A. Interdigital web contractures resulting from typical thermal-flash burns to dorsal surfaces of hands. **B.** Proximally based flap from radial side of middle finger rotated 180 degrees to correct transverse interdigital dorsal web contracture. A full-thickness skin graft from the hairless inguinal fold is used to repair the flap donor site. **C.** The postoperative results two years after repair by the transposition flap method.

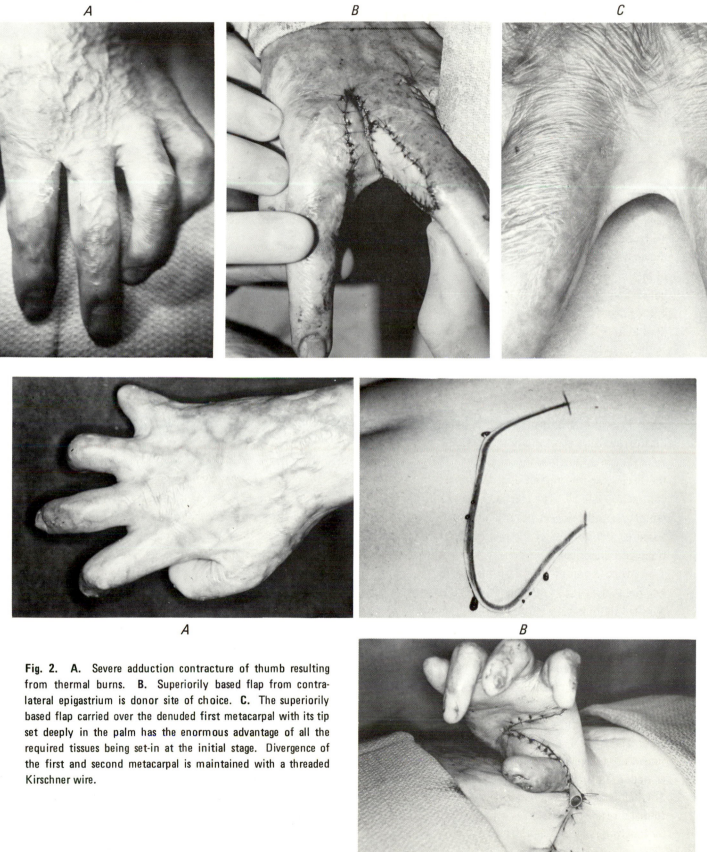

A   *B*   *C*

A   *B*

Fig. 2. A. Severe adduction contracture of thumb resulting from thermal burns. **B.** Superiorily based flap from contra-lateral epigastrium is donor site of choice. **C.** The superiorily based flap carried over the denuded first metacarpal with its tip set deeply in the palm has the enormous advantage of all the required tissues being set-in at the initial stage. Divergence of the first and second metacarpal is maintained with a threaded Kirschner wire.

C

deep "V" (Figure 2C). To close the wound, the edge of the dorsal skin remaining along the first metacarpal is sutured to the edge of the abdominal skin of the flap donor site. **This approach has the enormous advantage of suturing all the required flap tissues to their final location at the primary procedure.** None of the tissues of the pedicle of the flap are needed for the repair and, therefore, no delay in severing the pedicle is needed. Assuming primary wound healing, all of the implanted flap is receiving blood from the recipient site in two and one-half to three weeks, at which time the pedicle is simply severed. This usually

is done with local infiltration anesthesia on the ward. The resulting wounds on the hand are closed a few days later, after they have been prepared by frequently changed moist dressings. Morbidity is less if the resulting abdominal wound is permitted to heal by secondary intention, revising the scar later if desired. In long-standing severe cases, it may be necessary to sever part of the contracted thenar muscle for full release of the thumb. In such cases a tendon transfer through the reconstructed web to reinforce power of thumb adduction may be required later.

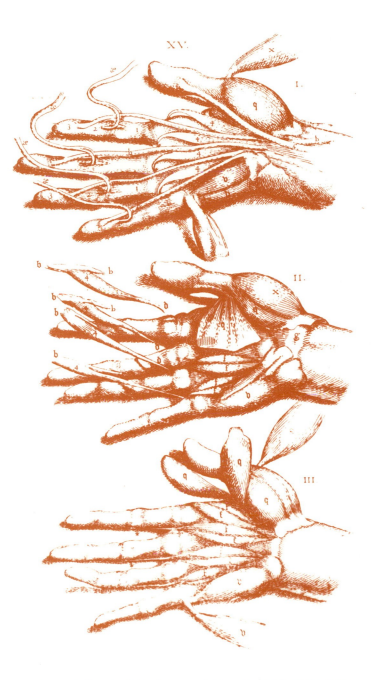

Anatomie der wtterlicke deelen van het menschelick lichaem, 1660.

95

FINGER RECONSTRUCTION

Irving Feller

The problems resulting from extensive burns to the hands are loss of function and amputation. Loss of motion results from tissue loss by scar formation and resulting contracture. Damage or destruction of tendons, joints, and bone also causes deformity and limits motion. When destruction is deep and extensive, amputation may be indicated. A serious concern of many patients is appearance of their hand.

Four specific problems seen are: (1) web space contracture, (Figures 1 to 5); (2) joint destruction resulting in deformity, (Figures 6 to 8); (3) palm or flexion contracture, (Figures 9 to 13); and (4) amputation of the fingers, (Figures 14 to 18). A method of repair for each of these problems is described.

1. WEB SPACE

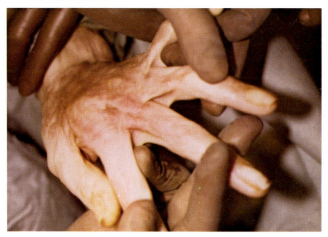

Fig. 1. Web space contractures result from burns to the dorsum or whole hand. When the contracture is severe, correction can be accomplished by a release and covering of the defect with thick or split-thickness skin grafts.

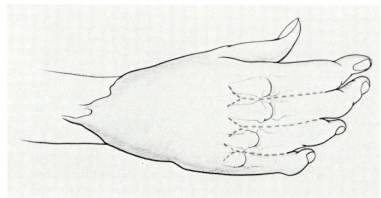

Fig. 2. The release is made as indicated by the dotted line.

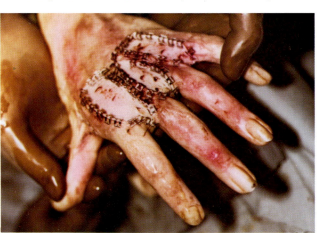

Fig. 3. When the contracture is released and the "Y" end becomes a rectangle, a large piece of skin is required to cover the defect.

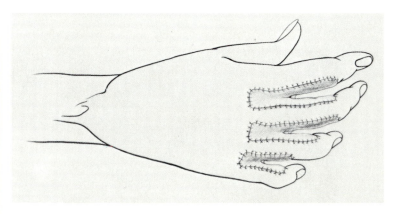

Fig. 4. The grafts are secured in place using sutures or metal clips and the appropriate dressings are applied.

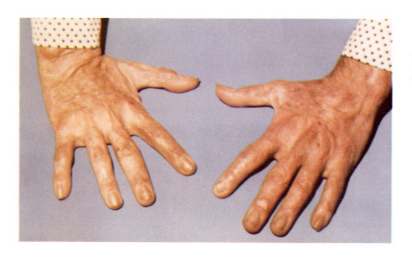

Fig. 5. The results of this procedure are seen several months after the operation.

2. JOINT DESTRUCTION

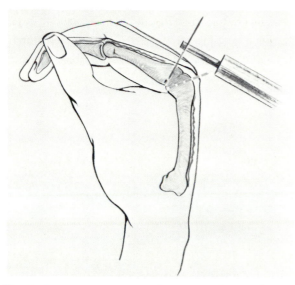

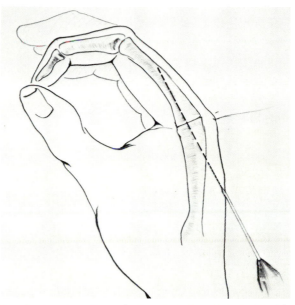

Fig. 6. Joint destruction results from a severe burn to the dorsum of the fingers. Not only is the skin destroyed but the tendon and the joint are burned. When skin grafting is complete, the final deformity can be evaluated for correction. In these cases tendon transplantation is not possible; proper positioning of the finger in a position of function is important.

Fig. 7. A wedge of bone (indicated by dotted line in Fig. 6.) has been resected to allow for the proper positioning of the finger. Flexion or extension contractures can be corrected by this system by varying the angle of resection. A threaded stainless steel wire is used to hold the ends of bone together for six weeks to allow for fusion. The skin is closed using sutures of choice.

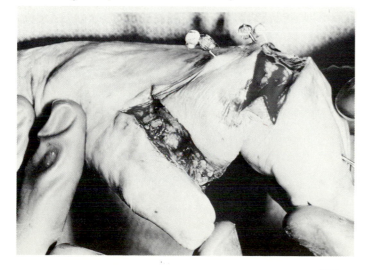

Fig. 8. At times both a release of contracture and fusion are necessary when a contracture causes an extension deformity. This case also illustrates correction of the first web space deformity.

3. SEVERE FLEXION CONTRACTURES OF THE PALM AND FINGERS

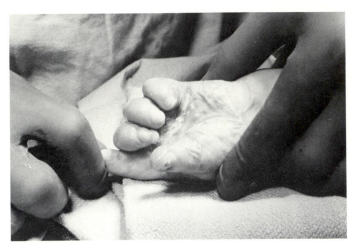

Fig. 9. Severe flexion contractures of the palm and fingers require correction by release and grafting with thick split-thickness autografts. These contractures are more difficult to repair than those that occur on the extensor surface. Adequate and timely splinting are important factors.

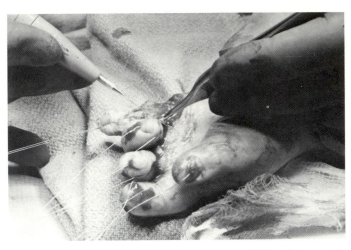

Fig. 10. When the contracture is severe in the child, stainless steel wires are inserted through the distal phalanges. The wires are used as retractors during the procedure and then become the cables for attachment to the splint. The contracture is shown as it is being released with the cautery.

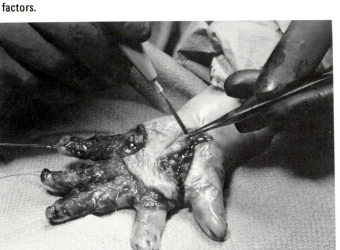

Fig. 11. The defect created by the release of the contracture is illustrated. In this case a small amount of scar tissue is also being excised to allow for a complete release.

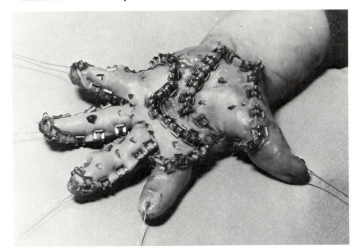

Fig. 12. Thick split-thickness grafts are placed over the defect and stainless steel clips used to secure the grafts. Small openings have been made to allow for drainage.

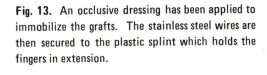

Fig. 13. An occlusive dressing has been applied to immobilize the grafts. The stainless steel wires are then secured to the plastic splint which holds the fingers in extension.

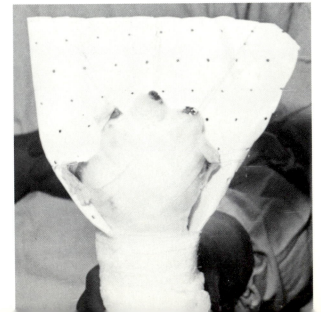

4. TRANSPOSITION OF PARTIAL FINGER

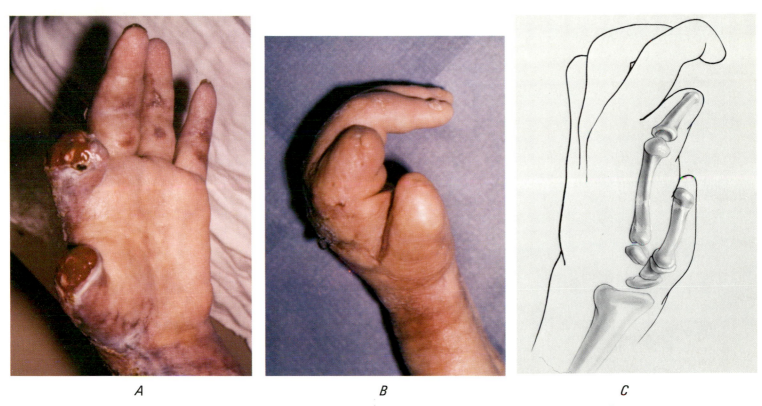

A   B   C

Fig. 14. When severe burns result in multiple partial finger amputation, parts of the remaining fingers can be used for reconstruction. **A.** Patient with loss of the thumb and the distal two phalanges of the index finger. **B.** The finger stumps are healed and the first web space has been deepened. **C.** Artist's conception of this problem.

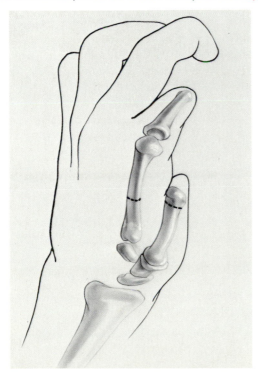

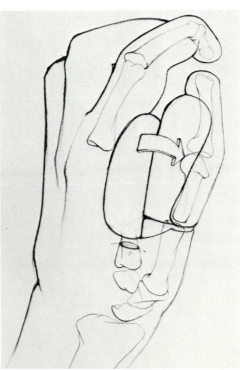

Fig. 15. The distal end of the first metacarpal is cut transversely to provide a base for the transplant. The second metacarpal is then cut at the same level as the first. Dotted lines indicate cutting line.

Fig. 16. The hand is incised to fashion a pedicle that includes the bone, tendon, blood vessels, and nerves. The pedicle is then rotated (arrow) to the first metacarpal base.

329

4. TRANSPOSITION OF PARTIAL FINGER (Continued)

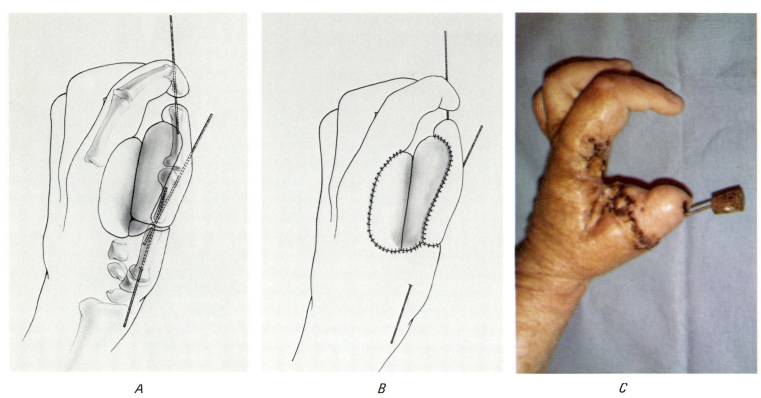

A   B   C

Fig. 17. Threaded stainless steel wires are used to hold the transplantation in place for six weeks to two months. **A.** Split-thickness skin grafts are placed over the open areas. Note the position of the wires. **B.** The grafts are sutured in place. **C.** Immediate postoperative view.

Fig. 18. The reconstructed thumb is functional with normal sensation. Stainless steel wires are removed.

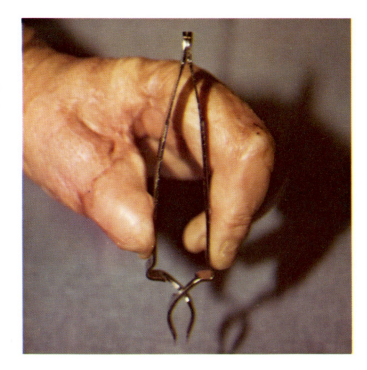

The form of an Hand made artificially of Iron.

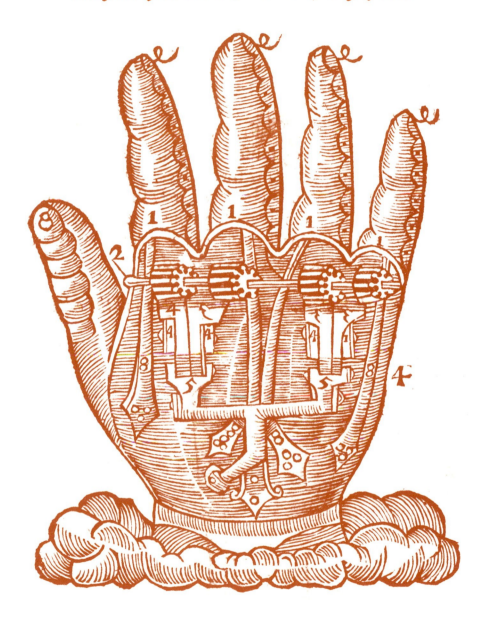

The Works of that Famous Chirurgeon: Ambrose Parey, 1678.

96

FINGER TRANSPOSITION

John M. Markley, Jr.

Restoration of a digit to oppose the remaining fingers in a hand which has lost its thumb can provide remarkable restoration of function and appearance. The radiating architecture of the digital rays with neurovascular and tendonous elements diverging from mid-palm allows multiple variations on transfer of portions of normal or partially damaged digits to locations of greater functional advantage.

Circumstances favorable for digital transfer to thumb position are infrequent in the burned hand but may occur when thermal injury has been relatively localized as in some electrical and blast injuries. Digital transposition should be withheld until primary healing and functional recovery of the remaining hand parts is complete.

INDICATIONS

The prime indication for digital transposition is loss of the thumb at any level between the carpo-metacarpal and the metacarpalphalangeal joints. If the metacarpalphalangeal joint and a portion of the proximal phalanx is intact, and if additional stable length with useful sensibility is required (a requirement not universally present in this situation), then reconstruction by either bone graft, skin flap, and neurovascular island flap or by metacarpal lengthening (Matev) should be considered. The digit or portion thereof to be transferred must be pain free, have useful sensibility, and a functional range of motion with stability. If a normal digit is to be transferred the index is preferred. If, however, a digital transfer is selected for a subtotal thumb loss with a portion of proximal phalanx remaining, the ring finger may be preferable due to the marked degree of recession necessary.

Patient selection requires great care. Consideration must be given to the patient's functional requirements, age, occupation, dominant hand, motivation for and understanding of the procedure, and willingness or desire to lose a finger to gain a thumb. Usually the advantages of transfer outshadow the disadvantages.

Toe to hand transfer utilizing microvascular and microneural techniques is an alternative approach to restoration of an opposing digit. It is most applicable in two uncommon situations: first, when only one digit remains on the hand; second, when the functional requirements of the patient demand a four-finger/one-thumb hand. A suitable recipient area with normal vasculature and available sensory nerve(s) is necessary. Microsurgical free toe transfer should be undertaken for the burned hand only with prior experience with microvascular composite tissue transfer techniques. Discussion of the technique is beyond the scope of this chapter.

SURGICAL REQUIREMENTS

Successful performance of digital transposition requires detailed knowledge of the functional anatomy of the hand and meticulous surgical technique. Tourniquet ischemia and optimum operating room conditions are mandatory. The procedure should only be undertaken by one schooled and experienced in reconstructive surgery of the hand. The price of failure can be functional or structural loss of a previously normal digit.

PLANNING

Preoperative planning is of utmost importance.

Provision must be made for durable skin and soft tissue cover at the transfer site. If this is inadequate, skin cover must be provided by local flaps at the time of transfer or by a separate preparatory operative stage using an appropriate selection of free skin grafts and local or distant skin flaps. Consideration is always given to the salvage of a partially damaged digit for transfer. If a normal digit is to be transferred, the index is usually best, except in cases of subtotal thumb loss as noted previously. Experience has shown that both function and appearance of a thumb reconstructed by digital transfer are best when the length after transfer is approximately ½cm less than that of a normal thumb. In most normal hands the thumb tip rests at the level of the index proximal interphalangeal joint when the thumb is adducted to the radial border of the index. Exact measurements are made preoperatively using 1:1 radiographs of the hands and by markings and measurements on the hands to determine the levels of skin incision and osteotomies. The arterial patency of the donor digit is determined by the digital Allen's test and by Doppler examination. Arteriography is usually unnecessary.

SURGICAL TECHNIQUE

I use the technique of J. William Littler[1], whose lucid and classic text and illustrations have not been improved upon. Hence the reader is strongly urged to become thoroughly familiar with these descriptions before undertaking digital transfer. However, certain points of technique deserve emphasis or elaboration:

1. The hand is thoroughly prepared and draped as for any reconstructive hand procedure. Pneumatic tourniquet ischemia is mandatory and is limited to two hours maximum duration.

2. When the index finger is transferred, care should be taken to preserve a dorsal vein in transfer to augment the multiple small veins accompanying the digital arteries. When the ring finger is transferred, a dorsal vein should be identified and transsected long enough to be transferred by microvascular anastomosis at the recipient site if any question exists regarding adequacy of venous drainage.

3. Soft tissues should be preserved surrounding the neurovascular bundles to preserve all venous and lymphatic vessels possible. The arteries and nerves should **not** be "skeletonized."

4. The flexor mechanism must be separated from the base of the proximal phalanx to allow proper freedom of transfer and direction of pull of the flexors.

5. The lumbrical muscle of the transferred digit should be excised.

6. The detached tendon of the first dorsal interosseous may be left free or may be inserted into the tendon of the second dorsal interosseous. If reinserted, undue tension must be avoided or the middle finger may develop an intrinsic plus deformity.

7. The transferred digit should be pronated 5 to 10 degrees at the osteotomy site when the thumb metacarpalphalangeal joint is absent.

8. Use of an interosseous wire suture of 22 to 24 gauge stainless steel across the fusion site has been found to increase stability and facilitate fusion.

9. Immobilization at the fusion site should be maintained for six to eight weeks, but distal joint motion may be started in four weeks.

10. Later transfer of flexor pollicis longus to flexor digitorum profundis of the transferred digit is advisable when the flexor pollicis longus is available.

Normal tactile sensibility should be preserved by this procedure. However, initially the patient identifies sensations from the transferred digit as arising in its original location. Spatial reorganization of awareness from "finger" to "thumb" is of variable rate and degree and may never occur. Incomplete spatial reorientation, however, is apparently seldom a functional detriment.

---

1. J.W. Littler, "Reconstruction of the Thumb in Traumatic Loss," *Reconstructive Surgery*, ed. J.M. Converse, 2nd Edition, Chapter 80 (Philadelphia: W.B. Saunders Co., 1977); idem, "Neurovascular Pedicle Method of Digital Transposition for Reconstruction of the Thumb," *Plast. Reconst. Surg.*, (1953), 12:303.

97

HAND SPLINTING

George H. Koepke

DORSAL HAND BURN

The dorsal surface of the hand is one of the most commonly burned areas of the body. Burns limited to the palm are much less frequent. The tendons and joint capsules of the dorsal surface are not protected, as they are in the palm, by thick skin, palmar fascia, and a thick pad of fat. The sequence of events following full-thickness loss of skin from the dorsal surface includes ensuing fibrosis accompanied by extension contractures of the metacarpophalangeal joints, flexion deformities of the interphalangeal joints and adduction of the digits (Figure 1). To lessen these deformities, a plastic or metal splint is applied during the acute treatment period (Figure 2). A delay in splinting the hand with full-thickness loss of skin until autografts have taken will often result in loss of motion. Whenever there is full-thickness loss of skin over the dorsal surface of the hand, with or without palmar burns, the hand is positioned over the splint with dressings to

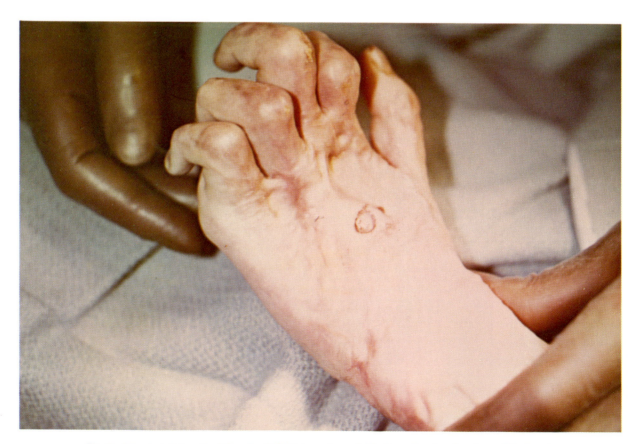

Fig. 1. A typical deformity following full-thickness loss of skin from the dorsal surface of the hand.

keep the metacarpophalangeal joints of the fingers in extreme flexion and abduction. The interphalangeal joints of all digits are extended and the thumb is abducted. The wrist is extended approximately 10 degrees. The angle of the medio-lateral axis of the metacarpophalangeal joints to the long axis of the hand and forearm is approximately 15 degrees. If the splint is constructed so that the angle of this axis is less than 15 degrees and nearer the angle of the normal hand, the small finger will probably curl under the dressings and develop flexion deformities of its interphalangeal joints. Should the proximal interphalangeal joints remain flexed, the central tendon of the extensor digitorum communis may be stretched excessively, and the lateral bands of the aponeurosis may slip. As a result, the extensor mechanism may be lost. If the fingers can be kept straight and the metacarpophalangeal joints flexed, remarkable joint stability and interphalangeal function can be preserved. The func-

tional advantages of full movement of the thumb are recognized and therefore the thumb is abducted and extended by the splint. If an adduction contracture can be prevented and full abduction maintained, one can anticipate good function of the thumb.

SPLINTS

A supply of paired splints in six different sizes may be stored for immediate use.* In keeping with isolation and aseptic techniques, the splint may be cleansed between dressing changes, during the time for hydrotherapy and exercises. Minor adjustments of stocked splints may be necessary to insure accurate fit. Experience at the University of Michigan Burn Unit with more than 1,000 burned hands has demonstrated the value of wet dressings changed two or three times daily, early hand splinting, and the application of split-thickness skin grafts as soon as the

*Splints available from ATCO Supply Co., Cuyahoga Falls, Ohio.

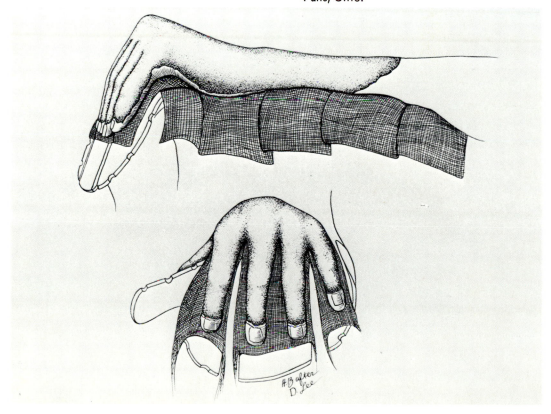

Fig. 2. A plastic or metal splint is indicated when there is acute full-thickness loss of skin from the dorsal surface of the hand.

recipient site has a clean granulating base. Hands with exposed interphalangeal joints and loss of the extensor mechanism will usually require subsequent internal fixation, but excellent functions may be anticipated if good motion is preserved in the metacarpophalangeal joints.

VOLAR SPLINT

A patient is seen occasionally with burns limited to the volar surface of the fingers and palm. If there should be full-thickness loss of skin from the anterior surface, a volar splint should be applied to hold the digits abducted and extended (Figure 3). If the palm is severely damaged or if there are fresh split-thickness skin grafts, a splint may be applied to the dorsal surface and the wrist held in about 20 degrees of dorsiflexion during the pre- and early post-grafting stages.

SKELETAL FIXATION

Skeletal wire fixation of the interphalangeal joints may be preferred to exoskeletal splinting during the acute treatment period if there are additional injuries to full-thickness loss of skin. Some of these include the loss of flexor or extensor tendons that are

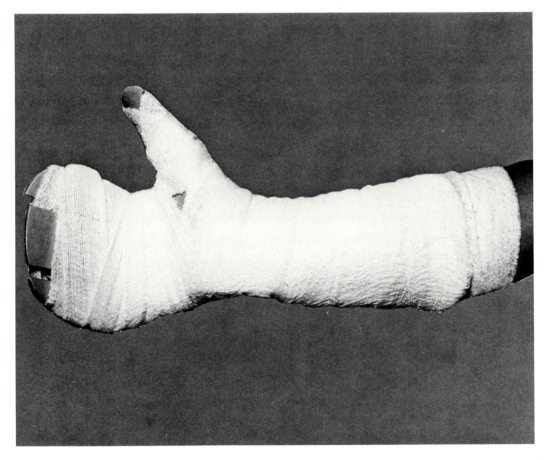

Fig. 3. Palmar splint is applied during the acute period when full-thickness skin loss is limited to the volar surface.

too extensive for tendon repair. Other possible indications for skeletal immobilization include peripheral nerve or plexus injuries, fractures, and loss of muscle. In these instances, muscle imbalance will often lead to dynamic contracture from the unopposed contraction of the antagonists. This potential deformity can be controlled by the insertion of pins through the digits. Appropriate position can be maintained by securing the ends of the pins in a splint of plaster. We have no experience using the "hayrake" splint during the acute treatment period but have found it helpful during the reconstruction period when contractures and deformities require a release of tendon, joint and/or capsule. Mild flexion deformities of the

metacarpophalangeal and interphalangeal joints may respond to the use of a combination of a dynamic knuckle-bender splint and passive exercises (Figure 4).

The location of full-thickness burns of the hand can serve as a useful guide during the acute treatment period in predicting the deformity, although surgical reconstruction is often necessary in the severely burned hand. Appropriate positioning with the application of splints during the pre- and post-grafting phase is a valuable measure to lessen hand deformity. Active and passive exercises help to maintain the rheologic properties of soft tissue and may be the only physical modality that is indicated in the treatment of partial-thickness loss of skin.

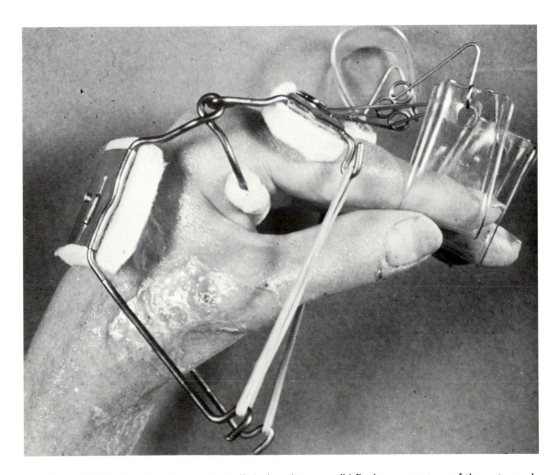

Fig. 4. Dynamic knuckle-bender may be applied when there are mild flexion contractures of the metacarpalphalangeal and interphalangeal joints.

98

AMPUTATION OF THE HAND AND ARM

George H. Koepke

Partial amputations of the hand may become disabling because adequate function cannot be restored by orthoses or reconstructive surgery. Traumatic amputation from an industrial accident is usually in a straight line through the phalanges or metacarpals; however, electrical and thermal injuries often result in digit or metacarpal stumps of unequal length.

The conservative approach is usually best in the management of a burned hand during the acute treatment period. With few exceptions, it is desirable to save as much length as possible. Regardless, it is important to provide adequate soft tissue over bone because adherent split-thickness skin grafts without an adequate bed of soft tissue over bone will often break down. A mobile split-thickness skin graft will mature if the pressure and shear requirements placed on it are slowly graduated. If a split-thickness graft on the hand is protected for the first few months by emollients and gloves it will become durable. No prosthesis is usually required if only one or two digits are amputated but if all digits must be amputated, function is best restored with the standard prosthetic socket, wrist unit and a functional short hook and harness. This will not prove cosmetically acceptable to some patients because the end of the terminal device is usually somewhat longer than the tip of the normal hand.

FINGERS AND THUMB

Each patient should be asked whether he prefers a functional or cosmetic device, or both. The physician should never insist on one rather than the other when it may not be the patient's interest. The prosthesis must be prescribed according to the vocational and functional requirements of each patient. Cosmetic fingers may be held on by special adhesives, suction or a cosmetic glove as shown in Figure 1. An alternative or substitute for the absence of all fingers is an orthosis that will provide a finger post for strong pinch between it and the thumb (Figure 2). Amputation of the thumb alone is relatively uncommon and a prosthetic thumb or post can be cosmetic and functional (Figure 3). A cosmetic hand in the shape of a mitt can be constructed for distal transmetacarpal amputation. The mitt is constructed of plastic material reinforced with glass roving to provide strength and to make it durable. If a portion of the thumb can be salvaged, an orthotic post can be quite functional.

WRIST

It may be better to amputate one and one half inches above the level of the ulnar styloid then disarticulate the wrist, especially if the circumference of the distal end of the stump should exceed the circumference of the more proximal portions of the forearm. In this instance, the prosthetic socket will have to be modified extensively to accommodate the width of the stump at the styloid process. The alternative is to cut a window in the socket near the styloid process. A wrist disarticulation stump may require a shorter hook or a small hand to provide length equal to the opposite hand.

ELBOW

For functional superiority, the normal elbow joint is preferred to an elbow disarticulation or a long

Fig. 1. A. Prosthetic finger for amputated middle digit with just enough proximal phalangeal stump to preserve lumbrical action.

Fig. 1. B. Prosthetic finger retained by adhesive cement.

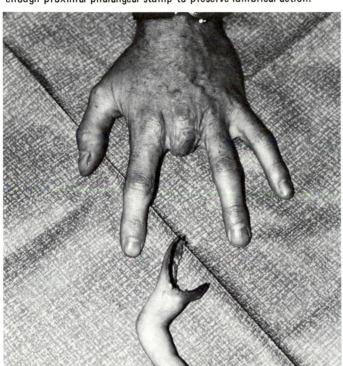

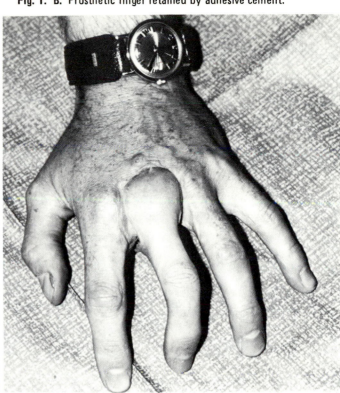

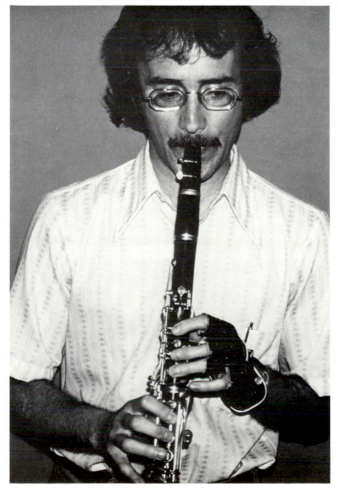

Fig. 1. C. Functionally competent as professional clarinetist.

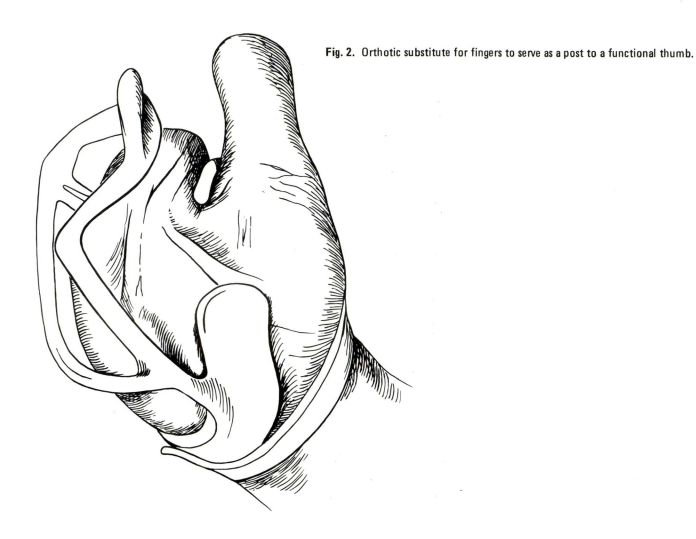

Fig. 2. Orthotic substitute for fingers to serve as a post to a functional thumb.

Fig. 3. Cosmetic thumb that may serve as a soft post to the index and mid finger for light pinch.

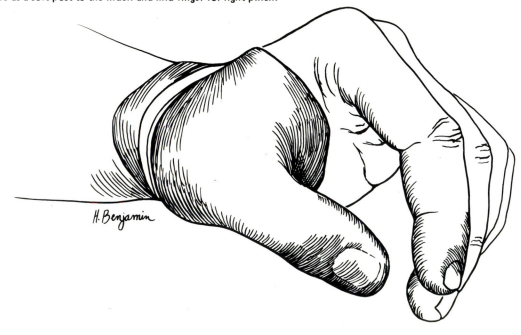

above-the-elbow stump. If the insertion of the biceps can be preserved, the resulting very short elbow stump is functionally much better than a stump at any higher level.

If the elbow joint cannot be saved, an elbow disarticulation is somewhat functionally superior to an above-the-elbow amputation especially for heavy laborers who use a prosthesis with outside locking hinges. The flare of the epicondyles creates some difficulty in donning the prosthesis due to the wide epicondylar portion of the socket. The prosthesis is wide because the hinges are usually on the outside of the socket. In these instances, tight shirt sleeves cannot be worn over the elbow joint. An additional objection to an elbow disarticulation or a very long above-the-elbow stump is that the necessarily long prosthetic socket will interfere with the use of the prosthesis at a table. For these reasons, a humeral amputation at a level approximately two inches above the medial epicondyle is cosmetically and functionally more acceptable than levels nearer the elbow joint because one can apply a standard above-elbow prosthesis. Amputations of the arm for burn injuries are rarely necessary at levels higher than the proximal 20 percent of the humerus.

The reason why so few good books are written is that so few people who can write know anything.

Bagehot

99

HAND PROSTHESIS

Denis C. Lee

HISTORY

Upper extremity prostheses have been used at least since the time of the Talmud. Although Putti (1930) did not consider the earlier prostheses as cosmetic, they rather faithfully reproduced the hand. Edwards (1972) cites first and 16th century upper extremity prostheses, the latter "cosmetic." Marks in his 1905 "Manual of Artificial Limbs" showed prosthetic hand parts made of rubber, aluminum, or silver (Figure 1).

Brown, in 1945, demonstrated a single and a four-finger prosthesis with a good aesthetic appearance. He thought cosmesis was important. Sooudi in 1973 reported construction of a cosmetic finger prosthesis to replace the incomplete loss of the distal phalanx of the left little finger in a 39-year-old female and made reference to some functional value.

References to cosmetic hands and hand parts are not extensive. Boyes (1970) states that in amputation through the hand, no prosthesis will be used if there are two remaining digits that can feel and work against each other in a prehensive way. If, however, there is only one remaining digit, a prosthesis will furnish the necessary broad hook with a flat surface against which to work. This is especially useful if the thumb remains and the fingers are off at the base of the palm. Hand parts are often discarded because of the lack of sensation. This does not consider the cosmetic aspect. Rank, Wakefield, and Hueston (1973) mention "improved cosmetic hands." Edwards (1972) considers satisfactory cosmetic hand parts important for psychological well-being in social situations and in occupations requiring a pleasing and normal appearance. He describes cosmetic prostheses with functional value.

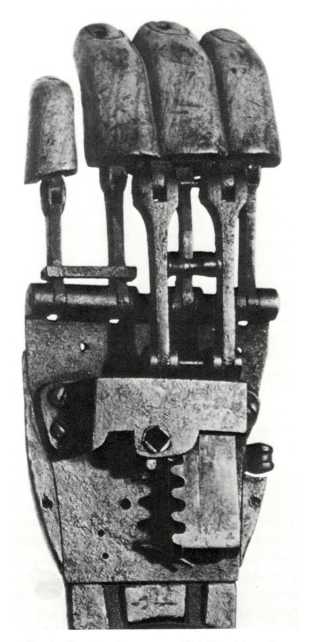

Fig. 1. Seventeenth century artificial hand from the Germanisches National Museum, Nuremberg.

A satisfactory hand part prosthesis should be well matched to the remaining hand in texture, color, and position. Ease of care and application of the prosthesis are desirable. Function of the part may be an added bonus. Ease of availability and reasonable expense are important.

Earlier prostheses made of latex and polyvinyl chloride had poor stain resistance and wearing qualities (Klopsteg et al, 1954), but had excellent color and matching characteristics. Schaaf, in 1970, described a method of color matching silicone facial appliances. With the recent development of silicone rubbers, the fabrication of prosthetic fingers and hands has become simplified, less expensive, and the parts are longer lasting with improved stain resistance.

No longer are complicated metal molds and heat vulcanization necessary. Prostheses can be prepared quickly in plaster stone molds with room temperature vulcanizing silicone.

At the University of Michigan Medical Center, I have developed a simplified method of producing cosmetic hand parts (Figures 2 and 3). The patient's physician submits casts of the opposite and involved hands with skin color selected from a swatch and the following technique is used.

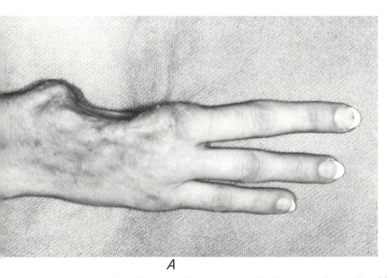

A

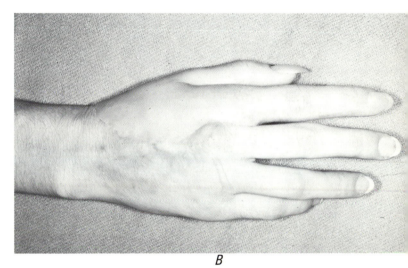

B

Fig. 2. Gunshot wound to the hand. **A.** Anterior before; **B.** with prosthesis.

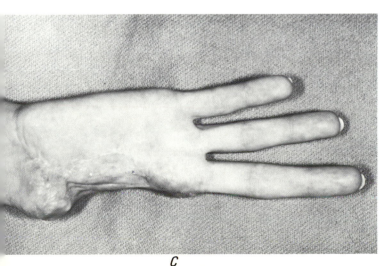

C

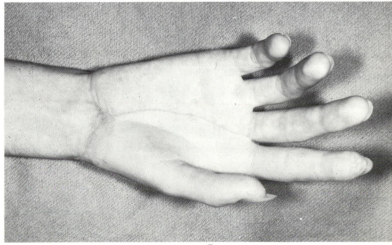

D

Fig. 2. C. Posterior before; **D.** with prosthesis.

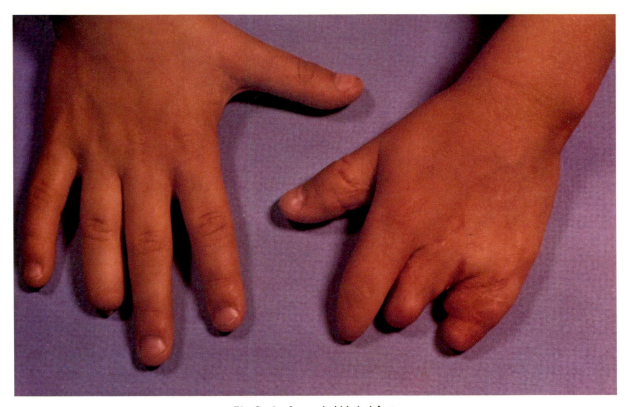

Fig. 3. A. Congenital birth defect.

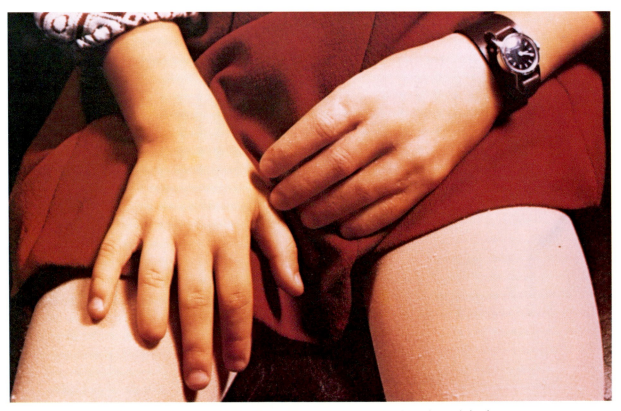

Fig. 3. B. Congenital birth defect with prosthesis; note matching tint and shaping.

TECHNIQUE

The most important step in preparation of hand prosthesis is sculpturing the missing finger or hand in clay.

When need for a prosthesis is indicated, a cast is prepared of both hands to include the defective hand and corresponding portion of the good hand. This is accomplished by using half gallon milk cartons filled with a flexible impression material such as dental hydrocolloid.

Have the patient insert his hand, holding it in a position that will totally record the missing parts. The impression is made with the hand in the position of function with the fingers in position while the hand hangs naturally at the side.

Hydrocolloid sets in three to five minutes. Mixing the hydrocolloid powder with cold water prolongs setting time while warm water hastens it. Room temperature water is desirable.

When the impression material has set up, move the hand to break suction and slowly remove the hand. Fill each mold with white stone plaster and vibrate to eliminate air bubbles which may be trapped.

The next step is to determine the patient's skin color; this is done by using prefabricated color swatches or mixing the color. Commercial inorganic pigments are used for coloring and mix readily with silicone.

Remove the plaster casts from the mold material, drill a small hole into the end of the stump of each missing finger and insert a piece of wire (coat hanger) dipped in epoxy glue. The next step is to reproduce the missing parts in clay on the surface of the stump or defect.

The detail in plaster molds may be diminished so one should exaggerate the details of skin texture, nails, and knuckles. The thickness of the clay around the stump should be no less than 1mm except where it is feathered at the seam. A cast of the normal hand is used for comparison during sculpture. Use of the cast of the corresponding part for the prosthesis or looking for a similar finger cast from another patient is undesirable.

After sculpturing in clay has been completed, all plaster surfaces of the hand model should be coated with a "separator" in preparation for making the final mold. A bed of plaster (stone) is poured into a box or suitable container and the reconstructed hand is placed, palm up, on the plaster. Gently tap or wiggle the hand model until the fresh plaster covers half of the hand and fingers. This may require some building up of plaster between the fingers if the fingers are curved more than normal. Registering holes are made in the plaster mold which is then coated with "separator." After the lower half has set, the second part of the plaster mold is poured, vibrating the plaster over the clay. The thicker the mold, the less the chance of cracking.

When the plaster has set up, separate the pieces of the mold and remove the clay. Clean all parts of the mold with xylene. Next, build up the areas that will make the prosthesis lighter, such as tips of finger stubs, with plaster. You should have a wire support to build the plaster on. This hollow space allows for tightness, better fit, and suction to help hold the prosthesis finger on the stump.

Next, on the plaster stump the area where the prosthesis fits on the finger is reinforced with nylon by coating a 3/8 inch wide strip of nylon with a tough silicone and wrapping it around the stump overlapping slightly before casting.

Another important step, especially in preparation of a prosthetic finger, is to measure the circumference of the stub on which the prosthesis will fit. This can be done with a jeweler's sizing ring obtained from a jewelry store. It is important to size the finger stump because the fingers have a tendency to swell slightly in the dependent position during the impression taking. To insure a tight fit, the finger stump of the model is merely sanded down to ring size.

There are different colors in the hand and fingers, and selection of the base color is difficult. If in doubt, the color should be lighter.

The base colored silicone mixture is catalyzed and brushed into the two halves of the stone mold filling the trough to slightly overflowing. The third part of the mold, the stump, is pressed on the dorsal half of the mold and pressed into place. The inferior section of the mold is squeezed into place and tightly held with a C-clamp. Keep some of the base color silicone for patching.

When the silicone has set, carefully remove the prosthesis from the mold and trim off the flashing and any other excess. The prosthesis is now ready to try on the patient.

If the prosthesis fits, it is ready for tinting. This is done by mixing pigment with silicone diluted with xylene and application with a small sable brush. Only once can the entire prosthesis be given a light spray of catalyst which bonds the color to the prosthesis. The prosthesis is then given a matting spray to remove the gloss left by the catalyst.

Often prostheses for patients with an even skin color can be pretinted by painting the colors into the mold. This type of prosthesis is the most ideal for longevity; however, aesthetically, external tinting is more realistic and the usual procedure.

A finger or hand prosthesis usually lasts about six months depending upon its care and use.

Most finger prostheses can be attached without adhesives if the stump is adequate. Available adhesives will hold the prosthesis securely to any part of the hand if there is satisfactory contact surface. A glove-type prosthesis is secured by a hidden zipper on the anterior or palmar surface.

Women tolerate cosmetic prostheses more readily than men, and persons involved in manual activities find prostheses less acceptable.

Desirable characteristics of silicone hand prostheses:

1. Light weight.
2. Natural color.
3. Comfortable and well accepted by the patient.
4. Easily reproduced.
5. Inexpensive.
6. Strong and durable.

Undesirable characteristics:

1. Must be replaced at least once a year (longer wearing than polyvinyl chloride or latex).
2. Easily stained by ink, grease, and dirt, but comparable to other materials.

SUMMARY

A relatively "rapid" and inexpensive method of fabricating hand part prostheses is described with a brief review of the literature.

The Form of an Arm made of Iron very artificially.

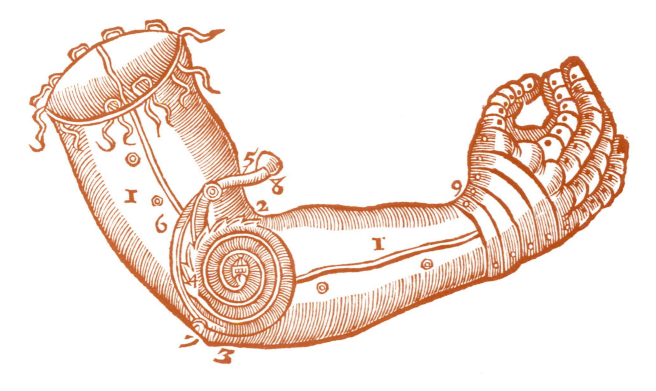

The Works of that Famous Chirurgeon: Ambrose Parey, 1678.

There are books in which the footnotes, or the comments scrawled by some reader's hand in the margin, are more interesting than the text. The world is one of these books.

Santayana

XV.

THE LEG

PRINCIPLES OF TREATMENT

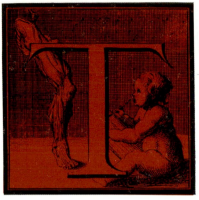

he deformities and functional impairments that follow deep burns of the lower extremity are usually amenable to reconstructive procedures. The approach to the problem should be conservative, expecially if the deformed extremity has an intact sensory nerve supply and an adequate blood supply, rather than hastening to more radical treatment that may include amputation. The chief considerations in reconstruction of the leg and foot are to provide good function, cosmesis, and durable skin coverage. A decision in the management of the deformity will vary with occupation, age, potential for growth, and the presence of other impairments.

The lower extremity reconstruction includes the inguinal region, thighs, knee, and leg. The most common problem in the inguinal region is contracture causing flexion deformity. A release of the contracture with a thick split-thickness graft repair usually suffices to correct the defect.

Horizontal, vertical, and spinal band contractures are the usual defects that deform the thigh. Release of the contracture with split-thickness autografts or Z-plasty repair are used to reconstruct the area.

Repair of knee contracture is often carried out by release with split-thickness grafts. When the skin over the patella is burned full-thickness, shaving and overgrafting of the initial autograft may be necessary to build up the skin to protective levels. All grafts around the knee should be splinted in the post-operative period for at least ten days. Some patients require splints for weeks and several months.

The only difference between leg and thigh grafts is that grafts to the legs require a longer post-operative period of observation than is required for the thigh. If the tibia has been exposed and grafted with autografts during the acute period, shaving and overgrafting may be necessary to provide good skin protection.

The problems that involve the foot and ankle are contractures with or without hypertrophic scarring, amputation and peripheral neuropathy. Reconstruction requires release of contracture with grafts, splints or braces for the peripheral neuropathy and special shoes for those patients who have had amputation of part of the foot.

George H. Koepke
Irving Feller

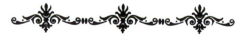

101

EARLY MANAGEMENT OF THE LEG AND FOOT

Irving Feller
Kathryn E. Richards

The principles for the early care of the lower extremity are similar to that of the upper extremity as described previously. Elevation, enzymes, and releasing escharotomy to minimize edema. Fasciotomy and heparinization for deep electrical burns (Figure 1); frequent dressing changes to keep the wound clean and provide gradual debridement, active and passive exercises to maintain good range of motion of the joint, and splinting to avoid or minimize contracture. These are the anticipated and observed similarities but there are significant differences that require additional attention.

Each lower extremity has approximately twice the surface area of the upper extremity. The debriding process can be hastened by grid escharotomy. Homografts can be used to effectively decrease the area of full-thickness burn and should be used on the thighs. The legs and feet should be autografted first because they require a longer period of immobilization with elevation following the application of the grafts. A ten day period for elevation is recommended to allow the arterioles and venous capillaries to mature. Lowering the legs sooner may result in rupture of these fine vessels due to the hydrostatic pressure caused by the standing position. Elastic dressings should be used to support the grafts when ambulation is started.

Peripheral neuropathy is a complication of severe burns over 40 percent of the body surface. Although the neuropathy may be present in both the upper and lower extremities, it is more prominent in the lower extremities. Foot drop is the earliest sign and should be treated with splints or casts to avoid serious deformity of the ankle (Figure 2).

Deep burns of lower extremities lead to exposure of bone more often than is noted in the upper extremities. Exposure of the anterior tibia is not uncommon, and when it does occur, gradual debridement of the bone is required to avoid removing or damaging normal bone.

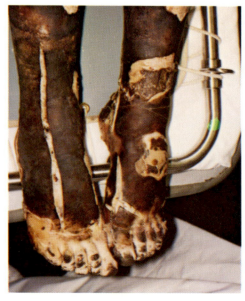

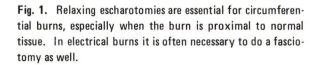

Fig. 1. Relaxing escharotomies are essential for circumferential burns, especially when the burn is proximal to normal tissue. In electrical burns it is often necessary to do a fasciotomy as well.

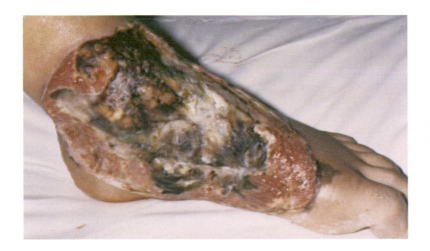

Fig. 2. A. This 19-year-old young man suffered full-thickness burns to his foot which included loss of tendon and bone.

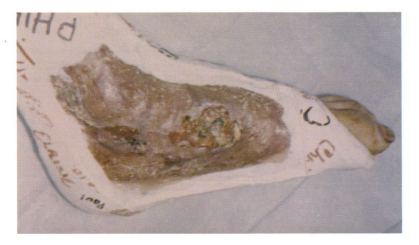

Fig. 2. B. A conservative approach to wound care is necessary in the acute period of treatment to save all viable tissue and to preserve good function. In this case a cast was used to maintain proper position of the ankle. The cast was windowed to allow for gradual debridement and skin grafting.

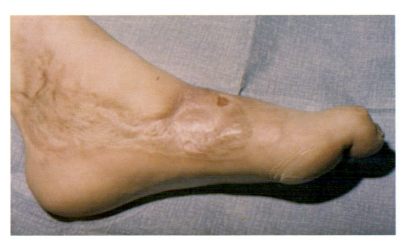

Fig. 2. C. The wound was closed with split-thickness grafts. Later a pedicle flap from the opposite leg was used to provide full-thickness cover so that a triple arthrodesis could be done to permanently stabilize the ankle.

102

RELEASE OF KNEE CONTRACTURE

Kenneth E. Salyer
William B. Nickell

Contractures of the knee frequently result from deep burns. When the knee is affected, burns of the adjacent areas, such as the ankles, feet, or other extremities, are also likely. We will discuss the release of burn scar contracture of the knee in isolation, but any treatment plan would naturally depend upon the other areas of involvement. The original extent of the burn dictates the depth and extent of the scarring. If deep structures, such as tendons, muscles, or bone are involved, then the reconstructive procedures become more complicated. Problems are further compounded if the patient forms hypertrophic scars.

If it is necessary to operate before six months or a year has elapsed since the injury, the wound will contain more reactive hypertrophic collagen. This influences both the surgery and the results. For any given contracture of the popliteal area, the simplest, most rapidly healing method, resulting in release of the contracture is the treatment of choice.

SPLIT-THICKNESS SKIN GRAFTS

Many contractures primarily involving the skin can be released by a single transverse incision crossing the midportion of the popliteal space creating a diamond-shaped defect when the leg is straightened during surgery. This diamond-shaped area is then covered with a moderately thick split-thickness skin graft from 0.016 to 0.018 inches thick. Whenever split-thickness skin grafts are used over concave surfaces, as in the popliteal area, they are sutured on with interrupted tie-over sutures. A layer of nonadherent dressing is applied next to the split-thickness skin graft and covered by a bolus dressing for pressure. The leg is immobilized with a plaster splint at the time of surgery and a large bulky dressing is applied

over this for added pressure. The dressing is then changed on the fifth day. Mobilization is initiated following primary healing of the graft.

When the scarring is minimal, a diamond-shaped incision can be preformed along the border of the popliteal area which is approximately 1½ to 2½ inches at its widest point. The incision is deepened throughout its entirety until the leg extends fully, then the resulting defect around the center diamond-shaped island is grafted. This prevents placing the graft in the irregularities and depths of the popliteal space itself.

In many cases, however, when there is ulceration of the popliteal contracture or an unusual amount of hypertrophic scar, the first two methods are not adequate. In these cases, the deeper lying scar as well as the overlying scarred skin is totally excised and the defect resurfaced with split-thickness skin (Figure 1).

LOCAL SKIN FLAP

At times, a local skin flap can result in release of the contracture, particularly in cases where there is normal skin adjacent to the burn contracture. Multiple Z-plasties are useful in cases where the burn has resulted in contractures as a linear band (Figure 2). In incising the Z-plasty, it is important to carry the incisions deep, including the scar tissue, to maintain vascularization of the Z-plasty tips. In cases where normal tissue is available on only one side, V-Y advancement of tissue from the unburned area has worked well. An incision through the scarred area is performed with advancement of normal tissue as far as possible, into the scar without tension on the flap (Figure 3). A light dressing is then applied to give

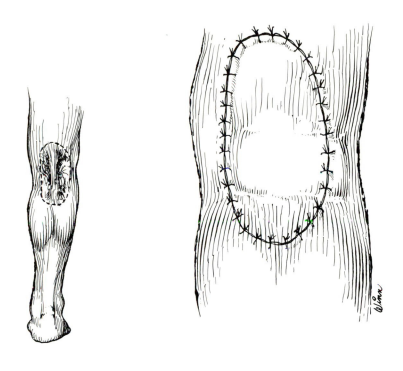

Fig. 1. Total excision of the scar with coverage by a split-thickness skin graft of the popliteal region.

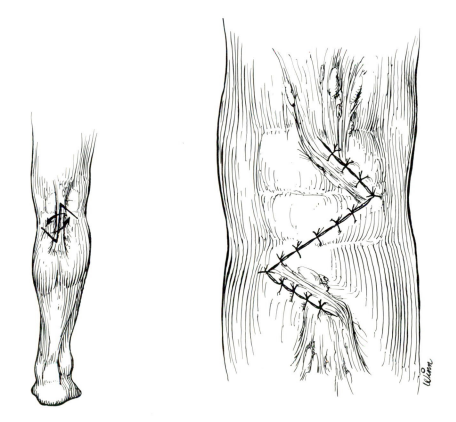

Fig. 2. Breaking up the lines of tension using a Z-plasty in the popliteal region.

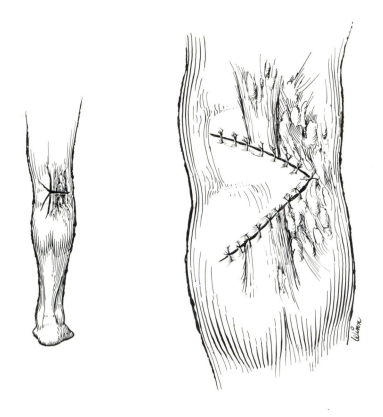

Fig. 3. Y-V-advancement for breaking up scar contracture of the popliteal area.

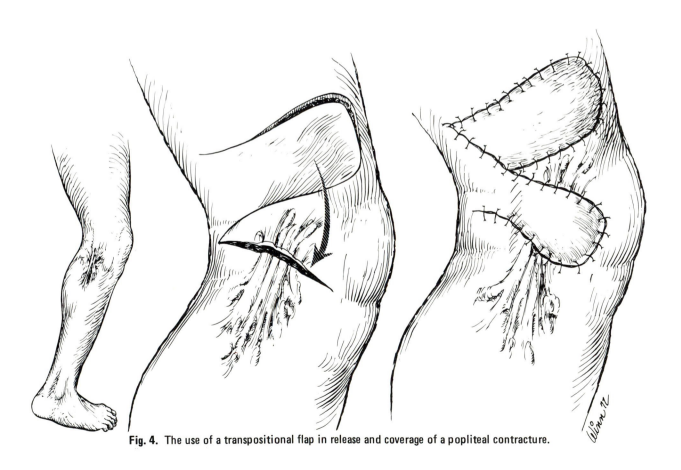

Fig. 4. The use of a transpositional flap in release and coverage of a popliteal contracture.

some compression for hemostasis. When more tissue is needed, a transposition flap may be of benefit (Figure 4). Instead of keeping the leg extended during the first few postoperative days, the leg is maintained in a flexed position to assure that there is no tension on the flap during healing. This is maintained by splinting with plaster or isoprene molded in the Operating Room. In the limited number of patients where contracture can be released without using a split-thickness skin graft, the duration of both hospitalizations and morbidity are decreased. Possible donor site scarring is eliminated.

MUSCLE PEDICLE TRANSPLANT AND DISTANT SKIN FLAPS

In deep burns, tendons, open joints, cartilage, or bone, tissue with its own blood supply is needed for resurfacing.

In a deep, localized burn which exposes bone or cartilage of both at the bottom of the wound, it is advisable to use a muscle pedicle transplant to fill the deep cavity and to then cover this with a split-thickness skin graft (Figure 5). This type of reconstruction has obvious advantages over standard skin

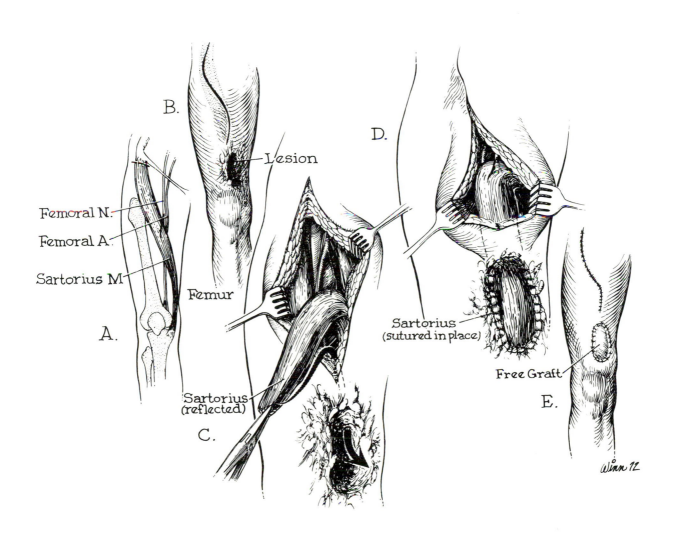

Fig. 5. The use of muscle pedicle graft for coverage of an isolated deep electrical burn of the anterior knee.

pedicle coverage. It will fill the deep cavity, which is difficult to do with a skin pedicle. In addition, it covers the exposed bone or cartilage, provides a suitable bed for a skin graft, acts as a vehicle for the distribution of antibiotics when required, and increases the vascular supply of that area which increases the rate of wound healing.

In unusual cases, a cross-leg or thigh flap may be necessary for coverage. When properly designed, it is possible to primarily elevate and suture it in the defect. After three weeks, the tissue is then transected and is set in two to three days after transection. If the opposite extremity is severely scarred, then tissue from another area is necessary. This requires further steps and time. We prefer the elevation of a vascular pedicle flap, usually from the groin, using the ipsolateral wrist as a carrier. Multiple steps are needed to obtain leg coverage.

POSTOPERATIVE CARE

Postoperative care is as important as the method of surgery. Where split-thickness grafts have been used, it is important to maintain extension for many months during the period of wound contracture. Once the area has healed, motion is started with the use of a splint, with complete extension of the knee at night. During the day, the patient is encouraged to use the knee to maintain mobility and strengthen the leg. The process of contraction continues, necessitating use of a splint for six months or longer. In the early postoperative period, when local advancement or transpositional flaps are used, it is important not to place them under tension. It is best to place the leg in a position of flexion for the first week. The knee can then be gradually extended.

Mobilization is easily accomplished later because the flaps do not contract. In areas where scar tissue remains once the wounds are healed, the continual wearing of a pressure elastic dressing (e.g., Jobst stocking) is of definite benefit in reducing scar tissue.

The use of triamcinolone by direct injection into the scar, 40mg/ml, utilizing up to 120mg at one time in an adult and 80mg or less in children depending upon the size of the patient, has been of definite adjunctive value in the treatment of scarring. If the patient is known to be a keloid former or hypertrophic scar former, it is sometimes elected to inject triamcinolone along the suture line at the time the contracture is released. Provided that it is used in the dosage suggested, there is no problem in wound healing, although the sutures are left in longer than usual. In patients that subsequently develop small areas of hypertrophic scar tissue, injections of triamcinolone are of benefit when repeated every three to four weeks for an extended period. As Ketchum has shown, triamcinolone, which has a collagenase-like activity, is effective in a large percentage of these cases. We have found this to be of definite help in approximately 80 percent of our patients.

ANTERIOR SCARRING OF THE KNEE

Problems of scar contracture and interference with mobility of the knee joint as a result of anterior scarring are unusual. There is usually enough padding of the anterior knee and sufficient vascularity so that the scar can be excised and a split-thickness skin graft applied with success. Again, in areas where there is interference with deeper structures of the knee joint, pedicle tissue from a distance or a muscle pedicle graft may be indicated.

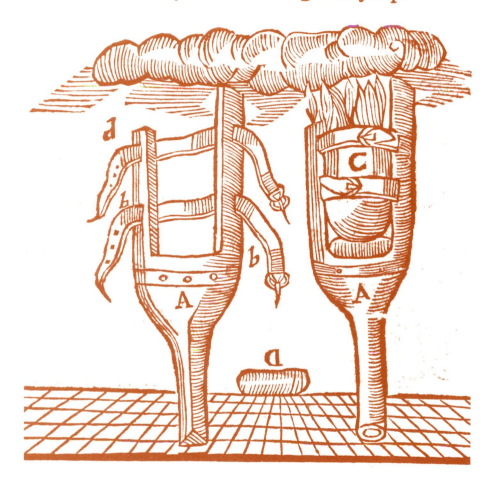

The Works of that Famous Chirurgeon: Ambrose Parey, 1678.

103

RECONSTRUCTION OF THE TIBIA

Irving Feller

It is not uncommon for all of the soft tissue and part of the bone to be destroyed in the anterior tibial area. It is advisable to allow for slow sequestration of the dead bone, thereby providing time for granulation tissue to form between the living and dead bone. Split-thickness autografts can be placed up to the margin of the dead bone before the patient is discharged to home care. If the defect is large a cast or splint may be necessary to avoid fracture. When the sequestrum begins to separate, he is readmitted for surgical removal of the bone and autografting. The autografts will grow very well on the granulation tissue. In some cases, younger patients may need a thicker layer of skin. This may be accomplished by dermabrasion and overgrafting of the area one or more times, as necessary. Pedicle grafts from another part of the body are rarely needed but should be considered when autografting is not sufficient.

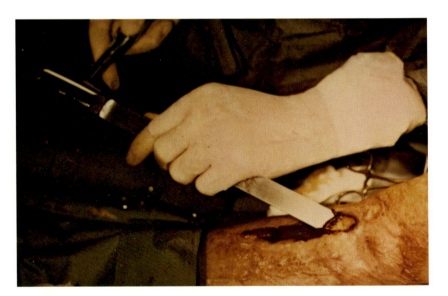

Fig. 1. The loose bone is chiseled away from the granulation tissue base that was forced between it and the underlying living bone.

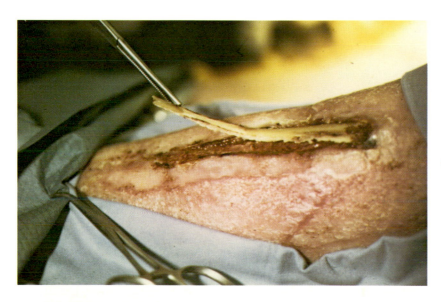

A

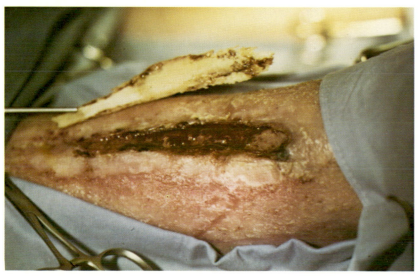

B

Fig. 2. A. The sequestrum is lifted away and the granulation tissue protected by dressings moistened in physiologic solutions. If the granulation tissue is not ready for grafting, the autografts can be cut, stored in the skin bank, and applied several days later. **B.** Split-thickness skin grafts are placed on the granulation tissue bed for the definitive cover.

104

AMPUTATION AND PROSTHESIS OF THE LEG

George H. Koepke

Amputation of the lower extremity is seldom necessary during the emergent treatment of the burned patient. It may be necessary, however near the end of the first day if massive muscle destruction should result in persistent gross hemoglobinuria. Occasionally either a crushing injury to a part of the limb or gas gangrene will warrant early amputation. It may also be necessary to amputate the limb when it is clear that tissues are not viable due to thrombi produced by electrical injuries, deep burns, or extensive sepsis. Additional but somewhat later causes for possible amputation are: extensive nerve destruction that is too large for a nerve graft, osteomyelitis, extensive functional impairment, and Marjolin's ulcer.

BELOW THE KNEE

Regardless of the time of amputation, potential function should be considered in determining the amputation level. There are several exceptions to the principle of saving as much limb as possible. The bone of the amputation stump should be short enough to insure adequate soft tissue at the end of the stump. When doing a below-the-knee amputation, the fibula should be at least one inch shorter than the tibia, and the anterior distal portion of the tibia should be beveled to avoid excessive pressure over this sharp point. Tarsal amputations that sacrifice insertion of the anterior tibial or peroneus longus muscles will usually result in dynamic plantar flexion contractures; therefore, it is usually better to perform a Syme's amputation.

ABOVE THE KNEE

An above-the-knee amputation may also be advisable if there is a history of impaired vascular supply to the legs, complications from burns (such as pyarthrosis of the knee), extensive tibial fractures, hemiparesis, or an extensive neuromuscular deficit of the severely burned leg.

KNEE DISARTICULATION

There are some functional advantages of a knee disarticulation over an above-the-knee amputation. Experience has demonstrated that split-thickness skin grafts on the end of the stump will tolerate graduated weight bearing and the sheer forces of a modern knee disarticulation prosthesis. A silicone gel lining at the end of a partially ischial weight-bearing prosthetic socket will help to distribute the pressure and sheer forces exerted on the split-thickness skin grafts that may cover tissues over the femoral condyles.

An amputation above the flare of the femoral condyles is preferred to an amputation through the lower levels of the femur because the prosthetic knee joint will not have to be longer than that of the sound leg. Further, if parts of the condyles remain, the prosthetic socket must be necessarily wide at the distal thigh. It will then be uncosmetic, and the wide femoral condyles cannot be inserted past the narrower supracondylar portion of the socket. Short above-the-knee stumps are less functional than supracondylar amputations. For practical use of an above-the-knee prosthetic socket, the shortest femoral stump should be no shorter than the ischial tuberosity. If the femoral stump is much shorter than the ischial tuberosity, the amputee will have difficulty keeping the short stump in the socket whenever he might sit. It will also become difficult for the amputee with a short stump to achieve knee stability at heel strike. For practical use of a prosthesis, an amputation stump that is shorter than the level of the ischial tuberosity will usually have to be fitted with a hip disarticulation prosthesis.

FUNCTIONAL CONSIDERATIONS

Additional functional considerations in the selection of amputation levels can be summarized as follows: (1) regardless of age, a unilateral below-the-knee amputee will usually walk with the prosthesis; (2) unless quite elderly, a bilateral below-the-knee amputee can be expected to walk with prostheses; (3) if a unilateral above-the-knee amputee can walk with crutches, he will probably become a successful wearer of an above-the-knee prosthesis; (4) a bilateral above-the-knee amputee past 40 years of age is not expected to find the use of prostheses practical; (5) the amputee over 50 years of age with an above-the-knee amputation of one knee and an amputation below the other knee is unlikely to find the two prostheses of practical value in walking.

PROSTHESIS

In most instances, an amputation stump with a split-thickness skin graft that is adherent to bone should be revised, but a prosthesis as shown in Figure 1 has proved to be superior to others in avoiding breakdown of the grafts. The rubber sleeve suspension offers a minimal amount of piston action, and the silicone gel liner of the prosthetic socket is known to distribute pressure and absorb sheer forces between the socket-stump interface. This prosthetic socket has also proved to be superior to other kinds of sockets for amputation stumps with immature split-thickness skin grafts.

ELECTRICAL INJURIES

In amputations resulting from gangrenous extremities produced by electrical injuries, it is common for the patient to have a persistently painful stump. There are several factors which explain this frequent complication. The density of bone offers a greater concentration of electric current than other body tissues, and so-called "bone atrophy" may occur at the distal portion of the amputated bone. In light of this, it may be well to amputate a bit higher than the first site of good bleeding to ensure that the circulation in the bone is adequate. Another possible explanation for persistent stump pain is the nerve ischemia that may result from the coagulation obstruction of small blood vessels supplying nerves. Another factor is damage to the sympathetic nervous system that may result in a reflex sympathetic dystrophy. Unfortunately, revision of the stump, sympathetic blocks, and other procedures often fail because the pain may become cerebrally "fixed." Last, it is necessary to consider that many electrical injuries are job related, and invalidism may be so rewarding among those receiving compensation that they cannot be rehabilitated successfully.

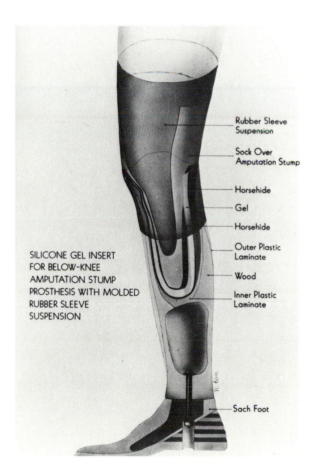

SILICONE GEL INSERT FOR BELOW-KNEE AMPUTATION STUMP PROSTHESIS WITH MOLDED RUBBER SLEEVE SUSPENSION

Rubber Sleeve Suspension

Sock Over Amputation Stump

Horsehide

Gel

Horsehide

Outer Plastic Laminate

Wood

Inner Plastic Laminate

Sach Foot

Fig. 1. Below-the-knee prosthesis with silicone gel "insert" in socket and rubber sleeve suspension.

XVI.

THE FOOT AND ANKLE

PRINCIPLES OF TREATMENT

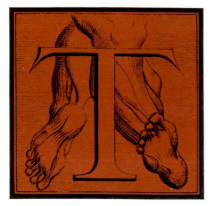

he complications resulting from foot and ankle burns are contracture, damaged or destroyed tendons, peripheral neuropathy, amputation of toes or part of the foot, and deep skin and subcutaneous skin loss to the plantar surface. Peripheral neuropathy can be observed with or without burns of the feet.

Essentially the treatment of contracture is release with or without excision, and covering the defect with thick split-thickness grafts. A period of internal or external fixation in the position of desired correction, or over-correction, is always necessary. Internal fixation can be accomplished by K-wires and Steinman pins. External fixation is carried out using casts, thick dressings, and/or splints. A combination of the two methods is possible using stainless steel wire through the toes attached to a splint.

When the deformity is primarily due to or includes peripheral neuropathy correction can be accomplished by serial casting. The deformity is cast in the closest position toward neutral for the joint. The cast is then changed at least once weekly during which time deformity is slowly corrected. Stretching of the muscle, tendon, and joint capsules is gradually accomplished by this system. In most cases the correction will be maintained after the serial casting is complete; in others a splint may be required.

In most instances repair of severe skin loss of the dorsum of the foot and the heel is accomplished using thick split-thickness grafts. If these are not successful then pedicle grafts are transferred from the opposite leg. Special fitted and padded shoes are necessary for the patient once operative procedures are completed.

Areas of tendon destruction are first covered with split-thickness or a pedicle graft and then tendon grafts may be added. Consultation with an orthopaedic surgeon and physiatrist should always be obtained.

George H. Koepke
Irving Feller

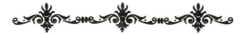

106

RECONSTRUCTION OF THE LEGS AND FEET

George H. Koepke

FOOT

Full-thickness loss of skin from the dorsal surface of the foot is often followed by hyperextension of the metatarsophalangeal joint and claw deformities of the toes. This deformity is accentuated with growth, and a conservative approach may provide a better functional result than amputation. If the toe flexor mechanism is intact, it is well to preserve the "push off" function provided by the toes rather than to risk the occasional complication of painful callouses over the metatarsal heads and the possible need for special footwear that may be required if all the toes are amputated. Excision of the limiting scar at the base of the toes and split-thickness skin coverage is necessary for the skin defect resulting from excision of the scar. The split-thickness skin grafts will allow limited flexion of the toes, but better correction is achieved if a wire suture is inserted in the nail bed. The wire can then be attached to a plantar foot plate. Immobilization of the toes in a flexed position will not only facilitate a "take" of the graft, but will also correct the muscle, tendon, and capsular contractures that form secondarily to the skin contracture on the dorsal surface of the foot. The foot is maintained in this position for approximately three weeks. It is kept elevated for the first ten postoperative days and, like all lower leg grafts, the foot and lower leg are wrapped with an elastic bandage before the foot is allowed to assume a dependent position. The patient may walk with crutches and after the plate is removed, full weight bearing is permitted with a slipper or soft shoe.

Figure 1 demonstrates septic infarctions of the feet in an infant boy who suffered facial burns and subsequently developed hematogenous osteomyelitis of a talus and its surrounding tarsal joints. This was treated by incision and drainage of the subtalar joint (Figure 2) as well as plaster immobilization of the ankle and amputation of a gangrenous great toe. Figure 3 demonstrates satisfactory position and function as a result of a spontaneous triple arthrodesis of the subtalar joint. Despite the boy's growth to more than 250 pounds, the foot has proved to be very serviceable in his work as a laborer.

ANKLE

If deep burns should destroy the tendons about the ankle, the foot should be supported in a splint or plaster in a position simulating mild contraction of the lost tendon. For example, if the Achilles tendon is interrupted beyond repair, the acutely burned foot should be maintained in 7 to 10 degrees of plantar flexion, and if the dorsiflexing tendons are lost, the foot should be dorsiflexed. These positions will result in better function than that given at 90 degrees because these deep burns often are accompanied by osteomylitis and pyarthrosis with pseudofusion. Of course, it is important to have a functionally balanced foot, so if appropriate positioning during the acute period is inadequate, it may be necessary to transfer tendons and fuse subtalar joints. In some instances it may be necessary to fuse the tibial-talar joints. As in cases of spontaneous fusion, a surgical fusion of the ankle at 5 to 7 degrees of plantar flexion is more functional than a right angle position. Further, the plantar ligaments of the metatarsal-tarsal articulation usually stretch a bit with the stress of walking and therefore some of the plantar flexion is lost.

ACHILLES TENDON

Skin contracture for deep burns over the Achilles tendon may limit foot dorsiflexion, but a contracture of the triceps surae is uncommon unless the dorsiflexors are weak. For this reason, "heel cord" lengthening is seldom necessary, it is usually a matter of releasing the skin contracture to provide a functional range of motion in the ankle. Split-thickness skin grafts often provide durable coverage, but may break down if the graft does not have a margin or soft or elastic tissue that extends to the surrounding skin. The graft must move freely with movements of the tendon during walking so as to avoid dehiscence or attritional changes in the graft. For these reasons, after a thick split-thickness skin graft is applied, the foot should be immobilized in a dorsiflexed position for approximately two weeks by either a splint or plaster shell. Occasionally, a full pedicle graft may be necessary.

SHIN

Pretibial split-thickness skin grafts may become vulnerable to trauma and breakdown. In these instances a plastic shin protector (Figure 4) may be applied during the rehabilitation stages instead of performing additional surgical procedures that may

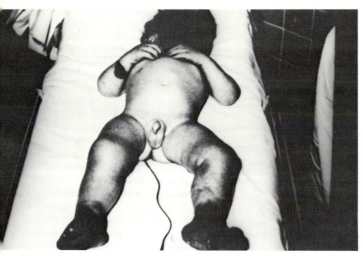

Fig. 1. Facial burns and septic infarctions of the feet and hematogenous osteomyelitis of a talus.

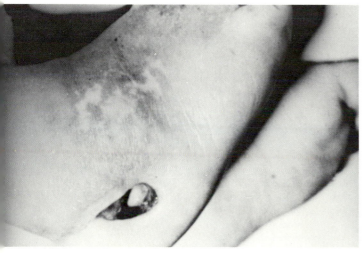

Fig. 2. Incision and drainage of subtalar joint with osteomyelitis.

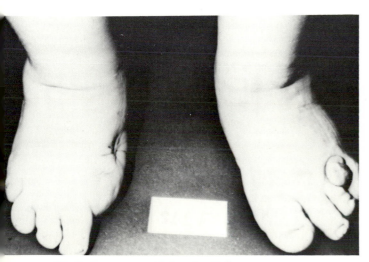

Fig. 3. Spontaneous triple arthrodesis.

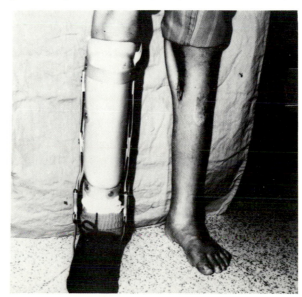

Fig. 4. Plastic protector for pretibial surface.

include a pedicle graft. Similarly, thin prepatellar split-thickness skin grafts may either break down or limit flexion of the knee. Ordinarily, resurfacing with thick split-thickness skin grafts is adequate if they are applied with the knee immobilized at about 90 degrees for approximately two weeks.

KNEE

Bridle scars of the popliteal space may cause knee flexion deformities. These usually respond satisfactorily to a simple Z-plasty, but a flexion contracture due to a broad scar may require a diamond shaped excision of the scar and additional split-thickness skin grafts for the skin deficit. Again, it is important to maintain extension of the knee during the postoperative period to facilitate a "take" of the graft and to ensure correction of the knee flexion contracture, thereby avoiding repetitive procedures. Flexion contractures of the inguinal and perineal areas should be followed by postoperative immobilization in a position opposite the deformity. Appropriate methods of positioning are splints, slings, or a padded and modified circumcision board for children to ensure immobilization and complete correction of the deformity.

The Form of little Boots, whereof the one is open and the other shut.

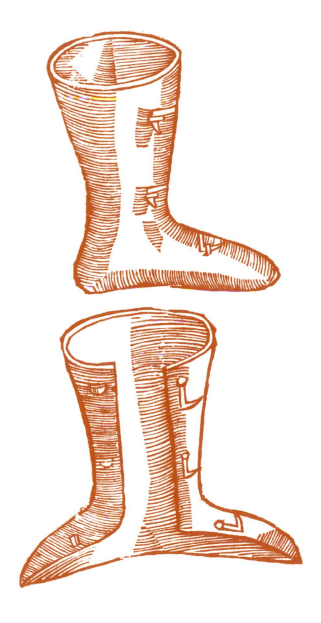

The Works of that Famous Chirurgeon: Ambrose Parey, 1678.

It is the manner of hypochondriacs to change often their physician . . . for a physician who does not admit the reality of the disease cannot be supposed to take much pains to cure it.

Cullen

107

ANKLE AND FOOT RECONSTRUCTION

Vincent R. Pennisi
Angelo Capozzi

The ankle and foot are specialized structures which require individual attention to maintain and restore function. In order to function properly, these structures must be stable, balanced, capable of bearing weight, movable, and have an adequate blood and nerve supply.

The ankle consists of the ankle joint with its surrounding ligaments, tendons, muscles, subcutaneous tissue, and skin. The calcaneal tendon stands out posteriorly. This skin is thin with little subcutaneous fat. Therefore, it is often the site of full-thickness burns following minimal thermal exposure.

The stability and flexibility of the foot result from its arched form and its system of curved joint surfaces. These are supported by ligaments, muscles, and tendons. The skin of the plantar surface is considerably thicker than the skin of the dorsum and is particularly thick over the weight-bearing areas of the calcaneus and the metatarsals. The heel bears 80 percent of body weight and the metatarsals 20 percent. The thick skin of the weight-bearing surface is infrequently involved in full-thickness loss, but the thinner skin of the plantar arch may be destroyed by the same trauma. Sensation of the foot is acute, as evidenced by the great discomfort caused by the smallest of pebbles in one's shoe.

CAUSES OF BURNS

Normally, the feet are so well protected by wearing apparel that full-thickness burns due to thermal trauma are uncommon. The dorsum of the foot and ankles are more easily damaged by heat, while the thicker skin of the plantar surface is less vulnerable but more critical. The Fakir Hindu sect whose religious practice includes walking upon hot coals are among the few groups of humans who are immune to burns of the feet. Their dispensation is probably the result of a heavy, cornified layer on the plantar surface of their feet. The depth of the thermal injury is directly related to the duration and intensity of the insult. Infants, the aged and body areas with thin skin (eyelids, ears, the dorsum of foot, and the hands) are more vulnerable to full-thickness loss by less intense heat and briefer exposure (Figure 1).

SECONDARY REPAIR

The majority of burns of the foot and ankle are restored to satisfactory function after the initial skin grafts have healed and matured. Occasionally, secondary repair will be necessary for breakdown of unstable skin, tender scars, contractures affecting the toes, and shortening of the heel cord. Unstable skin and tender scarred areas should be totally excised and covered by medium-thickness skin grafts applied in sheets. Although there are those who advocate pedicle grafts and full-thickness skin grafts for weight-bearing areas of the foot, these are usually unnecessary. A split-thickness skin graft of moderate thickness is quite adequate and the risk of graft failure is less.

Probably the most frequent cause for secondary repair is scar contracture over the dorsum of the foot, which results in the ankle and then the toes becoming dorsiflexed (Figure 2). Preservation of joint function and correction of toe deformity cannot be accomplished with simple excision of scar and replacement with thick split skin. The toes must be maintained in an overcorrected and plantar-flexed position by the aid of a plaster splint or cylinder cast. The splint is retained until the graft contraction has been overcome (Figure 3).

Fig. 1. An 18-month-old infant on the first day following thermal burn. The legs and feet sustained full-thickness skin loss.

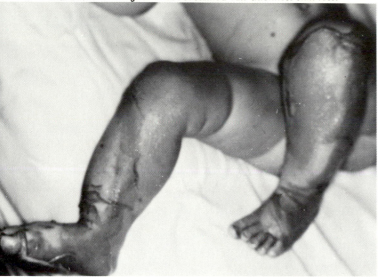

Fig. 2. Neglected contracture of the dorsum of the left foot in the infant in Figure 1, five years after the original injury.

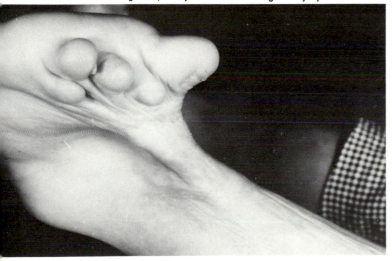

Fig. 3. Five years after, the contracture was corrected by thick split-thickness skin grafts.

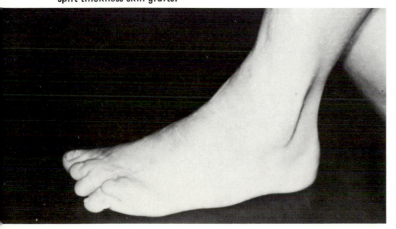

When the Achilles tendon has been completely exposed by destruction of the overlying skin, great care must be taken to keep the area free of infection. The tendon should be kept moist by wet compresses and autografted as soon as possible. **Every effort should be made to maintain the length of the heel cord.** If a tendon lengthening procedure becomes necessary, a distant pedicle flap may be required to eliminate the overlying unstable skin and protect the tenorrhaphy.

Hypertrophic scars of the feet and ankle can often be prevented by the immediate use of elastic stockings or elastic apparel. These elastic stockings are made to order and should be utilized as soon as the grafts have healed. They are worn constantly for 3 to 6 months and removed only when bathing and for minimal periods during the reclining sleeping hours.

When hypertrophic scars occur and do not improve by elastic compression, they then should be excised and grafted with medium or thick skin grafts. The grafts should be fixed with a stent dressing and a plaster splint or cast applied. When the graft has healed, the elastic apparel or stocking is fabricated and worn as described above. Intracicatricial injections of corticosteroids are **not** recommended unless one is certain that the scar is a keloid, in which case it will be painful and pruritic.

108

PLANTAR SURFACE RECONSTRUCTION

Irving Feller

Thick split-thickness autografts to the plantar surface of the foot are an effective wound cover in most cases. When destruction of subcutaneous tissue is complete, reconstructive procedures may be necessary, using serial dermabrasion and overgrafting or a pedicle graft from the opposite leg. Deep electrical burns of the sole of the foot have caused tendon damage or destruction with nerve loss. Such defects are small but very deep, and can at times be corrected by removing the bone from a toe and using the remaining soft tissue as a pedicle to cover the deep defect.

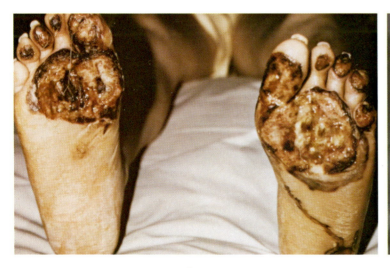

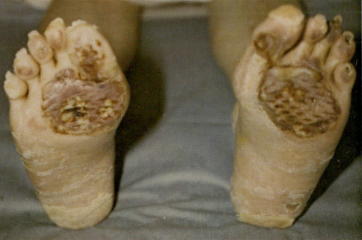

A

B

Fig. 1. A. An electrical burn caused this small but deep full-thickness loss to the plantar surface of the foot of this 40-year-old salesman. **B.** Split-thickness grafts were used first to close the defect.

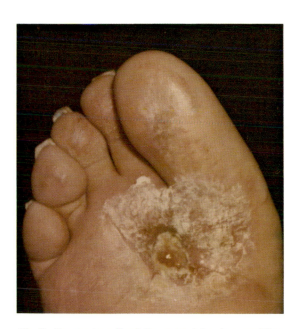

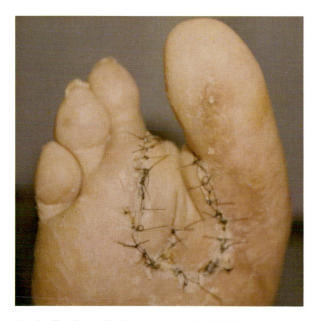

Fig. 2. Contracture fixed the second toe in a position which caused the patient pain when walking. The bones were removed from the toe and the soft tissue was used to cover the defect as a pedicle flap.

Fig. 3. The flap effectively provided full-thickness cover to the plantar surface.

109

TOE RECONSTRUCTION

Irving Feller

Frequently, the dorsum of the foot is burned resulting in extension contractures of the toes. The position leads to shortening of the tendons and tightening of the metatarsalphalangeal joint capsules. Also, the scarring has resulted in a marked shortage of tissue. These conditions prescribe the method of correction.

A simple release of the contracture in the proper location will usually allow the toes to be brought to the plantar flexed position. Excision of scar is usually not necessary, but covering the large created defect with a thick split autograft is important. When hypertrophic scarring and contracture are both present, excision of the scar, release of contracture, and grafting of the entire defect is necessary. Further fixation of the toes in the plantar flexed position is necessary for several weeks.

Immediate splinting can be accomplished by putting number thirty stainless steel wires through the nailbed distal to the phalanx bone. The wires are connected to a splint which keeps the toes hyperextended.

This splint is used until the skin graft has taken and is secure. In children it is advisable to next use a plantar cast for a month or more depending upon how the scar matures. Rapidly forming hard scars must be casted for a longer period of time.

This fixation can be maintained later by using standard shoes. The patient is instructed to use walking shoes during the daytime and a new pair of tennis shoes at night. This provides him with twenty four hour splinting in the appropriate neutral position. This case study illustrates these principles.

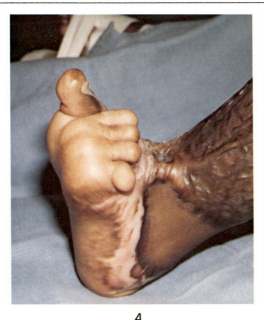
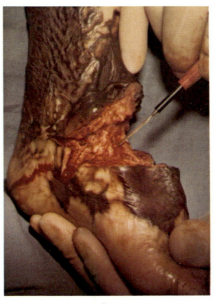
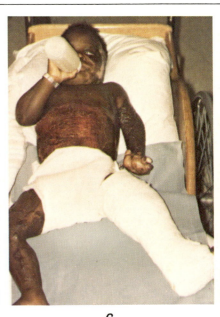

A	B	C

Fig. 1. A. Severe burns of this boy's left foot resulted in both ankle and toe contractures. **B.** Both the ankle and toe contractures were released by linear excisions without excising tissue. **C.** Split-thickness grafts were used to cover the defect and a planter cast was used for immobilization.

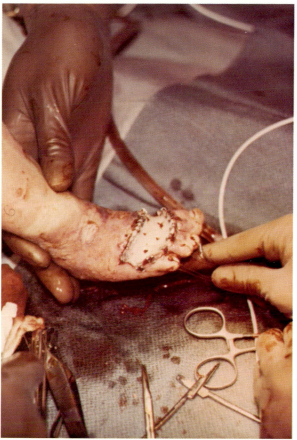

A

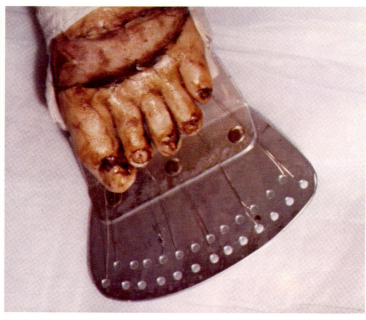

B

Fig. 2. A. A second method for immobilizing grafts and maintaining position after graft placement involves inserting stainless steel wires through the distal phalanges. **B.** The wires are then attached to a plastic or metal splint that has been molded to fit the patient.

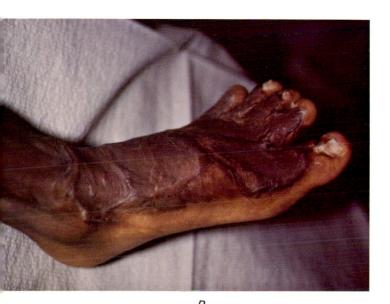

D

Fig. 1. (cont.) D. The repair is seen one year later with satisfactory reconstruction at that time. It is necessary to follow children to watch for recurrences of contracture as the child grows.

XVII.
REHABILITATION OF THE BURNED PATIENT

PRINCIPLES OF REHABILITATION

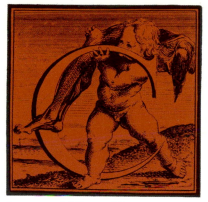

onceptually, emotional rehabilitation is achieved when the burned patient begins to feel good about himself. But, in practice this achievement is most difficult. Accidental injuries often leave scars and deformities which mark a person for life. When the head, face, hands, or breasts are involved, emotional adjustment may take a long and obstacle-laden path. Much guidance and direction are needed to reach an outcome of "feeling good."

The face is the "calling card" in our society. In fact, too much importance has been placed upon beauty, which at best is poorly defined where quality of life is concerned. Nevertheless, we live in this society and, can therefore serve our patients best by: (1) helping them strengthen their self-image, and (2) providing them with means of improving their appearance and function.

Self-image in the adult has been formed long before the accident occurs, probably during the first years of life; most likely the feeling about self is fixed by age four. The influence on the infant and child by the parents and other people provides that background. If a child develops with a good or healthy self-image, it will be easier for him to adapt to cosmetic deformity. If the opposite is true, he will have a difficult time and experienced counseling will be necessary. Most surgeons do not have the training to provide such counseling but should recognize where the need exists and have qualified therapists on the burn rehabilitation team. An experienced social worker, who has additional training in the newer methods for correcting emotional problems, is well suited for this work. Occupational and physical therapists are essential to assist the patient regain physical skills which in turn improves emotional outlook. When the therapy team successfully combine their efforts to support the patient in regaining physical function and strengthening self-image, the patient will be able to return to a productive role in society.

Patients who have adjusted emotionally to physical deformity have the best results from reconstructive procedures, prosthetics, and cosmetics. Reconstructive operations are designed to provide maximum improvement of function and appearance. At best, these operations can only partly improve appearance. The patient will never be able to look as he did before the accident, but that does not mean he cannot continue to have the same quality of life as before. Indeed, patients have stated that the quality of their life has improved following the burn injury. They tell us that the severe trauma, the threat to life, and the recovery process allowed them a period of introspection and insight into their problems combined with the skilled intervention of the burn team helped them improve their lives.

Irving Feller

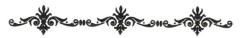

111

REHABILITATION FOLLOW-UP STATISTICS

Terrence N. Davidson
Michael H. James

The likelihood of survival for a severely burned patient has increased dramatically during the last fifteen to twenty years. It is certainly not coincidental that this same period has witnessed the creation and growth of specialized burn care facilities in this country. Both the dramatic decrease in mortality and the growth of these specialized facilities are due to the dedication of a group of highly skilled physicians, nurses, and health professionals, who through teamwork have applied a consistent plan of treatment to increase the burn victim's chance for survival. As improvements are made in survival for severely burned patients, a closely related question has begun to receive more attention: what about the quality of life of those who survive this traumatic injury? Because of the efforts of the burn team this question is receiving increased attention today, and because this team individually and collectively is equally dedicated to improving the life quality of the survivors, we can be reasonably optimistic that their efforts will also be successful.

How best might we study the effectiveness of efforts being made to improve the quality of burn victims' lives? There is no simple answer. However, we are certain that such efforts must involve follow-up throughout the rehabilitation period, which for many patients will continue for several years. With what frequency should such patients be followed? The answer must involve individual consideration of the patient's physical state, including age, type and number of complications, area(s) of body burned, type and staging of reconstructive procedures, and need for prosthetic devices, to name a few.

After the question of optimal follow-up has been answered, a more difficult issue emerges: namely, what high priority needs does the patient evidence at a particular point in time? These needs are likely to include aspects of the patient's occupational, educational, and family role, psycho-social adjustment, as well as medical care requirements. As the patient progresses through rehabilitation it is likely that these non-medical aspects of adjustment will assume even greater importance than his or her physical state. Also, complexities of adjustment will fluctuate greatly across time; their priorities (as seen by the patient) early on, may be unrelated to their priorities later in the rehabilitation period. From this we conclude that; (1) consideration of both medical and non-medical aspects is of utmost importance for successful rehabilitation, (2) such consideration must involve periodic follow-up of all patients, (3) the patient's perception of progress (or lack thereof) must be considered as well as the physician's observations regarding the patient's medical state, and (4) the rehabilitation period represents a dynamic time in which many important aspects of the patient's life undergo dramatic changes.

The situation just described presents a real challenge for the practitioner; it is complex, it involves factors not traditionally thought to be "medical," it requires careful consideration of the situation as seen by the patient, and it will likely necessitate frequent contact with the patient as well as relevant others in the patient's life. What is the optimal role for the burn team in this complex and challenging situation? At this time we can offer no specific answer; however, it may be helpful to imagine extending the team concept, the sharing of responsibilities among a group dedicated to a common goal — the patient's successful rehabilitation — to include the patient and relevant others in the life of the patient.

A brief review here of two past rehabilitation follow-up studies conducted by the Michigan Burn Center can shed some light on the importance to practitioners of such follow-up efforts. We then provide a brief description of two current efforts of the National Institute for Burn Medicine to develop, refine, and disseminate a model program for meeting the complex rehabilitation needs of the burn patient.[1]

EVIDENCE TO DATE

The Michigan Burn Center has completed two studies on the psycho-social, physical, and vocational adjustment of burn victims. In 1959, and again in 1969, extensive data were collected on hundreds of patients. Special emphasis was given to patients who had suffered especially severe burn injuries. Selection criteria included any patient who had a hospital stay longer than 30 days; (or) total area burn greater than 19% with a full-thickness area burn greater than 9%; (or) full-thickness burns of the face, hands, feet; or full-thickness burn of the breast area of young girls. Because such patients are likely to experience considerably greater problems during rehabilitation than would be likely for patients with more moderate injuries, the findings of these studies are especially important.

The 1959 study of 70 of the most severely burned patients admitted at that time was the forerunner of all our subsequent efforts. As the result of this study, the following modifications were made on the Burn Unit, they proved so valuable that they have become ongoing components of the Michigan Burn Center rehabilitation program:

- A weekly Burn Clinic was established for

more consistent follow-up for both medical and non-medical purposes,
- A full-time social worker was employed to deal with the patients' adjustment problems during rehabilitation,
- A part-time school teacher was employed to facilitate the educational progress of patients who were of school age when they suffered their burn injuries.

Evaluation of the existing rehabilitation program at the Michigan Burn Center was the subject of the 1969 study. Approximately 800 new patients had been admitted for treatment since the 1959 changes were implemented. Three-hundred of the most severely burned of this group were identified for study and over 80% of them were located and agreed to participate.[2] Information on each of these 254 patients was gathered from medical and social work records, staff interviews, and separate interviews with each of the patients and their families. Subsequently, the patient and family were seen by the medical staff. School personnel and staff of community agencies involved with the patients were also contacted and interviewed. In this 1969 study, all patients reported having had contacts with the social worker during rehabilitation follow-up periods (as opposed to 24% in the 1959 study).

When the data from the entire group of 254 patients were examined, 70% of them had post-burn adjustment indicators (in the categories of emotional, social, family, work, or school) which were essentially the same as their pre-burn adjustment indicators; 16%

---

1. These investigations are supported by the State of Michigan, Department of Education, Vocational Rehabilitation Service, and the Department of Health, Education, and Welfare, Office of Human Development, Rehabilitation Services Administration (Grant Number: 13-P-59197/5-01).

2. It may be worth mentioning a fact which is undoubtedly obvious to anyone involved in follow-up studies; such efforts are facilitated if accurate addresses for the population are maintained throughout the rehabilitation period. To meet the complex and varying rehabilitation needs of burn victims, especially children, return visits with members of the burn team are needed over extended time periods. Periodic follow-up contacts serve as a reminder that the well-being of the patient continues to be of paramount importance and at the same time provides an efficient mechanism for continual up-dating of the patients' address.

had indications of post-burn adjustment problems which were not in evidence before their burn injuries; and, remarkably, 14% provided indications of post-burn adjustment better than before their burn injuries. This latter provocative finding was explored in detai!. Although this group was not homogenous with respect to age, sex, or any other demographic factors investigated, each patient provided strong and credible explanations of their situation. All pointed to the importance of the contacts initiated and maintained with various members of agencies in the patient's community by the social worker on the Burn Unit. Very clear evidence was provided in the adjustment records of these patients for the efficacy of social work — community agency follow-up in the rehabilitation program.

In summary, the 1969 study outcomes added these important components to the rehabilitation program.

- All patients should be followed subsequent to discharge with special attention given to patients who are of school age when burned, have completed physical rehabilitation, and have evidenced problems in accepting help during their hospital stay. From the standpoint of the amount of staff time expended, following patients is a costly enterprise. Characteristics of the patient population (e.g. it is extremely mobile) suggest that such follow-ups require well planned, concerted, and persistent effort.
- Patients who resume their pre-burn roles as soon as possible (students, wage-earners, family members, and the like) have better adjustment levels than do patients who delay resumption of their previous functions.
- It is essential that patients establish realistic expectations concerning the types and duration of the treatment program (including reconstruction) and the likely outcomes of the program if successful rehabilitation is to be achieved.

- Utilization of a team approach to patient treatment and follow-up must incorporate the concept of each team member's role being recognized by the other members as important, and information must be shared among team members.

CURRENT STUDIES

The National Institute for Burn Medicine is currently involved in two studies which continue the effort to better understand and meet the rehabilitation needs of burn patients. The first of these studies involves systematically interviewing a sample of approximately 350 patients who were admitted to the Michigan Burn Center between 1959 and 1976. The sample consists of burn victims who were 16 or over at the time of the interview; the sample has been stratified by year of burn and severity of burn injury. These, unlike the earlier studies (1959, 1969) do not focus exclusively on severity of injury. Interviews, averaging about 75 minutes in length, were conducted by trained interviewers with each of the sampled patients. Interview topics include educational, occupational, social, and psychological adjustment, family-role activities, recreational and social activities, perceived social support, feelings of self-worth and fate-control, expectations for future treatment and treatment outcomes, satisfaction with past treatment, and future plans. Information provided by the patient is now being combined with data from the social worker's files, from relevant staff members of the Vocational Rehabilitation Service, the patient's medical records, and the files of the National Burn Information Exchange.[3]

Data from these efforts are currently being analyzed, and will become the basis for additional refinements in the patient rehabilitation program. In the near future, the study will be expanded to include children and their families.

This retrospective study also provides a springboard for another current rehabilitation study being

---

3. Feller, Irving and Crane, Keith H., "National Burn Information Exchange"; Surgical Clinics of North America, Vol 50, No. 6, December, 1970.

conducted by the National Institute for Burn Medicine. The study will represent a systematic effort to investigate the medical and psycho-social rehabilitation needs of burn victims. Some of the important characteristics of the study are:

1. It is prospective in its design. The patient population of primary concern consists of all patients admitted to the Michigan Burn Center for emergent/acute care during a three-year period beginning in 1979.

2. It is multidisciplinary in its approach. The conceptual framework underlying the study draws upon previous and current work in the several areas of medicine, public health, sociology, psychology, and education.

3. It utilizes a multiple indicator approach to rehabilitation and adjustment. One of the most difficult problems faced in past studies concerns the great variety of methods used to measure adjustment. In this study, several well-established measures, to be supplemented by new measures currently being developed, will be utilized.

4. It is longitudinal in its design. Several follow-up contacts with each of the patients will be made during the period of study. Each of the indicators of the patient's rehabilitation will be monitored across that time period, and

5. It directly involves the patient, family members, burn team members, and members of community service agencies in systematic data collection efforts. Comparisons between and among these several information bases will provide for more discriminating analytic efforts than have been possible in past studies.

IMPLICATIONS OF REHABILITATION FOLLOW-UP FOR THE PRACTITIONER

Improvements in the medical treatment of the burned patient has been impressive; our ability to meet the psycho-social rehabilitation needs of these patients has not kept pace with the dramatic gains made in improving the survival. Evidence suggests that follow-up efforts, though expensive, provide important benefits for practitioners involved in meeting the rehabilitation needs of burn patients. Such follow-up efforts should actively involve contacts with the patient by various members of the burn team—not focus exclusively upon the physical reconstruction of the patient, but include emphasis on the patient's educational, occupational, and psycho-social needs as well. Periodic contact with the patient, with family members, and with representatives of community service agencies will directly offer and thus increase the benefit of the patient's compliance with home care plans and scheduled return visits.

The unexamined life is not worth living.
Socrates

112

PREPARING THE PATIENT FOR DISCHARGE AND FOLLOW-UP

M.L. Bowden

Returning home after a long hospitalization is a major transition for individuals who have been severely burned and for their families. Happiness and anticipation are coupled with anxiety and distress. All too often this stress and its effects are minimized, and the opportunity is lost to use this transitional phase for growth and change. However, like other transitional periods in life, such as adolescence and marriage, the post-discharge period can be used by burn victims to assess their situation and decide on new ways of dealing with life. We have identified four phases that individuals who have been severely burned pass through after they leave the hospital. Each can be seen as a stage where intervention can occur that will facilitate a new level of adjustment.

PHASE ONE: DISCHARGE PLANNING

The first phase is the period immediately following the discharge from the hospital. During this period, which may last from several days to several months, the individual and his family remain highly focused on physical condition and physical levels of functioning. Energy levels are low, and affect usually is somewhat depressed. Psychologically, there are three significant tasks facing the individual. **The major task is relinquishing the role of patient.** The individual must give up the sick role and assume primary responsibility for the time structuring and physical care no longer provided by a medical staff and facility. **The second task is dealing with the unfinished emotions that surrounded or were related to the circumstances of the injury.** Examples of this are accidents that resulted in the death of a family member, a destroyed home, or a suicide attempt. Not so apparent are situations in which there was

conflict within the family prior to the accident that went underground during the period of acute stress of injury and hospitalization. These conflicts again surface when the individual and family are reunited and old patterns are reestablished. **The third task involves the resumption of social and familial roles** that were disrupted by the injury and long hospitalization. Roles of spouse, wage earner, parent, son, sexual partner, etc., again confront the burn victim upon return to home and family. Concerns about the ability to resume these roles, or stress over any initial inability to resume these roles, will quickly surface at the point of returning home.

The role of the social worker during this phase is primarily preparatory. Prior to discharge from the hospital, the social worker, using information about the patient and family obtained during the hospitalization, begins discussing these psychological issues with patient and family. The patient is helped to anticipate his response during this first post-hospitalization phase. Discussing with family their plan of returning to a community—having friends over, role resumption, responsibility for the children, sleeping arrangements—provides valuable information about and insight into family attitudes and opinions about what will or will not happen during this period. Family members are also helped to establish and focus on both short- and long-range goals. The social worker will need to be very directive with some families to help them establish reasonable goals (some families set up unrealistic expectations, others establish few expectations for improvement). With others, the social worker may only need to support and reinforce the steps the family is taking.

During this discharge planning stage, those community agencies that will be a part of the rehabilitation team are identified. With patient or family permission, or both, the social worker contacts the community agencies, informs them of patient discharge plans, and helps them anticipate the needs of the patient and family.

PHASE TWO: SOCIAL FUNCTIONING

Once the individual is home from the hospital and attention and energy become less focused on physical needs, the second rehabilitation phase begins. The time spent in wound care, baths, and skin treatment becomes nominal and physical therapy activities are incorporated into daily routine. This period can begin several days or several months after discharge. As energy is freed from attention to physical care, it can be invested in social functioning. The individual will begin to assign tasks to self, and the family ideally accepts and encourages this independent activity. Role resumptions become readily apparent as homemaking, child care, and family maintenance tasks are assumed. During return visits to the clinic, individuals will begin talking about work-related roles, and many will report establishing phone contact with employers or fellow workers. Resumption of social activities, such as attending church and shopping, will also be discussed.

Psychosocial tasks during this phase center on interactional issues either within the family or within the community. Potential or actual problems will become apparent as individuals attempt to deal with real or imagined inability to resume certain roles previously held within the family or community and the emotional impact of real or imagined physical loss. Delayed grief reactions and situational anxiety are not uncommon during this phase.

The social worker's task during this phase is to assess the adjustment levels and identify the problems or potential problems of individuals and families as they return to clinic. Communicating difficulties to the medical members of the team greatly facilities a unified approach to patient care. Patients and families experiencing emotional distress may need frequent return clinic visits. Other patients and families may need a break from the intense focus on

physical and medical problems so that they can direct their energies to social-emotional problems. Referring families to agencies for counselling and communicating medical information to and planning with involved community agencies is also an important role of the social worker. This facilitates continuity of patient care, and enhances the transfer of primary care from the Burn Center to the community.

It is during this phase that the rehabilitation team needs to formulate a plan for job retraining or reemployment that meshes with the physical rehabilitation plan. This is in preparation for the third phase and is shared with the individual.

PHASE THREE: RETURN TO WORK

The third phase begins as the individual becomes physically ready to resume at least part-time work. This may be a return to previous employment, transitional employment with the previous employer, or it may be education or job retraining. Initiation of the third phase depends on the severity of the initial injury and on the post-burn adjustment. The patient may indicate his readiness to return to work, or the members of the burn team may raise the question.

Unresolved emotional issues from earlier phases will continue or surface during this time. New problems that arise usually center around reluctance to return to work, or societal blocks, or both. Reluctance can be caused by a previous pattern of never or only sporadically holding a job, a fear of returning to a dangerous situation, or emotional problems related to physical loss. External blocks occur when social systems require a return to full employment rather than a gradual return on an as able basis. (The gradual return also alleviates the emotional stress of the return as well, especially when the burn victim must deal with a changed appearance.) Societal blocks are caused by insurance systems that stop benefits upon return to work, disregarding ability or level of return except full-time employment. They are also raised when employers are reluctant to employ accident victims because of increased insurance rates even when the accident was job- or company-related and not the fault of the individual.

The social worker's task during this phase is to evaluate with the individual and the involved community agencies the causes of any individual or social problems and to seek their resolution. An interagency meeting between community personnel and the burn team may be needed to fully assess the problem and come up with solutions. A return admission to the hospital for reconstructive surgery may be used to reestablish contact with the family. In some instances, individual or family counselling must resolve significant emotional problems before effective strides can be made in reemployment, rehabilitation, or both.

Timing is an important factor in this phase of rehabilitation. Allowing too much time to pass between hospital contacts can mean the patient becomes lost to follow-up both physically and emotionally. They content themselves with less-than-satisfactory physical corrections because they fear rehospitalization and surgery and do not know how to deal with these fears—or even know that someone might be available to help.

PHASE FOUR: INDEPENDENCE

The fourth phase begins when the individual has completed all surgical reconstruction and no longer needs medical care for his initial injury (the burn victim may need medical care for residual or secondary complications for the remainder of his life) and an assessment of any physical limitations can be made. From this time on, only nominal contact with the burn team can be anticipated. This usually occurs one to three years after discharge. At this time, individuals will either be fully employed (within their physical and educational capacities) or difficulties related to reemployment will be clearly discernible. It is at this time that the medical team will be called upon to make decisions about patients' ability to resume work that may affect their ability to continue to draw insurance benefits. It is also a time when some individuals who have been hoping for change and improvement may reach an awareness that it won't happen.

A major task for families during this phase is separation and acceptance. For some, that means giving up hopes and dreams that weren't fulfilled. For others, it is only a moment out of a busy, active life. For a few, it is the beginning or continuation of an unemployment or underemployment career that, without significant efforts on the part of social agencies (and social policy change), will afford little or no opportunity for change.

The community social worker is more involved in this phase than the burn team worker since, by definition, only nominal contact will be had with the patient once this phase is reached. Helping those people who still have unresolved problems from the other phases of the rehabilitation process by counselling, referral to appropriate agencies, or consultation with involved community agencies continues. Spending time with individuals who need to deal with their grief over loss of function or disfigurement may also be important during this phase.

SUMMARY

Working with the severely burned patient and his or her family requires a thorough evaluation of their social and emotional resources and problems. This process begins on the day of admission and continues throughout the hospitalization and the rehabilitation period. It requires a working knowledge of the medical and physical aspects of a severe burn, the treatment process, and the psychosocial tasks that need to be mastered during the process of recovery. Rehabilitation follow-up can be divided into four phases of cumulative psychosocial tasks which confront the burned patient and his or her family.

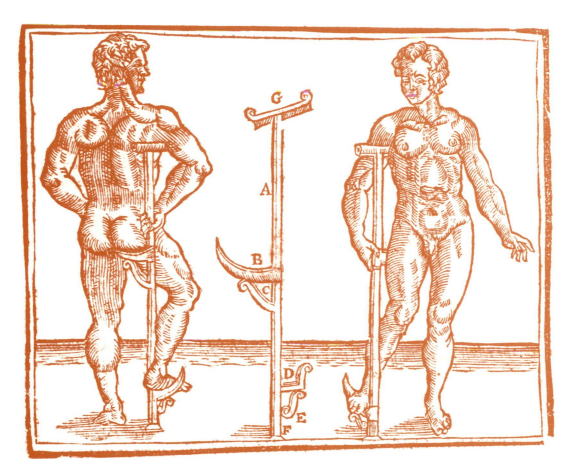

The Works of that Famous Chirurgeon: Ambrose Parey, 1678.

Science commits suicide when it adopts a creed.

Huxley

113

DISCHARGE PLANNING AND FOLLOW-UP

Irving Feller
Mary E. Haab

Preparing the burned patient for return home and a useful place in society begins at the time of admission and continues throughout the hospital course into outpatient visits. Each patient is evaluated as to physical and emotional status prior to the accident as well as prior to discharge. A plan is then formulated as how best to provide the guidance and intervention required to meet his particular problems.

INITIAL EVALUATION

Evaluation of patients emotional status prior to the accident is necessary to determine how he responds to pain; was he a dependent or independent person; what was his involvement with family, friends, and community, etc. By understanding the patient and how he functioned prior to the accident, it is possible to make a discharge program geared to his personal needs.

All care, regardless of severity of burn, is provided on a positive level, directed toward returning the patient to a useful place in society. A positive goal of survival not only encourages the patient to live but also speeds recovery.

DEPENDENCY TO INDEPENDENCE

The accident has suddenly placed the patient in a position of dependency from some previous level of independence based on age and emotional status. Normal daily activity is no longer possible. The patient becomes dependent upon the burn team's help with body hygiene, excretion of body wastes, ambulation, and feeding. Added to this is the wound care necessary to heal the burned areas. The period of dependency varies with the severity of the burn and the part of the body injured. It is obvious that burns of the upper extremities, face, and feet will prolong the rehabilitation process.

One of the first steps toward self help is to encourage and assist the patient to resume normal activities as circumstances permit. Then teaching him how to assist in wound care which may well continue after discharge from the hospital. The occupational therapist can be very helpful by providing adoptive devices to assist the patient in carrying out such tasks as brushing teeth, eating, shaving, and combing hair. The nursing staff should encourage the patient to assist in removing dressings as soon as the patient is capable.

As areas of the wound, including skin grafts and donor sites, no longer need special care by the nursing staff, they should become the responsibility of the patient. The patient should apply the skin lubricating creams, ointments, and lotions as well as antibiotic ointments to small open wound areas. When the use of elastic bandages is indicated, he should be taught to apply these. The longer the patient has the opportunity to perform his own wound care under supervision by the nursing staff, the more comfortable he will be when he is home.

STEP-DOWN

One important aspect of inpatient rehabilitation is to physically move the patient from the area of intensive care to intermediate and then to a rehabilitation area as his condition improves. This step-down system not only encourages the patient reinforcing the recovery process as he is being moved into lesser care areas, but also provides efficiency and economy for total care.

DISCHARGE EVALUATION

When the approximate day of discharge can be determined the patient, his family, and his community should be alerted to participate in the transition.

The patient is "checked out" to be sure he can perform the basic activities for body hygiene, feeding, and dressing. If he cannot perform all of these, a family member should be taught to assist the patient until he is independent. The patient should be able to care for small wounds, to apply medications and dressings, apply devices such as splints for contracture control, and taught to take whatever medications are prescribed and learn expected outcome as well as contraindications and reactions. When small children and severely handicapped patients are involved, more family assistance and visiting nurses are indicated.

A discharge form (Figure 1) has been devised to provide the patient with written instructions. This form also provides a record of discharge orders for

Fig. 1. Discharge Instruction Form.

IRVING FELLER, M.D.
KATHRYN E. RICHARDS, M.D.
P.C.

200 NORTH INGALLS, ANN ARBOR, MICHIGAN 48104

313-761-3666

NAME _____

DATE _____

DISCHARGE INSTRUCTIONS

SKIN CARE:

___ 1. Take a bath once a day.

___ 2. Shampoo hair_____ a week.

___ 3. Apply Nivea cream, baby oil or _____ to ALL HEALED areas including donor sites and skin grafts.

___ 4. Apply _____ ointment to any open areas _____ times a day. Always wash off the areas with soap and water before applying a new thin layer of the ointment.

___ 5. Wear a clean white T-shirt over any open areas on the **upper** trunk.

___ 6. Wear clean white cotton pants or shorts over any open areas on the **lower** trunk.

___ 7. Wrap **one layer** of Kerlix (or use sterile 4" x 4" gauze) around any open areas on the legs or arms.

___ 8. **If your legs were burned:** Wrap your legs with ACE wraps from the base of the toes to the knees. If there are open areas wrap one layer of Kerlix before using the ACE wraps. Remember that the ACE bandage can be washed. Have an extra pair so that you can always have a clean pair while one is being washed.

___ 9. If your legs have not been burned wrap your legs with just ACE wraps from the base of your toes to the knees.

SUPPLIES:

Dressings: _____

Solutions: _____

Medications:

    Vitamins: _____

    For Itching: _____

    For Pain: _____

    For Sleep: _____

    Other Medications: _____

ACTIVITY: _____

SPECIAL INSTRUCTIONS:

    Next outpatient visit: _____, _____ p.m. Office _____ Clinic _____

    Visiting Nurse: _____ Phone No. _____

If you have a problem that must be answered before the next visit, please call 1-313-761-3666. The office address is 200 North Ingalls, Ann Arbor, Michigan 48104.

(Notes on back if necessary)

385

the treating physician, the referring physician and visiting nurse. This form decreases the confusion that can take place by misinterpretation of verbal discharge orders.

A few days before final discharge date, the patient should be encouraged to visit the "outside world" for short periods to start reentry into society. Emotional and physical changes have their place during a long and difficult hospitalization and it may be necessary to have professional emotional help during the first part of the reentry process. This can best be provided by the social worker who has been working with the patient during the entire hospitalization. The same professional will be available during the outpatient follow-up period.

During these final days the patient and his family should be told about the process of wound healing in general, continued care of donor sites as well as the wound, and review the patient's ability for activities of daily living. Emotional concerns should be discussed and responded to individually. If the burn has been severe enough to require a change in the persons activity as compared to the preburn period, the need for and availability of vocational rehabilitation services should be emphasized.

On the day of discharge, the patient is provided with a copy of the discharge form, wound care supplies, and prescriptions. The visiting nurse should be notified if her services are required and a copy of the discharge form should be mailed to the patient's family physician. In many cases the family physician becomes an important part of the team after the discharge.

FOLLOW-UP

Essential to discharge planning is a program for outpatient follow-up. The first outpatient visit should be one or two weeks after discharge and then continued according to the patient's needs—both emotional and physical—until rehabilitation is complete. The problems of cosmetic and functional reconstruction as well as emotional and vocational rehabilitation should be attended by the team of professionals who have cared for the patient from the outset.

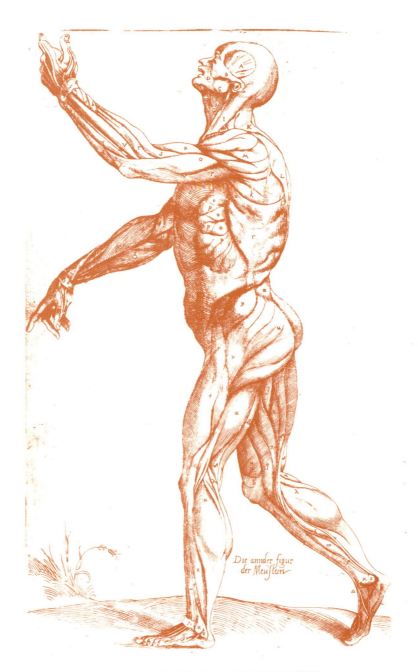

Anatomia viri in hoc genere princip, 1617.

Fashions in therapy may have some justification; fashions in diagnosis have none.

Herrick and Tyson

114

SUPPORTIVE FOLLOW-UP AFTER DISCHARGE

M. Phyllis Hill

Supportive follow-up after discharge remains important if goals accomplished during confinement are to be maintained and progress continued toward the achievement of long-term rehabilitation goals. Transition from the protective environment of the hospital, back to the familiar family and social environment, can create new stresses and adjustment needs different from those experienced during confinement. Concerns shift from those related to survival to the reality of returning to the real world and eventually resuming pre-burn roles. Because the family has usually become dependent on the staff and has had little responsibility for physical care, feelings of insecurity and uncertainty about their ability to properly provide for the relative can be anxiety provoking. In addition, there may be concerns about the relative's readiness to go home or community acceptance of a disabled or cosmetically disfigured relative. Although adequate preparation may already have been given, the reality of discharge can leave both the patient and family with many feelings of ambivalence.

Knowing that they are "not alone" and will have some continued linkage with the medical center tends to help many families feel more comfortable during this transitional period. The awareness of appropriate community resources also lends support. Many families require reinforcement of their ability to manage without over-dependence on the institution. Helping them to utilize resources among their own extended family is also important. A mother, for example, who is not able to effectively care for her child's burn may find that a grandmother is less threatened by the child's outburst and can relieve the mother of her frustrations experienced in wound-cleaning or dressing change.

The family members often raise questions about how to treat the relative when home, fearing that they may do or say something that will be detrimental. By helping them accept that the patient is not necessarily "different" and their approach to him should be the same as pre-burn, with no special treatment required, anxiety and conflict can be avoided. It can often be difficult for families to accept the patient as "normal" but easier for them to accept that if he is treated differently he then will be different. Also, of importance in on-going contacts with families, in some cases, is to help them to realistically recognize that all adjustment problems developed after the burn are not necessarily related to the burn itself. A parent, for example, may require help in understanding developmental behavior or behavioral problems related to management or other family stresses, and not caused by injury.

An educative approach does much to heighten supportive services. Families have a need to know about their relative's prognosis and long-term medical treatment plans and either anticipated or actual changes in their relative's condition. Their questions should be answered in non-medical terminology to prevent further confusion. Questions asked while the relative was an inpatient can often be repeated on an outpatient basis. Many families often need repetitive information in order to understand. Questions can often center around treatment of the burned skin as families tend to be over-protective fearing that touch or activity may cause further damage. Reinforcement of the return to full activity, when medically indicated, needs to be an on-going focus. Parents may be reluctant to re-enter a child in school or a relative may delay return to work if

388

education and support is not on-going.

Concerns relative to sexual issues may not always be openly verbalized by the patient or spouse, but are usually areas of concern. When not verbalized, it should be anticipated that there are questions and appropriate responses made. Mr. A., for example, who had been home several weeks following confinement returned for outpatient follow-up jokingly stating "I guess I'll have to get myself another wife." Mrs. A. expressed concern that she and her husband had not been "as close" as before the burn and she feared that they were headed for some serious marital problems. In exploring the "joke" of Mr. A. and the serious concern of Mrs. A., it was revealed that Mr. A. felt his wife was rejecting him because of his appearance, while Mrs. A. had resisted his sexual advances because of fear of inflicting additional injury to her husband's skin during periods of closeness. After reassurance, the couple returned for their next clinic visit more relaxed and volunteering that "everything is fine again." Although not being able to directly state what problems they were experiencing in their sexual relationship, they were able to indirectly relate this as a definite concern. Providing ample time to listen to what the family is saying, and not saying, is very important.

Contact maintained, either on an on-going or as-needed basis, is very important in helping families resolve many of the practical concerns that follow discharge. The relationship established during a long-term inpatient confinement is beneficial in helping the family feel comfortable in relating most concerns. Interim telephone contact with some very anxious families can be tremendously supportive and also allow an opportunity to reinforce or clarify instructions received in clinic. In addition to families being aware of a consistent course of help, an on-going relationship also provides an opportunity to help them deal with their overall adjustment needs and, can often, contribute to the resolution of stressful situations before they reach crisis proportions. As previously mentioned, with families who have difficulty verbalizing their questions or concerns, support includes anticipating and responding to their need for informa-

tion and guidance. Observing family behavior by supportive personnel can also be important in assessing adjustment problems and may give clearer diagnostic clues to behavior than verbalized feelings.

Mrs. W. returned to clinic with her two year old daughter and verbalized that she and the child were doing well since she returned home. Mrs. W. had difficulty handling her guilt around the child's accident as she had been injured while the mother was momentarily out of the room. At the time of clinic return she felt she had resolved her previous guilt and needed no further intervention in handling adjustment or emotional problems. In observing Mrs. W. she appeared tense and her facial expressions contradicted her verbalization of good adjustment. Although the weather was warm, the child was over-dressed wearing two bonnets which completely hid the burned area on her face, long sleeves and pants in addition to a dress and coat. Upon questioning, Mrs. W. revealed that she had not taken the child out of the home since discharge and was discouraging visits from extended family members at this time. It was obvious that Mrs. W. was endeavoring to completely cover the child and prevent any exposure of the burned area. Mrs. W. quite clearly was not adjusting adequately nor had she resolved her guilt about the child's accidental injury.

In order to facilitate rehabilitation, the family needs to be involved in and aware of both intermediate and long-range medical and social rehabilitation goals. They further need to understand and accept the importance of their roles in the overall rehabilitation process. A realistic appraisal of the relative's capabilities at any given time is important with the family helped to understand that improvements in all areas come with time. They can often become discouraged or impatient because of the time element and need reassurance that positive changes are occurring and goals cannot be reached immediately.

Adjustment patterns established during confinement to help the family cope usually have to be again altered as the injured relative begins to regain independence. Help that was required upon discharge should decrease as the patient is able to assume more responsibility and families often need assistance in permitting the patient to assume more independence and give up the sick role. By having adequate information and support, they are more comfortable in reinforcing to the relative that he "can do it himself" and thereby avoid unintentional impeding of progress. For some families, conflict can be minimized if instructions and expectations are written so they are accessible both to the patient and family. Role reversals and modification of life-style which were necessary during the relative's confinement may become problematic if a family member is unable to relinquish a role position as a relative regains functioning and is able to resume his pre-burn roles. Intervention directed towards restoring the family to its pre-burn position considers the nature of this type of conflict and, often, can prevent its becoming an unmanageable problem. Again, through contact with the family over time they are helped to understand and gradually prepare for required adjustments.

Families need preparation for disruptions in their lives which will be necessitated by additional hospitalizations for reconstructive procedures. This provides them an opportunity to plan ahead and prepare. Interruptions in work routine or school can be distressful but easier to accept if it is understood how this relates to the overall rehabilitation plan. If possible, supportive services during these short-term rehospitalizations should be made available for those patients and families who require it. Mr. G., for example, who seemed to have adjusted adequately during his initial hospitalization later revealed that the emotional impact of rehospitalization was a surprise. It "brought back" to him all of the sadness, anxieties, and fears he experienced at the time of his original hospitalization. The death of two daughters in the fire was very vivid and he felt he mourned their death again.

It is extremely important that both the patient and family have a realistic understanding of the procedures to be performed upon rehospitalization and the anticipated outcomes. It cannot be overemphasized that they need preparation for both the immediate and long-range anticipated results. They can thereby maintain a positive outlook, within realistic limits, and both emotionally support and realistically reinforce ultimate rehabilitation goals to the relative. With the continued availability of both medical and supportive services, and the utilization of community resources, families can better accept and participate in the rehabilitation process and accept total rehabilitation as a reachable goal.

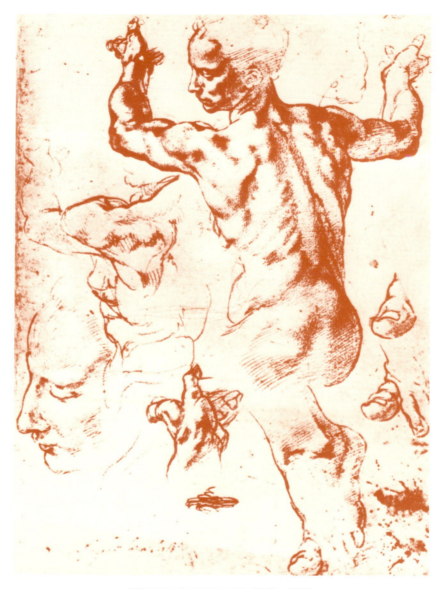

Michelangelo Buonarroti, 1475 — 1564.

115

GROUP THERAPY AND REHABILITATION

Sheryn S. Dungan

Catastrophic illness creates tremendous stress for patient and family. The severe burn cannot be underestimated as one of the most traumatic of these illnesses. It causes an immediate loss of equilibrium, both physically and psychologically. Regression is often rapid, and normal defense mechanisms break down. The patient may be isolated for long periods of time and, out of necessity, may become totally dependent. The complete sense of dependency often becomes incorporated into the patient's whole behavior pattern. Even after dependency is no longer necessary, the need for dependency may remain.

Because of the normal regression which takes place, many patients feel they are completely alone in their experience. Self-centeredness and concern about disfigurement persist and often make realistic discharge planning difficult. Observation of numerous patients in the Burn Unit has led us to a greater understanding of the patients' difficulties in making the transition from hospital to home. Patients who beg to go home often become increasingly anxious, depressed, or withdrawn when finally given a discharge date. Numerous excuses to remain in the hospital appear, as the anxiety level rises.

In trying to meet the predischarge concerns, we have come to realize that dealing with detached and dependent patients is often difficult solely on a one-to-one basis. For this reason, we began using the group experience as an additional therapeutic tool in helping make the transition from hospital to home more realistic.

THE PREDISCHARGE GROUP

The groups consisted of adult burned patients who were approaching discharge in one to two weeks.

The sessions were conducted daily by the Burn Unit social worker. The idea of the group as part of the burn care program was introduced to patients individually by the social worker, and the decision to participate was voluntary. It should be emphasized that individual counseling with the patients and families continued. The overall purpose of the group sessions was to realistically prepare the patients for discharge.

We established three main objectives for patients participating in the group encounter. The first was to decrease the patients' sense of isolation and detachment. We wanted to begin the patients' social experience with people who do understand their fear and who are probably most tolerant of it. The patients would know that they were not alone in their feelings. In addition, since members could actually see others go home the message was clear that people really do leave the hospital.

Secondly, we wanted to increase the patients' ability to form more realistic expectations for themselves in dealing both with concrete problems and more intangible concerns. For example, one particular male patient, who was married, had regressed a great deal and sincerely thought that rather than go to his own home, he had better recuperate in his mother's home, since he would need very "careful attention." Rather than dispute his reasoning, the social worker tried to focus the groups attention on the feeling behind his statement and on recognizing that it was common to everyone. A consensus was reached that fear can motivate all of us to do many things, if we allow it to. After hearing empathetic statement from other patients, the man was more able to go on to the next step—realizing that fear made him see something as necessary, when it was in fact what he *wished* were necessary.

The third major objective was to expose patients to the various ways other members had learned to deal with their experience. How had others been coping? We hoped the various strengths of group members would become the group norm. Role play was sometimes used to demonstrate problems. The patients acted out how to handle curious stares and questions from the public, or how to reassure an overprotective relative. This led to a free exchange of ideas among the patients about handling these and other stressful situations.

In general, the results were gratifying. We found that the group seemed to provide an equalizing influence on members. The more depressed patients did not set the tone of the sessions, as we feared they might. In fact, the group norm seemed to help dissipate these feelings in the more depressed or dependent patients. We also observed that patients do not really like to rehash the acute experience. Although it is a very easy thing to fall into, the patients said they no longer found it helpful. Obviously, the effect of a group experience was more beneficial to some patients than others, but we did observe a gradual decrease in withdrawal for many patients. The short-term nature of the groups, as well as the need to keep concerns focused on discharge, convinced us that the social worker's role during the sessions should be an active one.

OTHER USES FOR GROUPS

Experience with the predischarge group has led us to believe that there are many possibilities for the use of groups with burned patients. Besides the counseling nature of the predischarge group, there are educational and instructional benefits that can be gained from the group situation in an inpatient setting. For example, a group discharge meeting which would include the various burn team members, can be held with the patients. Instruction on good

aftercare by nursing, physical and occupational therapy, and other staff members can be given. The patients can also have their concerns answered in a concise and accurate way.

Or, individual patients can meet with the team just prior to discharge. The patient can receive his instructions from the physician, as well as from other team members. It is also beneficial for close relatives to be included in the conference. This is an excellent way to improve communication between the patient and medical staff and offers good continuity between the in- and outpatient settings.

If many patients return to the setting for reconstructive surgery, this can be a good opportunity for group contact. As these return hospital stays are often brief, an ongoing, open group is most useful. Patients come and go, according to their schedules, but the basic group discussion continues. The reconstruction patients have returned to their home setting, and now bring new kinds of experiences and feelings to share.

Finally, the outpatient setting has almost unlimited potential for developing treatment alternatives, including groups. Group treatment can involve a large, open group of patients and relatives. The group can also be designed for a specific population, such as parents of burned children, or burned adolescents, who do particularly well in a peer group atmosphere. These patients are totally involved in life outside the hospital. From experience, we have learned that this is often where the real adjustment begins.

The type of treatment approach naturally depends a great deal on the particular burn care facility and the staff available. The focus of any treatment measure is to aid the patient in reaching his or her maximum rehabilitation level. The group approach is designed to supplement individual therapy, not to replace it. It is not a better approach, but a different one, utilizing specific objectives to help steer patients toward sound, overall rehabilitation.

116

THE PSYCHIATRIST AND REHABILITATION

Joseph M. Meadows, Jr.

Further emotional damage to patients already severely emotionally traumatized by a burn injury, can be minimized by providing competent psychological management throughout the recovery process. Staff awareness of the patient's emotional state and needs is the first requirement in dealing with emotional problems which become manifest during the early stages of somatic treatment. Their harmonious and willing care provides a measurable assurance and facilitates emotional recovery. Effective psychiatric involvement in returning the patient to a useful place in society will require:

(1) Continuation of coping mechanisms begun during inpatient management;

(2) support, guidance and counselling for the family; and,

(3) continued outpatient psychiatric supervision as needed.

Thus, the role of the psychiatrist in the return of the patient to a useful place in society is appropriate in all phases of treatment. Attention is directed not only to the needs of the patient, but also to the psychological stress on the staff and family.

PREPARING FOR DISCHARGE FROM HOSPITAL

As soon as the patient is reasonably stabilized and minimal rapport established, the psychiatrist must approach the subject of leaving the hospital. Preparations for leaving must begin early, as there will be many fears and many resistances in both the patient and the family. During the hospital stay, family attitudes and dynamics must be assessed and appropriate intervention made to prepare all members for post-hospital problems associated with the trauma.

Later in the burn patient's recovery, when longer interviews are conducted, prompt recognition of common fears will develop. Anticipating questions not only enables the psychiatrist to get the patient's confidence, but also facilitates freer discussion. In general, females will be more concerned with looks while males will be more concerned with their ability to function; both men and women will fear rejection by their families or by society.

FAMILY INVOLVEMENT

In discussions with patients, the reality of the injury and its effect on the patient's life cannot be glossed over or minimized. This holds equally true during consultations with the patient's family. Family members too are involved in the treatment and in the sequellae of the trauma. As early as possible they must be made aware of the long, arduous task of treatment, including surgery, rehospitalization, and rehabilitation. **One must be frank without pessimism and supportive without giving rise to false hope.** Conferences with the family should begin at once. Family members are as in need of support and reassurance as the patient. At these conferences, information can be obtained to anticipate and avoid problems in the hospital as well as after discharge.

Active and on-going involvement by the medical social work department is a necessity for proper hospital treatment as well as post-hospital management. Families must be prepared to adapt to more "togetherness" than prior to the burn. Except for vacations or long weekends, couples or families are rarely in one another's company for long periods of time. The burn patient frequently cannot pursue former individual interests or diversions due to the physical trauma.

Several weeks after her husband returned home, the wife of one burn patient developed anxiety attacks and began episodes of hyperventilation. A somewhat obsessively-compulsively oriented person, she ruminated on actions of the third parties responsible for her husband's injury, as well as on the changes in her husband's physical appearance. His job had always required long hours away from home and he had no hobbies. He was further prevented from household maintenance tasks due to burn deformities of the hand. As she was helped to verbalize her anger and adjust to the reality of permanent change in her husband's appearance, tension in the family decreased. The patient himself found diversion in exploring for antiques, an activity that took him away from the house for several hours each day.

The frustration of being idled, helpless, and dependent on the spouse and others can strain the most stable marriage and family relationships.

Another woman was finally able to get her husband to agree to psychiatric consultation after he began uncontrollable weeping while in the hospital. The patient had worked the night shift for years, enabling the two of them to avoid one another. Obsessed with order and cleanliness, he was constantly at odds with his wife and teenage children because of their untidy habits. His underlying depression could not be avoided in the hospital. After discharge, weekly conjoint sessions over an extended period were needed to temper this man's demands on his family and on himself to a tolerable level. Further tension reduction was achieved when the patient became agile enough to return to his only diversion.

Litigation, unfortunately, may hinder a patient's recovery or return to work. Legal complications not only add to the patient's difficulties, but also create a dilemma for the psychiatrist. An attorney will sometimes advise the patient that any return to work will lead to a loss of claim or will compromise his legal position.

For example, one attorney warned a patient that photographs could be taken if he did the limited lawn work permitted by his injuries. The attorney feared that photographs could be used to "prove" that the patient was not disabled. The patient's hands were indeed severely deformed by burns, and his ability to tend his lawn, although severely restricted, would have provided a much needed outlet.

LONG-TERM FOLLOW-UP

Long-term psychiatric treatment is seldom needed, and flexible attitude toward the needs of individual patients must be maintained.

One 52-year-old man, burned in a plant explosion, was discharged after several months of hospitalization. As is common, a return to the hospital for more surgery was needed. On readmission, tachycardia developed in the operating room before anesthesia. The cardiologist ruled out cardiac pathology, but she prudently requested further exploration of nonorganic etiology of the tachycardia. During psychiatric evaluation, it was discovered that during the patient's first hospital stay, the squeaking of the wheels and the carts themselves became associated with death and the removal of dead patients from the Burn Unit. Therefore, the patient's trip to the operating room on a cart with squeaking wheels was extremely traumatic; the resulting tachycardia was, therefore, not surprising. An approach combining desensitization, ventilation of apprehension, and exploration of the original trauma enabled this man to return to the hospital to continue reconstructive surgery.

Alcoholics, recognized and unrecognized, present difficult problems. The alcoholic, whether he has burned himself or suffered an industrial accident, may have such a poor self-image and such strong self-destructive drives that obtaining cooperation is nearly impossible. Since the burn patient frequently has a poor appetite and may suffer from depression on return home, one must be careful to not overlook alcoholic gastritis as a cause of weight loss. In my experience, alcoholics are best handled by those specifically trained or specialized in their treatment.

Regression is routinely observed in the burn patient. The burn team readily accepts it as a phase of adjustment. The markedly regressed patient can be a severe problem, sorely taxing the endurance of the staff.

One psychotically withdrawn young man began soiling willfully to anger the staff, as well as to obtain the secondary gratification of being cleaned. Psychotropic medications were of no apparent value. Staff conferences were needed to permit the burn team to ventilate their anger, as well as to discuss management problems. It became obvious that discharge to the care of the family would be the best treatment possible. After grafts had healed, discharge was effected and arrangements made for physical rehabilitation at his local hospital. Consultation two months later revealed the soiling had stopped after two days at home. His family reported a return to normal behavior after one week. An interview with the patient failed to indicate any reference to the psychotic behavior previously observed.

Attemped suicide, consciously planned or unconsciously determined, will be observed from time to time. Occasionally suicidal patients will be chronically or acutely psychotic, but at other times only acutely disturbed and irrational.

One very pretty young female from a Middle Eastern culture, unaccustomed to the freedom of women in this country, met and married a fellow student against strong family opposition. Her husband was a very immature, abusive, irresponsible person. Rejected by her family and abused by her husband, she decompensated and set fire to herself, suffering severe burns to her chest that destroyed her breasts. During her hospital stay, she divorced her husband. After discharge, she returned to college, was reaccepted by her family, and became a nurse. Her brief psychotic episode and self-mutilation effectively removed her from the threat of freedom.

A young black male from a rural southern area

moved north with his wife. Two children were born in quick succession. Financial pressures mounted after a layoff. Marital separation resulted, and the patient moved out. Unable to cope with the accumulated tensions, the patient set fire to himself with lighter fluid. Burns were severe enough to permanently remove him from the work force.

During the post-hospital phase of treatment, the development of a work phobia or extreme anxiety in a work situation is a frequently observed complication.

The owner of an asphalt paving company was burned in an explosion during equipment cleaning. Asphalt paving had been his only occupation since age 16 and he had 20 years of success in the business. As owner of the company, he was not actually needed to do the work and could successfully run the business by estimating costs and checking completed jobs. Nevertheless, he was so depressed and fearful of being reinjured, it was difficult for him to even discuss his work. Unfortunately, due to his fears, he resisted all attempts at treatment. His irritability was intolerable to his wife and disruptive to the family. He would not keep his appointments and contact was lost. This man was indeed very frightened and very depressed.

Another young man burned in a freak explosion experienced such apprehension upon return to work that his attention could not be focused on his job. Moving him to areas of the plant where fire or explosions were not possible proved useless. Counselling him out of that particular factory job and retraining into another job enabled him to readapt to work.

The psychiatrist must not only deal with the burned patient's emotional and physical trauma, but must also consider the stress on all persons involved in the burn victim's treatment. The burned patient has some problems common to anyone severely traumatized. Other problems are unique to the burned patient. **Careful attention to the burn victim's emotional needs is an essential part of the recovery process.**

1.Msc. Die Seite der Stirn entspringt aus dem obern teil des Kronformigen Beins, und endiget sich über die Augenbraun Meuslein.

2.Msc. Der Rand der Augenbraun, welcher die ganze Höle, oder den Umkreis einnimt, und die Augen zuschließen hilft.

3.Msc. Das Schlafbedeckende Meuslein entspringt aus dem Schlaf, mit einem Anfang eines halben Mond. Kreis, und fahret fort unter das Jochbein, endiget sich in dem untern Kinnbacken.

4.Msc. Das Eß-Meuslein hat seinen Ursprung von dem Joch Bein, endiget sich in dem Winckel des untersten Kinnbackens, und hilft zugleich mit dem Schlaf Meuslein gedachten Kinnbacken in die höhe heben.

5.Msc. Beweget die obere Lefzen, und entspringt bey dem Anfang des Jochbeins, genau bey der Nase.

6.Msc. Trucket die undere Lippe nieder, entspringt von dem Grund des undern Kinnbackens.

7.Msc. Das Trompeten oder Backen Meuslein, hat seinen Anfang von dem obern Kinnbacken, hänget sich an dem untern an, und hilft die Lippen gegen das Ohr ziehen.

8.Msc. Die Zwey-beuchige Meuslein entspringen in denen Dutten-förmigen fortsätzen und endigen sich in dem untern Kinnbacken solchen nieder zu trucken.

9.Msc. Die duttenförmige Meuslein entstehen aus der Höhe des Brustbeins, und Anfang des Schlüs. selbeins, endigen sich in dem Duttenförmigen fortsätzen, genau bey dem Ohr, helfen das Haubt biegen.

10.Msc. Die Raben-Schnäbel-förmige Meuslein, entspringen aus dem Rabenschnablichten fortsatz, und gehen fort unter dem duttenförmigen Meuslein, endigen sich in dem Zungen oder Kehlbein, helfen die Bein und die Zunge hinunter drucken.

11. Die Schildförmige Krospel, welche auf der Höhe des Brustbeins entsteht, endiget sich unter dem Kinn.

12. Die Blut-Puls- und Senn-Adern, welche zu dem Haubt hinauf steigen.

43.Msc. Das beugende Meuslein des Daumens, entsteht aus dem Handgelenk.

44.Msc. Das abziehende Meuslein des kleinen fingers entsteht aus der flachen Hand.

45. Das Ringförmige Band.

65. Ander Band des fusses.

66. Msc. Das ableitende Meuslein der grosen Zehe, entspringt genau bey dem fuß-Solen Bein.

67. Ein ander Band.

L'Anatomia dei pittori, 1732.

117

THE OCCUPATIONAL THERAPIST AND REHABILITATION

Leslie Kamil-Miller

The goals of the occupational therapist (OT) are multifold. The OT works to: (1) prevent deformities, (2) increase function and facilitate independence in activities of daily living (ADL), (3) provide psychological support, (4) involve the family in treatment to assist in carry-over of goals both during hospitalization and after discharge, and (5) provide follow-up care.

PREVENT DEFORMITY

Formation of contracture is an ongoing problem that must be dealt with on a consistent, long-term basis. Splinting, positioning, exercise, and pressure are the most prevalent measures used to prevent deformities.

Splinting may be used post-grafting for stabilization of an extremity, in the latter aspects of treatment during hospitalization and at home both to control contractures and to improve function, and following reconstructive surgery for maintenance of range of motion (Figure 1).

The purpose of the splints, in rehabilitation, is: to increase function; to maintain and increase range of motion; and to correct deformities when surgery is contraindicated due to hyperactive scar tissue. Sometimes function has to be slightly compromised because positioning opposite the direction of the anticipated contracture is mandatory.

The roles of the OT in splinting are: (1) to assess, with the physician, the need for splinting and the type of splint to be used, (2) initial application of the splint, (3) routine assessment of the fit and the patient's ability to function with the splint, (4) modification of the splint, when necessary, to achieve maximum fit, and (5) education of patient, family

and staff in properly applying and fitting the splint. In most institutions, splint fabrication is also the responsibility of the OT.

There are various types of splints. Static and three-point extension splints are used routinely for positioning to maintain either a functional or maximum range. A dynamic splint is frequently used to simultaneously correct range limitation and provide active exercise. The function of the conformer splint is to maintain range while applying even pressure to a site of hyperactive tissue.

Positioning during rehabilitation is done primarily to maintain the existing range of motion and to maximize independent patient function, through instruction in compensatory motions and/or alternative methods of performance. Contracture formation has already been established, so extensive positioning to increase range could lose some effectiveness. However, once range has been achieved following reconstructive surgery, an external force such as splinting is the most efficient approach.

Exercises are necessary to maintain present active range of motion, function, and to increase strength. A resistive exercise program can be utilized to achieve these goals. One of the media utilized is theraplast. This resistive media, through proper positioning, can strengthen hand musculature and achieve active range of motion (Figure 2).

To evaluate the effectiveness of an exercise program, prehensile strength and coordination must be continually assessed. Results help the therapist determine future treatment goals and media (Figure 3).

Routine performance in ADL is also considered a form of exercise. Participation involves range of motion of both upper and lower extremities and

Fig. 1. Splints can be used as a method for increasing function and increasing or maintaining range of motion. **A.** An axillary splint can be used post-grafting for static positioning of an extremity and to maintain range. The same splint with slight modifications can be used to maintain range after reconstructive surgical release.

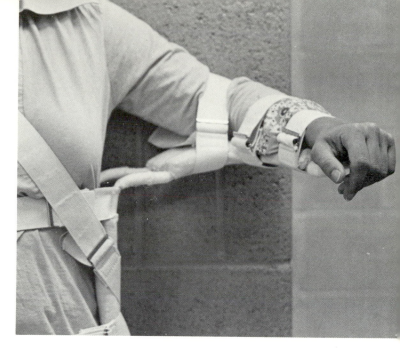

Fig. 1. B. A knuckle bender is utilized to increase metacarpophalangeal joint flexion. Since this splint is dynamic, functional activities and exercises can be performed with the splint on. Flexion can be increased by regulation of resistance applied with rubber bands. **C.** A reverse knuckle bender can assist to increase proximal interphalangeal joint extension when a flexion contracture is present. External resistance to increase extension can be regulated with rubber band tension.

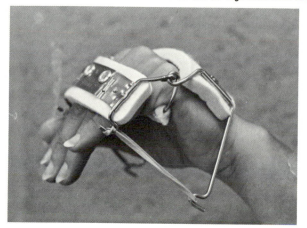

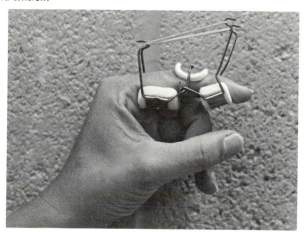

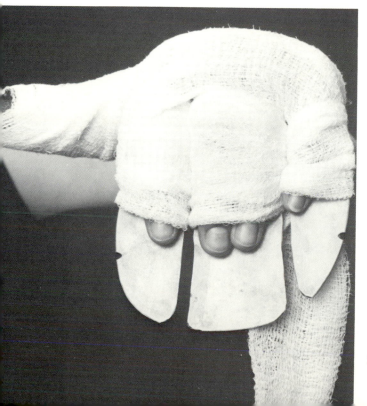

Fig. 1. D. Palmar burn splint with slits. Although a dynamic splint might be worn during the day, the standard palmar burn splint is frequently applied at night to maintain correct positioning while the patient is at rest. Positioning: MCP joints 90 degrees of flexion; PIP and DIP joints full extension; thumb-abduction; wrist—30 degrees hyperextension. The slits are to separate the web spaces and maintain pressure over PIP joints for a secure fit.

Fig. 2. Theraplast, a resistive media, can be utilized to enhance an exercise program, to increase strength and achieve active assistive range of motion. The theraplast was cultured after use, for bacterial growth, and results were negative. **A.** Gross finger flexion.

Fig. 3. Hand dexterity and prehensile strength, respectively, are evaluated. Results are compared with norms of standardized tests and prior results. In this way, a baseline is established for future treatment planning. **A.** Nine Hole Peg Test to evaluate dexterity.

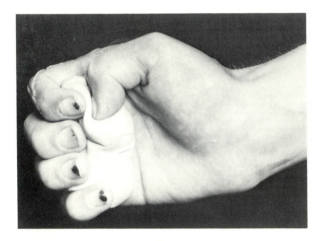

Fig. 2. B. Thumb interphalangeal joint flexion.

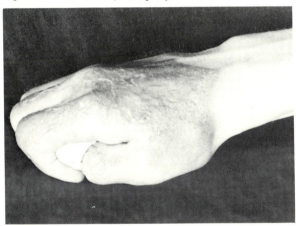

Fig. 2. C. Three jaw chuck prehensile pattern.

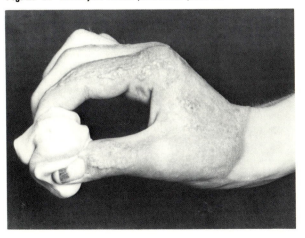

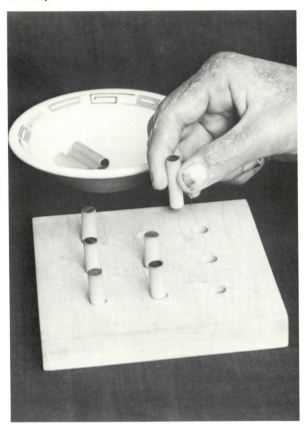

Fig. 3. B. Pinch gauge to assess prehensile strength.

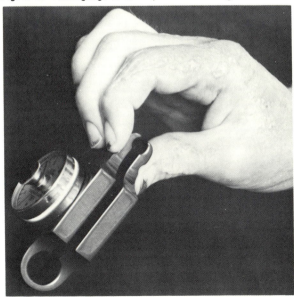

Fig. 4. Neck wrap or conformer. This neck wrapping assists to maintain the neck range, while evenly applying pressure to the hyperactive scar tissue. The wrapping is done with one layer of kerlix, ½ inch foam and a three inch ace wrap. Lower mandibular contour can be maintained if the wrapping extends above the lower jaw. This can be done with the above type of wrap or with an isoprene neck splint.

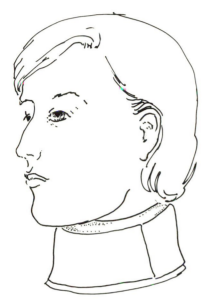

Fig. 5. Writing and typing skills must be evaluated prior to discharge. Often times, a limited grasp, due to decreased range and/or strength, can hinder independent performance. Built up utensils can enhance this independence.

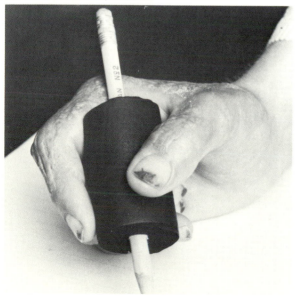

integration of these motions into completion of a meaningful activity. Emphasis of performance without adaptive equipment helps to maximize exercise benefits.

Many centers believe that pressure wrappings help to control contractures and the process of hypertrophic scarring. The constant pressure assists in maintaining the collagen in a more parallel pattern, reduces the inflammatory response and controls the blood supply to these vascular areas. Pressure wraps must be constantly worn, until the scar tissue is mature (Figure 4).

INCREASING FUNCTION AND FACILITATING INDEPENDENCE IN ACTIVITIES OF DAILY LIVING

Often the patient and family question the patient's ability to perform tasks done prior to admission. Thoughts of inability to perform permeate the patient's mind. Can I dress myself? Can I cook a meal?

Therefore, an extensive evaluation encompassing the patient's present ability to perform self-care, household, and communication activities is completed prior to discharge. Management of standard equipment necessary to perform these activities should be evaluated and compensatory methods of management should be taught, if a contracture inhibits performance (Figures 5, 6, and 7).

Various simulated job activities can be evaluated in regards to gross upper extremity and fine hand function. Again, compensatory motions, adaptive equipment, or reorganization of a work area can be recommended to increase the feasibility of performance (Figure 8).

As a patient goes home and resumes participation in leisure-time activities, it is important to evaluate the patient's ability to function in these areas. Once the patient can perform an activity, education on achieving range of motion through participation should follow. This enhances the exercise program and allows the simultaneous completion of a meaningful task, thus increasing the patient's self-esteem.

These leisure-time activities can be employed to increase physical tolerance by increasing the intensity, duration, resistance, and type of activities performed.

An electrical injury or full-thickness burn may lead to amputation. An upper extremity amputee, while in the hospital, is routinely instructed in one-handed techniques, so independence in all the above areas is feasible. If the dominant extremity has been amputated, activities to increase strength and coordination of the nondominant extremity would also transpire. A discussion on prostheses, their components, fit, and function is necessary to provide the patient with a realistic idea of the function to be obtained from its use. Once stump shrinkage has been achieved, often after discharge, a prescription for the appropriate prosthesis is written, and the patient then trained in grasp/release activities, self-care, ADL, vocation, and prosthesis care (Figure 9).

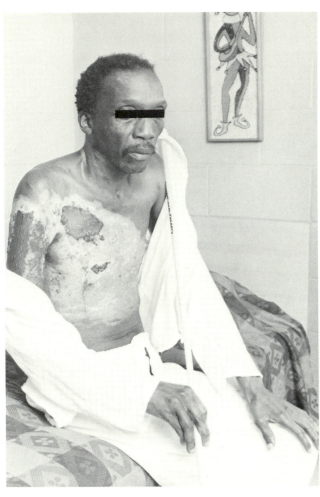

Fig. 6. Returning to independence. Limited range of motion due to contractures can foster dependency in self care skills. **A.** A dressing stick is utilized to help don and remove shirt, due to axillary contracture. Patient presents inability to maneuver shirt, as all parts of his trunk cannot be reached.

Fig. 6. B. A stocking device can increase independence in dressing, when hip and knee contractures limit ability to reach feet.

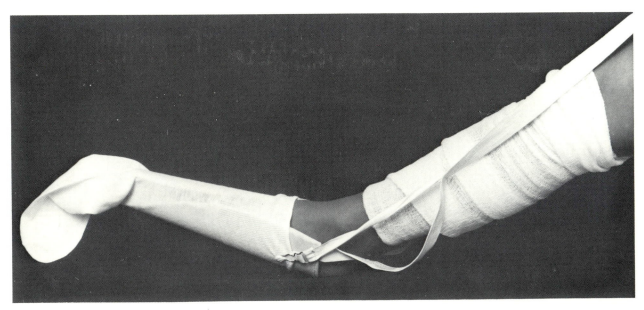

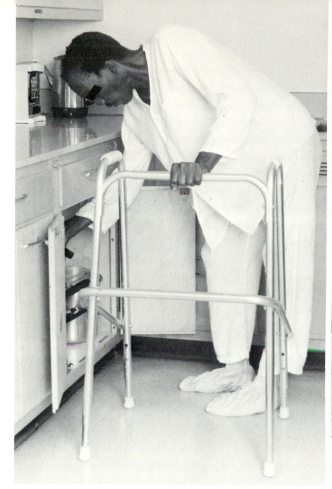

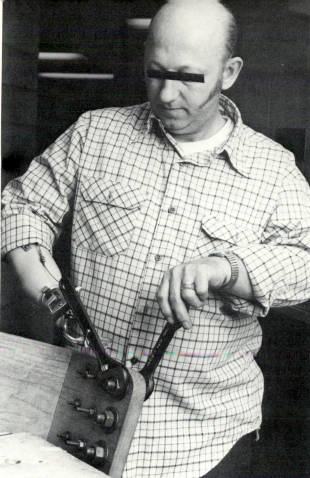

Fig. 7. Independent functioning relating to patient's previous home responsibilities must be evaluated. Instruction in kitchen activities with use of walker and compensatory methods of performance due to limited range must transpire.

Fig. 8. Vocation. Simulated job tasks can be used as an effective measure of the potential of patient's returning to previous vocation.

Fig. 9. When a patient has an upper extremity amputation secondary to a burn, evaluate patient education regarding the components most suitable to patient's life style. **A.** Training in grasp/release activities and pre-positioning hook. **B.** Self-care training regarding use of prosthesis in functional activities.

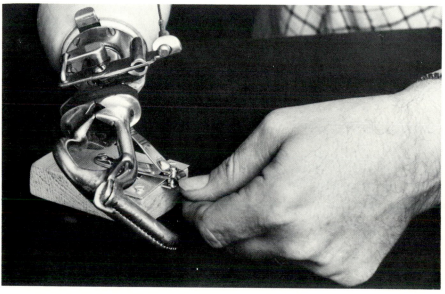

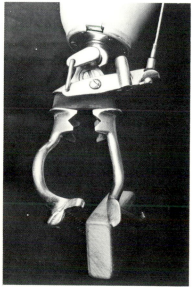

PSYCHOLOGICAL SUPPORT

The OT should be constantly aware of the patient's great needs for psychological support. Adjusting to new methods in performing activities often contributes to frustration. Without constant support, cessation in performance can result. Frequently, when scarring is present, a change in self-image occurs. Early interaction with others not involved in burn care provides the patient with the opportunity to adjust to their reactions. Support regarding these changes is necessary prior to discharge, so that isolation from friends and social events does not occur. A community trip prior to discharge to help eliminate some of these problems is a meaningful addition to an occupational therapy program.

Family Involvement. The therapist should be sensitive to the injury's impact on the family. Explanation of the program, as well as the family's role in its implementation, is an essential part of the program. The responsibility for completion of treatment programs cannot rest with the patient alone. The physical and emotional contributions of family members are crucial in treatment effectiveness and patient attitude.

FOLLOW-UP CARE

Each patient is sent home with a written program. Although these are individualized, all comprise exercises, activities, ADL tasks, and instructions for their performance.

Reevaluation of physical and functional status is assessed on an outpatient basis. Recommendations regarding performance in a difficult task, use or change in splinting, or exercise are explained at this time.

SUMMARY

The functions of the occupational therapist in the rehabilitative phase of burn patient care are multifold. They are to prevent deformities, increase function, provide psychological support, and follow-up care. In order for the patient to achieve maximum previous function, it seems apparent that an OT's contribution to the patient is crucial.

It is imperative that the therapist considers the patient as a "whole person" and that all aspects of their lives be considered in their treatment program.

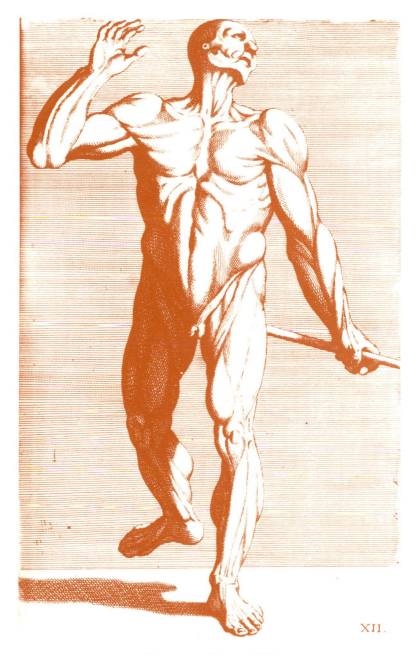

L'Anatomia dei pittori, 1732.

By nature's kind disposition, most questions which it is beyond a man's power to answer do not occur to him at all.

Santayana

118

THE PHYSICAL THERAPIST AND REHABILITATION

William L. Combs

The rehabilitation phase begins, by definition, when the burn wound is decreased to less than 20 percent of the total body surface; it continues until the patient reaches his or her maximum level of physical and emotional independence. Nevertheless, this rather strict definition does not preclude planning and goal setting by the patient and the physical therapist shortly after the time of admission. The physical therapist's role during the rehabilitative phase is to work with the patient to plan and implement a treatment program which will assist the patient to regain muscle strength, range of motion, and gait. Methods employed by the therapist cannot be strictly assigned to the emergent, acute, or rehabilitative stages of recovery. Rather, methods carry over from one stage to another. The success of the patient's rehabilitation depends not only on correct program planning and the diligence of the physical therapist during and after hospitalization, but also on the patient's willingness and determination to follow through with treatment programs both in the hospital and at home. Therefore, the more the therapist can motivate a patient to strive for functional independence, the more successful the rehabilitation will be.

INCREASING JOINT RANGE OF MOTION AND MUSCLE STRENGTH

One goal of the physical therapist is to assist the patient in regaining his preburn range of motion. An aggressive program of preventing or decreasing joint and skin contractures is continued from the emergent and acute stages into the rehabilitative stage. Although their complete prevention is occasionally impossible, minimizing contractures and deformities is essential. Three major methods are employed by the therapist to achieve this goal: activity and exercise, positioning, and splinting.

Activity and exercise are the most natural methods for maintaining range of motion. The activity and exercise program either can be done by the patient alone or with the aid of the therapist or a family member, who has been instructed by the therapist. Using the involved extremities to perform prearranged activities and activities of daily living, such as, eating, drinking, and ambulation, does much to maintain and increase the patient's functional range of motion. Also, the patient's ability to perform everyday tasks independently results in less reliance on other persons for assistance and usually facilitates the emotional adjustment following discharge.

Passive exercise is often needed to maintain and increase range of motion. Passive range of motion exercise is performed in the following manner. Generally, the exercise is repeated only three to five times. The joint is taken to the maximum available range, then gently stretched and held for one to two minutes. The next repetition takes the joint to the maximum range achieved in the previous motion and then a bit further, and so on, until the maximum range of motion for that exercise session has been attained.

Following grafting over joint surfaces, all range of motion exercises are discontinued for approximately five days to facilitate grafting success. As healing progresses, gentle, active motion is encouraged and employment of active-assistive range of motion is utilized to decrease skin contractures. Passive stretching can be utilized for patients unable to achieve full active range following grafting, but the therapist must be certain that the grafts are sufficiently healed to withstand stretching.

Positioning can reduce the formation of contractures, and should be stressed by the therapist and the Burn Unit staff during the patient's hospitalization. It should be continued by the patient and family after discharge. While resting or sleeping, any affected joints should be placed in a position that facilitates motion away from the potential or actual contracture or deformity. For example, if a patient has a knee flexion contracture, he or she should keep the knee in as much extension as possible and should rest or sleep without a pillow under the popliteal fossa.

Splinting is also used to prevent or decrease contracture and deformity. With the materials available today, virtually any type of splint can be fashioned for the patient, be it static or dynamic. The turnbuckle splint is one of the most effective splints for reduction of contracture at the elbow or knee. A turnbuckle splint over the joint facilitates serial splinting. This splint is easy to apply and remove, and, after sterilization, can be used repeatedly on different patients. It can be converted to a dynamic splint by replacing the turnbuckle assembly with an elastic material. When the elastic is attached, the splint offers a constant pull. A schedule for wearing the splint is generally devised, for example, two hours on, one hour off. This schedule allows the patient both time to rest and time to work for motion opposite that effected by the splint (Figure 1).

The rehabilitative stage is also the time for the physical therapist to assist the patient in regaining lost strength. By this time, the energy demands placed on the body in surviving the burn injury have decreased sufficiently to allow more energy expenditure in exercise.

Resistive exercise is employed to increase the patient's strength. Isometric, isokinetic, and isotonic exercises can be used in the treatment program either separately or in combination, depending on the patient's needs. Isometric exercise, such as quadriceps setting, is useful for decreasing atrophy while joints are immobilized following grafting.

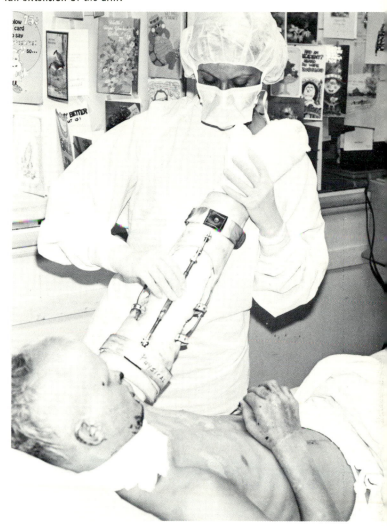

Isokinetic exercise requires equal resistance throughout the joint's range. It is best accomplished at the bedside, with the therapist offering manual resistance. Working with weights is an example of isotonic exercise. Because isotonic exercise offers varied resistance through the joint's range, it is not as effective as isokinetic exercise.

The therapist should demonstrate the excercises to be done at home prior to the patient's discharge. Patients and their families, if possible, should be made aware that maximum results depend on adhering as closely as possible to the program. To obtain maximum patient compliance, the program should be thorough, but not overly tedious or lengthy. Alternate methods of exercise, such as exercise games, are very useful, especially with children.

GAIT TRAINING

Normal-gait training begins in the acute stage and continues into the rehabilitative stage. Patients should briefly stand at the bedside as soon as their condition allows, even though they may still require nasogastric tubes, IVs or catheters. A Circolectric bed can be used to gradually accustom the patient to the standing position if orthostatic hypotension is a problem. Once standing tolerance is achieved, the patient can step off the end of the bed and begin to ambulate. The walking distance is increased with each session, until the patient is able to ambulate independently. Instruction in associated activities, such as the transfer from sitting to standing and standing to sitting, must also be incorporated into the ambulation program to assure total independence (Figures 2 and 3).

Prior to standing or ambulating, all burn patients should be provided with elastic bandages or stockings for the lower extremities, even if the lower extremities are not burned. The bandages will increase tissue turgor and decrease the possibility of venous stasis. If the lower extremities are involved, they should be wrapped to the level of the burn. If lower extremities are grafted, sitting, standing, and ambulation must be discontinued for 10 to 14 days. When ambulation is reinstituted, the elastic supports are applied as they were before the grafting.

The patient may require assistive devices, such as the tilt table, parallel bars, walker, cane or crutches, to aid in ambulation. The first two devices require that the patient be able to go to the Physical Therapy Clinic; the others may be used at the bedside.

During ambulation, any deviations from a normal gait are corrected. If the upper or lower extremities are injured, the patient generally will exhibit an antalgic gait. With injuries involving the legs, the patient will tend to favor the more

Fig. 2. Prior to ambulation the patient can be put in the standing position using the Circolectric bed for a few minutes daily to achieve standing tolerance.

Fig. 3. Once standing tolerance is achieved the patient can step off the Circolectric bed (as shown) with help to begin ambulation.

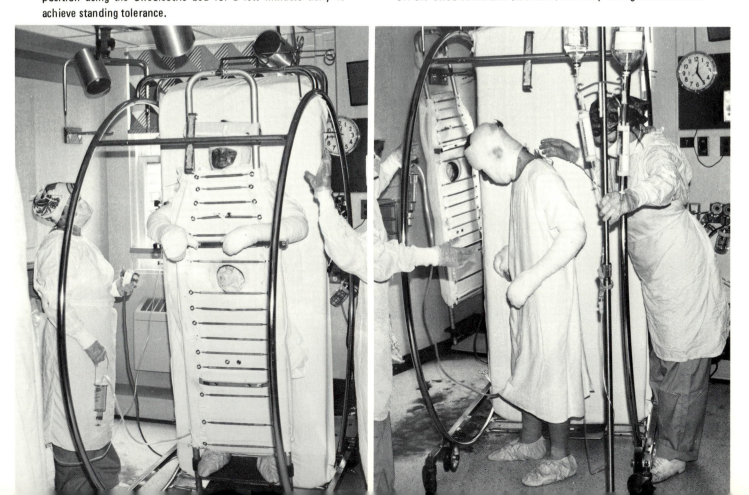

painful extremity. When the upper extremity or trunk is involved, any resultant splinting may cause deviations in motions associated with a normal gait, such as reciprocal arm swing. The patient should be encouraged to disregard pain as much as possible and to strive for the preburn gait. Having patients watch themselves in a mirror is particularly useful because it provides constant feedback regarding gait deviations.

A structured program for increasing ambulation tolerance should be included in the home program given to the patient at discharge. Patients should be encouraged to ambulate as much as their tolerance allows, but they also should be cautioned not to exceed this tolerance.

Assistive devices are occasionally necessary for patients whose burn injuries are complicated by tendon loss or peripheral neuropathy, for example, a short leg brace with a dorsiflexion spring assist for a patient with deep burns of the dorsum of the foot involving dorsiflexor tendon loss. These devices are best fitted by the orthotist or prosthetist.

Occasionally, a lower extremity is so severely insulted that it must be amputated. Initially, the treatment program for patients with amputations consists primarily of upper and lower extremity strengthening preparatory to gait training with the prosthesis. As soon as the majority of the stump is covered with skin, and any revisions have been done, instruction leading to independent stump wrapping is begun. After the prosthesis ordered by the physician is fitted by the prosthetist, the physical therapist instructs the patient in proper gait using the new limb.

Stump wrapping and wearing of the prosthesis on grafted areas must be explained to the patient. The patient should be instructed to check the stump for even wrapping several times daily and should also occasionally remove the prosthesis and check the weight-bearing and other surfaces of the stump in contact with the prosthesis.

RE-EVALUATION AFTER DISCHARGE

When the patient returns for routine visits following discharge, the physical therapist should re-evaluate the patient's status. Has the patient been following the activity, exercise, ambulation program since discharge? If so, has there been improvement? If not, how can the patient and his family be sufficiently motivated?

CONCLUSION

The physical therapist is an essential member of the rehabilitation team. The therapist's knowledge concerning prevention of deformities, therapeutic exercise, ambulation and gait training, and orthotics-prosthetics is invaluable to the overall effort to help the patient regain the maximum level of physical and emotional function.

The sooner patients can be removed from the depressing influence of general hospital life the more rapid their convalescence.
Charles H. Mayo

119

REHABILITATION OF THE BURNED CHILD

M.L. Bowden

Developmental stages and the family system profoundly influence the rehabilitation of children. The ability of a child to relate, understand, and maintain emotional and psychological resources is closely connected to developmental stages. A one-year-old cannot be involved in a rehabilitation program in the same way as a 12-year-old. One may opt for postponing hospitalization because the yearling's attachment to the mother is more significant than cosmetic revision of burn scars, while the opposite might be true for the older child. In addition, rehabilitation needs must be constantly reassessed with respect to changes brought about by physical, emotional, and intellectual adjustments.

Secondly, the child as a member of the family group is significantly influenced by the behavior and attitudes of that family. Inherent dependency upon the parents for all rehabilitation effort demands that the rehabilitation team consult and work not only with the child but with the parents.

Major problems which seem to influence childhood rehabilitation are (1) failure to return for medical follow-up, (2) unresolved regression and increased dependency, (3) unrealistic future planning, (4) family and emotional problems. Each will be briefly explored and suggestions made as to how to counter these problems.

MEDICAL FOLLOW-UP

Children recovered from severe burns need reconstructive procedures to correct residual problems from the initial injury. In addition, functional reconstruction for problems secondary to rapid growth, and cosmetic reconstruction can only be done when growth is complete. Losing these children to follow-up before completion of these procedures is not uncommon. In a ten-year follow-up study by Withey (NIBM, 1972) where burned children were called back, of those that returned, 50 percent required corrective surgery.

An outreach approach must be employed to ensure that children return for clinic appointments and necessary surgeries. Families need help in dealing with problems that may prevent their involvement in an ongoing program. These include ignorance—some parents may not know that the rehabilitative treatment is needed; lack of resources—some parents do not have the financial resources to get transportation to the visits, or fear their ability to finance hospital expenses; and emotional problems—parents may have difficulty bringing the child back to the hospital in the face of the child's obvious emotional distress at returning, or parents themselves want to avoid dealing with new encounters that reactivate their own feelings about the initial injury and hospitalization experience.

REGRESSION AND DEPENDENCY

Regression and increased dependency is a frequently observed phenomenon in the severely burned. If it continues for too long it can significantly impede rehabilitation efforts. Regression has been most common in families where the parents reinforced the child's behavior either because of their guilt or because the maintenance of the behavior was adaptive to the family system. An example of this is the case of an adolescent whose mother had been having difficulty with the teenager's independence prior to the accident. The burn injury was a convenient excuse for not resolving the conflict.

Every effort should be made to deal with regression and increased dependency in the hospital prior to discharge. Patients and parents should be encouraged and rewarded for their efforts at independence and a return to at least a pre-burn level of functioning. In discharge planning, include a projected schedule of return to activities that were part of the patient's repertoire prior to the injury. (Self toileting might be a goal for a three-year-old, and return to school for a school-age child.) A combination of education and counseling seems to be effective. In addition, utilize community resources such as public health nurses and teachers/counselors to reinforce the program. Finding ways to help family, friends, and community resources help the patient that do not encourage dependency and regression is a challenge, but in the long run the effort can assist the child to develop behavior patterns that can be later mobilized to plan education and career goals.

REALISTIC PLANNING

Lack of realistic planning for the future has several causes. For some children and families, it is not a part of their behavior. They do not plan for the future and would not even if they had not been burned. Some parents and children assume that the patient cannot return to school, will never have a job, and will not marry or have children (the fear of negative information may keep patients from discussing their future). Some parents are unfamiliar with community resources and services available to help them and their child in planning and preparing for the future. In some instances the community agencies that are identified to help children and families are influenced by their own ignorance and prejudices. For example, agencies may counsel adolescent girls to consider secretarial training rather than seeking training in a technical trade, or discourage disfigured persons from seeking jobs in which they might have considerable social contact.

The provision of information to families and to agencies assigned to help children and families is an ongoing process for the burn team. The sharing of current information on the child's abilities must be placed in context with his or her potential. If a family and/or child seem to be having difficulty in making realistic plans, they may need extra attention from the team or from others within the community. Care must be taken not to impose our own values and judgments upon clients, while at the same time encouraging them to maximize their potential. Intervention may include exposure to others who have successfully established social relationships and are successfully employed, the use of group therapy for socialization purposes, and individual counseling.

An area not often mentioned in assisting the severely burned to plan realistically for the future is sexual functioning. While this has been more extensively explored with other handicapping conditions, it is an area that begs mentioning because of the lack of attention in burn care. Conversations with parent and child should include a discussion of the impact of the injury upon capacity for sexual functioning and child-rearing. Both males and females may have questions about their ability to attract a mate, perform sexually, and conceive children. Others, because of physical limitations, may need instructions in behavior that will maximize sexual satisfaction.

FAMILY AND EMOTIONAL PROBLEMS

The family must constantly be considered in dealing with the child's rehabilitation. In some cases the family presents special problems that significantly impede progress for the child. Some families are so disorganized that they cannot manage care and rehabilitation of a severely burned child. Psychotic parents, problems with abuse and neglect, and intellectual limitations that interfere with following anything except basic day-to-day functioning are all examples of serious problems. The rehabilitation team may have no recourse except recommendation of placement in a setting which will facilitate the child's rehabilitation. In other situations the family might be significantly impaired in its functioning. Crisis-prone families require continual community support and monitoring to maintain a child in a rehabilitation program. Mobilization and maintenance of this support system can require considerable effort on the part of the burn team because, predictably, staff members in community agencies become angry and fatigued by the demands made upon them by these families.

Emotional problems of the child might also interfere with rehabilitation. The need to mourn a lost parent and resolve a depression may be necessary before a child can focus energy upon physical functioning and future planning. The provision of supportive or intensive counseling, individually or as a part of the family unit, may do much to help the child resolve problems. With younger children, the use of play therapy or special assistance from the expanding infant mental health programs can also be valuable to problem resolution. On occasion, hospitalization in a children's psychiatric facility may also prove useful as an intensive healing experience.

Unlike grownups, children have little need to deceive themselves.
Goethe

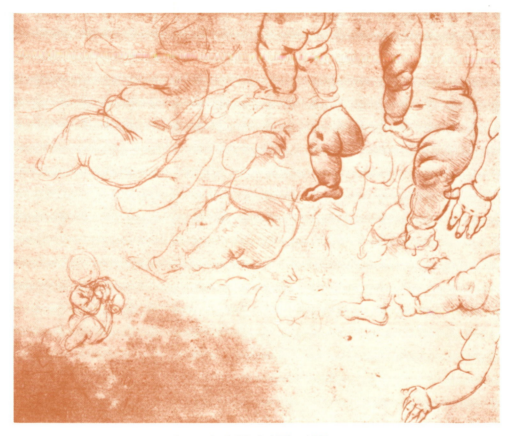

Leonardo da Vinci, 1452 – 1519.

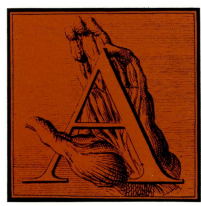

AUTHOR INDEX

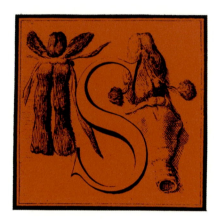

SUBJECT INDEX

The Figure of Teeth bound or faſtned together.

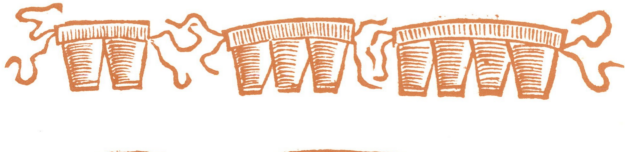

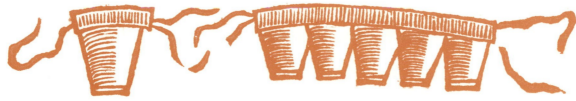

The Works of that Famous Chirurgeon: Ambrose Parey, 1678.

HISTORICAL ILLUSTRATIONS

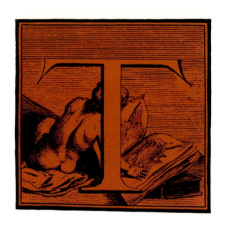

he Crummer and Pilcher Collections of Rare Books of the University of Michigan Medical Center Library have provided most of the woodcuts and engravings which illustrate historical practices preceding our present knowledge of burn medicine and reconstruction. These are included to allow a look into the customs of the past which have brought us to our present state of the art and science of burn medicine.

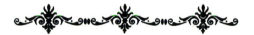

Barton, John K. "Observations upon the Treatment of Deformities Resulting from Severe Burns." *Dublin Journal of Medical Sciences* 32 (1861):1-12. . . . . 39, 237, 239

Bauhin, Kaspar. *Vivae imagines partium corporis humani aeneis formis expressae.* Frankfurt: J.T. de Bry, 1620. . . . . front end paper

Cesi, Carlo. *L'Anatomia dei pittori.* Nuremberg: 1732. 397, 405

Cowper, William. *Myotomia Reformata: or an Anatomical Treatise on the Muscles of the Human Body.* London: Robert Knaplock, 1724. . . . . all display initial letters

Paré, Ambroise. *The Works of that Famous Chirurgeon Ambrose Parey.* Translated by T. Johnson. London: Mary Clark, 1678. . . . . 35, 47, 109, 125, 131, 211, 229, 281, 331, 347, 357, 367, 383

Tagliacozzi, Gaspare. *De curtorum chirurgia insitionem.* Venice: Apud Robertum Meiettum, 1597. . . . . 19, 99, 163, 263

Van der Gracht, Jacob, comp. *Anatomie der wtterlicke deelen van het menschelick lichaem.* Rotterdam: Handrick de Bruyn, 1660. . . . . 13, 325

Vesalius, Andreas. *Anatomia.* [Engravings by Johannes Crieger of drawings from Jan Stephen van Calar]. Venice: I.A. and I. de Franciscis, 1604. 79

Vesalius, Andreas. *Anatomia viri in hoc genere princip.* Amsterdam: I. Ianssenius, 1617. . . . . front fly leaf, 69, 309, 387, back end paper

Reconstruction and Rehabilitation of the Burned Patient, a monumental compendium of knowledge, represents the state of the art of reconstructing and rehabilitating the severely burned patient as it existed in the 8th decade of the 20th Century. This book took 10 years to complete and added a wrinkle or two to William Grabb. However, Irving, Claudella, and Sandra all agree you will find the wait worthwhile.

Book about the burned, reconstructed and rehabilitated in which is contained not only all which was once known by very learned men, but also [that which] has been recently discovered, in the most blessed year of our Lord, 1978. Begun 10 years ago, [it is] finally finished, not without plowing a few wrinkles into the forehead of Dr. William Grabb. However long the time, dear reader, we, Irving, Claud and Sandra agree you will find it worthwhile.

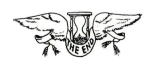